The Camelid Care Handbook for Alpaca & Llama Owners

Foundations of Care (Volume 1)

Claire E. Whitehead BVM&S MS
DACVIM FHEA MRCVS

The Camelid Care Handbook for Alpaca & Llama Owners
Foundations of Care (Volume 1)

ISBN: 9781068357206 Paperback

Published by: Inspired By Publishing

The strategies in this book are presented primarily for enjoyment and educational purposes. Every effort has been made to trace copyright holders and obtain their permission for the use of copyright material.

The information and resources provided in this book are based upon the authors' personal experiences. Any outcomes or other results are based on the author's experiences and there is no guarantee that your experience will be the same. There is an inherent risk in any business enterprise or activity and there is no guarantee that you will have similar results as the author as a result of reading this book.

None of the medicines listed in this book are licensed for use in llamas or alpacas. Doses and recommendations described have been used by the author, her colleagues, or taken from published literature. The author does not accept responsibility for the accuracy, efficacy, or safety of any of these drugs, dosages, routes of administration or adverse reaction that may occur as a result of the use of these drugs. They must be used under the direction of your veterinarian.

The author reserves the right to make changes and assumes no responsibility or liability whatsoever on behalf of any purchaser or reader of these materials.

Dedication

I dedicate this book to my mother, Joy Whitehead, without whom I would never have discovered the joys of working with camelids!

Acknowledgements

There are so many people to thank!

First, I'd like to thank my husband Damion and my daughter Grace for putting up with the endless hours I hid away in the office on weekends, evenings and even on holiday!

I'd like to thank my mum and dad for supporting my ventures and adventures over the years. This project would never have come to be if Mum hadn't first thought alpacas might be fun!

I'd like to thank my cousin, Mary-Jo, for helping me get good photos and videos for training purposes with the alpacas on the farm. I'd also like to thank all my clients who have contributed their stories to this book or whose animals' stories appear within.

Whether your stories appear in this book or not, I want to thank all my clients for allowing me to work with them and their animals. My patients always teach me and help me become a better vet. They have also helped me develop my skills, allowing me to write this book and help others.

Lastly, I cannot end this section without thanking my mentor, David Anderson. David taught me with patience and trust. He taught by example, through his hard work and passion for his craft, and encouraged me to teach. He taught me everything I know and was fantastically supportive in an environment where some thought I was a bit odd to be specialising in camelids. To David – thank you.

Foreword

It is my great pleasure to write a foreword for this new and exciting textbook focusing on the health care of alpacas and llamas. I have known the author, Dr. Claire Whitehead, for over 22 years. Claire first contacted me when I was a professor at The Ohio State University's College of Veterinary Medicine. She reached out to me because she had an intense interest in advancing her knowledge and skills in health and management related to South American Camelids. At the time, I was building an international program, the International Camelid Initiative, which was focused on accumulating and sharing knowledge regarding llamas and alpacas. At the time, these species were rapidly increasing in popularity in the United States and Europe – a trend that has continued over the last 20+ years.

Although these animals have been domesticated for thousands of years in South America, veterinarians in other parts of the world have relatively little knowledge and experience with the species. Owners of alpacas and llamas were eager to learn everything they possibly could about the management, health and vitality of these magnificent animals. Throughout the late 1990s and early 2000s, we were rapidly building a veterinary and scientific community exploring all aspects of camelid management and discovering new information in medicine, surgery, reproduction, nutrition, herd management, and a wide variety of other topics, including genetics, textiles and adaptation to highly variable environments that differed significantly from their native lands.

As a young veterinarian whose family was intensely involved in the alpaca industry in England, Claire had an insatiable thirst for knowledge, an intense desire to gain expertise and a boundless curiosity to know everything possible about the species. Due to her tremendous dedication and interest, she reached out to me and asked if she could spend time at The Ohio State University to learn from our clinical experiences, interact with our clients and their herds, and develop skills that would enable her to not only help her family's alpaca farm but also to serve as an authoritative resource for the growing industry in England and the international community outside of South America.

As a result of Claire's drive and determination (which extended far beyond the short-term experience she could gain under my mentorship), we created the first veterinary residency focused on camelid internal medicine. Claire was extraordinarily successful in her residency and became a board-certified specialist with the American College of Veterinary Internal Medicine.

During her residency, she completed a master's degree in which she explored the dynamics of vitamin D metabolism, specifically its relation to the fetal-maternal transfer of vitamin D. Her master's work was ground-breaking in understanding the role that colostrum and milk play in ensuring that newborn llamas and alpacas have sufficient vitamin D to support their metabolism until they can maintain it independently.

Claire also became intensely concerned with healthy nutrition, internal parasites and the role farm management plays in preventing, treating and managing parasites. After she completed her residency, she stayed at The Ohio State University as a clinical instructor of camelid medicine. She helped us teach our students, train other veterinarians and educate our clients, while also providing critical clinical support for the growing needs of the industry. Building on her expertise, Claire and I jointly edited a periodical text, *Alpaca and Llama Health Management*, for the Veterinary Clinics of North America series. We also collaborated with Dr. Toni Cotton on a self-published book, *Camelid Neonatology: Breeding to Birthing to Weaning.*

I am extremely excited to see Claire sharing her knowledge and thoughts by writing this resource textbook. This project provides her with an opportunity to put her thoughts to paper and share the tremendous knowledge that she carries around with her every day. This includes insights into medical diseases, parasites, infectious diseases including tuberculosis, and a wide variety of reproductive disorders. Her experience in managing critical problems for the betterment of the camelid industry has made her a highly respected international authority in camelid medicine and management. The readers of this book will be able to gain valuable insights that would otherwise not be readily available or easily obtained, and I am confident that this book will have a profound benefit for the many people entrusted with the care and management of llamas and alpacas around the world.

David E. Anderson, DVM, MS, DACVS

Professor and Associate Dean for Research and Graduate Studies
Founding Director, International Camelid Initiative
ACVS Founding Fellow of Minimally Invasive Surgery (Large Animal Soft Tissue)
Fellow, American Association for the Advancement of Science
Fellow, Food Systems Leadership Institute (Cohort 17)

Contents

Introduction

It was early December 2015. I had just met a lovely couple from France attending a Reproduction & Neonatal Course at my clinic in Oxfordshire. The couple were winemakers who worked in a vineyard in Bordeaux. The winery's owner had decided to buy 32 alpacas, import them from the other side of the world, and had asked his winery staff to look after them. The seller told the owner they were easy to look after and that, as owners, they "didn't need to do anything special." In fact, if they were to have any problems, they should just give them a call. The alpacas had arrived in France in the spring of 2015. All went well until October. This was when their problems began...

Twenty-four females were due to give birth between October and January. A male had been running with the females until mid-October when he had raped a pregnant female, causing the premature birth of her cria that subsequently died. The female died 24 hours after her cria. Following those deaths, and up until the time I met the winemaking couple, they had lost their stud male and five more females. Two crias had been stillborn, and seven more had died. There were also seven premature births.

One of the females had died while en route to see the vet. Post-mortem, they found 10,000 eggs per gram of strongyle-type eggs in a faecal sample. The vet had noticed that the stud male had anaemia, but his egg count had been very low. The herd had then all been treated with a combination wormer from another country under the instructions of the breeder 12,000 miles away. No other control measures had been put in place. The deaths continued into 2016. Their vet had thrown his hands in the air in that very French *laissez-faire* style, declaring, "This farm is diseased!" He did not know how to help. The couple were desperate by this stage...

I first visited the farm in the middle of January 2016. The remaining alpacas were in an extremely poor state by this time, and the couple were exhausted from bottle-feeding twelve crias day and night. The alpacas were in poor body condition and had overgrown toenails. A female had died shortly after my arrival with severe anaemia. I had minimal equipment for a post-mortem examination, but I set to with a scalpel in the most bizarre of settings. The alpaca was elevated onto a pallet makeshift table with a board on top. We were surrounded by rows of lifeless vines extending into the early morning fog. My crude post-mortem examination confirmed a large number of *Haemonchus* worms in her third stomach compartment. I walked the farm with the couple, checked all the alpacas, trimmed their toenails and collected blood and faecal samples that I brought back to my clinic.

Essentially, I identified extremely poor nutrition in the animals. The couple had been given no guidance on feeding the alpacas and was unable to provide forage or supplementary feed to match the requirements of the late pregnant females who were giving birth in the autumn and winter months. They had minimal knowledge of routine husbandry and lacked facilities, including appropriate trough space, hay feeders, and accommodation to house the animals that needed extra care. The alpacas were heavily parasitised, and the crias had rickets.

I initiated a parasite control plan for the couple to treat the alpacas and how to manage this moving forward. I gave clear instructions on how to improve their facilities, feed provision and general husbandry. There were no more deaths from parasitism and only a single further death in a cria that died from an unrelated issue. I returned to Bordeaux on a beautiful sunny day in May to find a much happier and healthier herd and a couple that, despite all their increasing work commitments on the winery, were much more relaxed and finally in control. As for the alpacas, their health was much improved. Their body condition scores rose from an average of just 3.7/10 (ranging from 2 to 6/10) to a healthy average of 5.5/10 across the herd.

This couple had been faced with a circumstantial perfect storm. This led to an absolute nightmare that was entirely avoidable had they received the correct advice and guidance from the start. Despite not having personally chosen to get into alpacas, they cared about the animals but felt completely unequipped to deal with the situation in which they found themselves. Since the non-resident owner had bought pregnant animals that moved from the southern to the northern hemisphere, they were due to give birth in the entirely wrong season of autumn without appropriate nutritional planning or herd management. The seller had utterly failed in his duty to prepare them for this. The herd was sleepwalking through the pleasant Bordeaux summer into a firestorm of metabolic disease, vitamin D deficiency, immunosuppression and uncontrolled parasitism all in one go. The problem had been exacerbated due to the numbers they had opted to take on simultaneously.

If you have alpacas or llamas (or are thinking of getting some, given that you are reading this book), if you follow the strategies within, I can assure you that you will not find yourself in this situation. This book is all about camelid care for owners of alpacas and llamas and preventing problems from occurring in the first place. I start with a chapter entirely for those merely thinking about taking the plunge and testing the waters to see what it's all about. I will provide useful information about camelids and answer some commonly asked questions. I cover some key areas that you should address right at the start and provide a checklist of questions to ask yourself to see if you are ready to take the next step and purchase your first alpacas or llamas.

Over Chapters 2 to 4, I cover everything you need to know about camelid husbandry and the 10 non-negotiable herd health activities that will get you well on your way. Nutrition, covered in Chapters 5 and 6, is one of the most fundamental features of any herd health plan and is crucial to understand. It forms the basis of everything that ensures your animals are fit and healthy, develop sufficient immunity, breed successfully, grow to their potential, and produce sufficient quality and quantity fleece.

In Chapters 7 and 8, I move on to discussing the types and sources of potential risks to your animals' health from disease, how to prevent disease outbreaks on your holding and how to minimise the impact of any disease events that occur. Thinking about this can sometimes seem a little scary, but the point is awareness so that you can do everything you can to prepare for and prevent problems from occurring in the first place.

From Chapters 9 to 13, I deal with the most common problems you will likely encounter when keeping camelids. Some topics are so important that they have chapters dedicated to them, namely parasites, skin problems and neurological problems. In Chapter 13, I cover most other potential problems you might encounter in your animals. You can use this as a reference guide by going to the main clinical signs that you are observing, such as anaemia, colic, dental problems or weight loss. When discussing these problems, I talk about what you might see as an owner, what diagnostics are available and what solutions or treatments there might be to help you and your vet decide what to do.

Chapter 14 is a guide to dealing with emergencies. I will explain how to do a basic health check and give you some pointers about what you can do as an owner if you find a sick animal. You may need to relay specific information to your vet ahead of their visit to help them determine what they may need to bring with them. In this chapter, I also share valuable information about available diagnostic options and the importance of these diagnostic tests in helping your animals. I also cover field therapeutics, what you need to know about using medicines in camelids and how valuable intravenous fluid therapy can be in sick camelids.

The final chapter is a guide to being a responsible owner of alpacas or llamas. I have developed a five-point model to help you remember the key areas of responsibility for meeting your legal, ethical, and animal health obligations regarding camelids.

You will notice that I'm not covering any reproduction topics or cria care in this book. I have intentionally not included this because I realise there are people out there who aren't interested in breeding and don't need that information. Regardless of whether you wish to breed, you first need to know how to look after camelids, how to feed them right, protect them from disease and what to do if they have problems. I will write a second volume of this book covering reproduction, breeding management and cria care.

Now, why have I written this book? How did I get here, and why should you listen to what I have to say? These are excellent questions... To explain, let me tell you a little bit about myself.

When I was 15 years old, my mother told me that she'd seen a programme on television about alpacas and was interested in getting some. I thought that sounded great, so I accompanied her up to the Lake District to look at some that were to be sold at auction. They were absolutely gorgeous! We went to the auction, and my mum bought five alpacas – four females and one male. Their names were Totora, Palpa, Chimbote, Anna and Macchu Picchu. The females were aged between two and five years and had never been shorn in their lives! They literally looked like big black pom-poms! You can imagine our surprise when we had them shorn that first spring – they looked so tiny afterwards!

When we bought the alpacas, there were fewer than 3,000 camelids in the UK, mostly llamas. Nobody knew much about them, so we learned as we went. Our veterinarians knew nothing about them either, so they approached each case using basic principles and what they knew about other species. It really was a case of jumping in with both feet and feeling quite out of our depth!

A few years after we got the alpacas, Chimbote got sick. We brought her into a shed bedded with fresh straw and called the vet. He examined her. He didn't know what was wrong with her but gave her a few medications based on what he thought might be going on. Soon, she was dead. You can imagine how devastating this was. We only wanted to help her, but had only succeeded in killing her. One of the medicines she'd been given was called "Lutalyse," and I later found out that this can be toxic to alpacas.

A few years later, I decided to go to vet school. I was determined to be the best vet that I could possibly be. I learned a huge amount, but unfortunately, I learned only one thing about camelids during the entire five years of my course! This nugget was that there was once a case of halothane-induced hepatitis in an alpaca, and I learned this from my anaesthesia lecturer, Eddie Clutton. (Thank you, Eddie!) So, I left vet school still poorly equipped to work with camelids, and in my first job, I found myself off to visit a collapsed llama that I had no idea how to help. I had to put him down, and the experience didn't sit well with me. I felt utterly useless. Nothing in vet school had prepared me for dealing with these cases.

After a year in practice, I had the opportunity to go out to Peru to help with an alpaca selection for my mother, Joy Whitehead. By this time, Josef Kuonen, a Swiss breeder, had established new protocols with the authorities to enable the import of top-quality alpacas from Peru into Switzerland, as they were not allowed to enter the EU directly. The first alpacas were imported into Switzerland in 1998, and our share had to spend a year in Switzerland before entering the UK. I went out to Peru in 2000 with Josef and Steve Knoblock, an American breeder who had also come to help with the selection. Josef and Steve looked at the animals from a phenotypic perspective, and I evaluated them from a veterinary perspective. Steve told me about some university-based veterinarians doing lots of work with camelids. In particular, he recommended Chris Cebra at Oregon State and David Anderson at Ohio State. I wrote to them both.

When I first wrote to Dave, I asked about opportunities for internships or residencies. He said those weren't available, so I asked about just coming out and spending time with him. This is what we would call "seeing practice" in the UK. He replied that while I would be welcome to come and visit, the university had a somewhat inflexible policy of charging for this. I was appalled – I'd never paid to see practice in the UK! In return, I asked if there was a way around this, like being a research slave for a while… In response, he asked how long I'd like to come for. I suggested six months, as I knew I could get a visa for that period, and I set off to Columbus, Ohio, in March 2002.

When I arrived in Columbus, everything was grey. The sky was grey, the grass was grey, the buildings were grey – and it was cold! It was the most uninviting place you could imagine. I wondered if I would make it the month, let alone six months! Fortunately, what I found at the Food & Fibre Animal Section astounded me. I couldn't believe the quality of the farm animal medicine and surgery being practised there, not just with camelid patients but for cattle, sheep, goats and pigs! Animals were receiving IV fluids and having orthopaedic injuries repaired surgically – I hadn't ever seen this in the UK! They had mobile chutes for cattle and were being wheeled around the hospital to radiology and surgery. You could get bloodwork results within the hour, and there was round-the-clock care. At the end of those first few weeks, it happened that the International Camelid Health Conference was being hosted at Ohio State. All the big names were there – Murray Fowler, LaRue Johnson, Chris Cebra, David Pugh, Walter Bravo. The information shared was extraordinary – my mind was opened. Around that time, Dave told me that he had funding for a residency in camelid medicine or surgery and asked if I was interested.

Soon after that, the sun came out in Columbus, and the grass turned green again. It was as if God had switched life back on! Following the conference and the revelation about the knowledge to be learned, and my eyes opened to the untapped possibility of farm animal medicine, I realised that this residency was an opportunity that couldn't be missed. I applied for the position. I believe it was one of those opportunities where I was in the right place at the right time. I was already putting IV catheters in patients and helping with the camelid caseload in the section, so they knew what they could expect from me.

My residency started in July 2002, and I chose medicine as my speciality. At the start of the residency, I remember being told that we weren't entitled to any holiday but that "out of the goodness of his heart," the department chair *allowed* us to take 10 days a year. This was quite a shock to someone from the UK, where a minimum of 20 days' holiday was standard on top of public holidays! Also, it transpired that even when we weren't on call for new case arrivals (we were on call for a whole week out of three for the first year of my residency), we were still on call for our hospital inpatients. Sometimes, this could be quite intense. I remember on my first week on call, I took in a very sick premature cria on a Saturday night. This cria required frequent observations and treatments, plus calls to me each night that it was hospitalised. By Tuesday night, I was exhausted, had several new case admissions and got home at about 4am. ICU called me about 30 minutes later. I answered one or two questions about the cria very sleepily. The next thing I knew was I woke up at 5:30am with my phone still attached to my face!

Despite working about 70-80 hours per week *and* taking master's classes alongside a research project, I soon found that this was a recipe for an incredible learning experience. We were responsible for our cases from when they arrived at the hospital until they were discharged. This meant that you really understood how your case evolved, knew that the tweaks you made were your success or otherwise, and felt a real connection with the patients and owners, many of whom thought we didn't sleep! True enough, sometimes, we didn't! It was hard work, but I learned more than I ever thought possible. Dave was the most incredible teacher. He had a way of helping you find your own answers rather than simply giving solutions. He even let you make your own mistakes – not patient-harming ones, I might add – that improved the learning experience. I also highly valued the amazing Equine Internal Medicine clinicians Steve Reed, Ken Hinchcliff, Catherine Kohn and Jeff Lakritz when he joined the Food Animal section. Without them, I would never have passed boards!

After three years of my residency, I sat and passed my exam boards for the American College of Veterinary Internal Medicine (Large Animal Speciality) and became a Diplomate of the College. I also obtained my master's degree with a thesis on the effect of maternal vitamin D supplementation on transplacental and trans-mammary transfer to neonatal llamas and alpacas. I was lucky enough to be asked to stay on at Ohio State as a clinical instructor. This was a worthwhile year as it helped me to consolidate my skillset in a familiar environment before moving elsewhere.

I moved home to the UK in October 2006. I spent a few months travelling and competing in my first Ironman triathlon in Western Australia, and then I returned home to start at the Royal Veterinary College (RVC) in London, where I became a lecturer in farm animal medicine. I started the Camelid & Farm Animal Hospital on the hospital campus in Potters Bar. This was a frustrating experience because there was a complete lack of facilities or aspiration to help me provide the hospital-level care for farm animals that I was used to. Funding promised to renovate a wartime barn evaporated, leaving me to spend four years working in an unheated, leaky barn. I used an ultrasound machine I had purchased with my own money and worked hard to build a caseload. Fortunately, colleagues in other areas of the veterinary hospital were terrific to work with and always enjoyed the opportunity to work with us on our unique cases. However, at the end of 2010, the department heads showed how little they valued farm animal teaching by decimating our section in the higher education funding cuts that followed the global financial crisis of 2008.

I left the RVC at the end of 2010 and set up practice on my own in the spring of 2011. I realised that the pressures of teaching and fighting for resources weren't that fulfilling, as they had been taking me away from my passion for working with camelids and helping their owners. I was now liberated to work solely with camelid patients and to focus entirely on providing for their health and welfare. Providing consultations and teaching owners and veterinarians has been something I've done throughout my time in the US and in London, and I have continued to offer these services since. Nothing gives me more pleasure than teaching people who light up when talking about their animals and who appreciate the wonderful creatures that camelids are.

I wrote this book for you, camelid owners, because I believe in improving the health and welfare of camelids. I didn't have access to a resource like this when I started working with camelids, and I don't want to see you having to learn the hard way by making entirely preventable mistakes. I see many people with sick animals or having lost animals, either because of something they simply didn't know or didn't do. I want to make what I have learned available to you, wherever you may be in the world, so that I can help you optimise the health and productivity of your animals and help you avoid making the mistakes that others have made. I realise that you want your animals for various reasons, but I know that without exception, you want to spend time enjoying them rather than worrying about an animal that is sick and whether you're doing the right thing. Following the strategies in this book will help you do just that.

I hope you enjoy this book – *and* your animals!

Disclaimer

A little note about medications: none of the treatments discussed in this book are licensed for use in llamas or alpacas. Doses and recommendations described have been used by the author or others known to her. Claire Whitehead does not accept responsibility for the efficacy or safety of any of these drugs, dosages, routes of administration or adverse reactions that may occur due to the use of these drugs. They must be used under the direction of your veterinarian.

1

What to Know Before Getting Alpacas or Llamas

"All things are ready, if our minds be so."
- William Shakespeare (Henry V)

Are you considering getting alpacas or llamas but haven't yet taken the plunge? If so, then this chapter is written entirely for you. As a prospective owner, *before* taking the leap, there are some things you need to know to ensure you have the right facilities, provide proper care for the animals and make the most of your investment in alignment with your goals.

Why?

The first thing to ask yourself is, *why?* Why are you getting these animals? People have different reasons for doing so, and no reason is better than another. But those reasons should guide your decisions about the type of animals you choose to buy. Some people are interested in high-quality fibre, in which case you should be looking at alpacas rather than llamas. Some people like to run trekking operations with llamas, as they are great trekking animals and were domesticated to carry burdens. Others run businesses based on camelid experiences and walking with camelids, which can involve both alpacas and llamas. Just remember that alpacas will not be interested in carrying anyone's stuff! Still, other people are simply interested in having intriguing and wonderful pets. While camelids have a unique charm and are beautiful to look at, with their huge eyes and fabulous cuddly-looking fleeces, they are not the sort of animal that enjoys being hugged constantly like a dog or cat! They prefer to maintain their personal space.

Understanding and clarifying your reason for getting camelids will help you focus on where to look for your animals and what sort of animals you are after. It is all too easy to get carried away and get talked into buying the loveliest breeding animal with a cria at foot when, actually, you might not want to be responsible for dealing with breeding animals and would rather just have some healthy companion animals. The price difference could be quite significant, and you'll have frittered away money that could have been better spent on infrastructure such as good fencing.

Key Camelid Facts You Should Know

1. Llamas and alpacas have never been "wild." The Incas domesticated them around 6,000 years ago from their wild predecessors, the guanaco and vicuña, respectively. All four New World (or South American) camelids are part of the camelid family, including Old World camelids (dromedary and Bactrian camels). The llama was bred to be a beast of burden, and the alpaca a fibre producer. Both come in a wide range of natural colours.

2. Llamas are larger, typically weighing 110–200 kg (240–440 lb). Since they were originally intended for carrying things, less attention went into selecting for colour. So, you'll see a lot more mixing of colours in llamas, with multicoloured and "paint" forms quite common. Alpacas, on the other hand, tend to be single-coloured more frequently, presumably because they were used for fleece production, and this made it easier to process, even by hand. Llamas also have a lot more guard hair, the longer wispy hairs extending beyond the main fleece. The guard hair is more coarse and not as desirable in fleece-producing animals. A llama's face also has much less hair than an alpaca, and they have Roman-shaped noses and long banana-shaped ears.

3. Alpacas weigh 55–90 kg (120–200 lb) as adults but can weigh up to 100 kg (220 lb, although I've seen fat ones weigh more!). They have straight noses, short straight ears and a lot more fleece around the face and down their legs. Breeders primarily look for density, coverage and fineness in the fleece. The fleece can be very fine; uniformity is desirable. You can collect fleece samples to investigate various statistics, with key indicators being the average micron count (the diameter of the hair fibres) and the standard deviation. If the standard deviation is small, the fibres are more uniform across the sample, which is a good thing. Alpaca judges will be able to teach you a lot more about fleece assessment than I can ever hope to know!

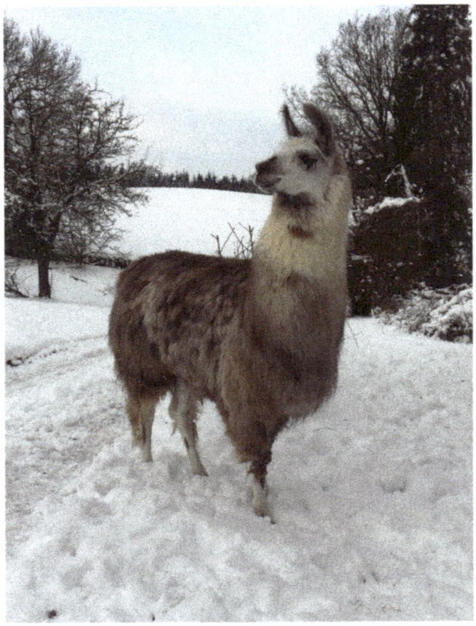

Figure 1. An adult male llama
Photo: Lisa Fox, Briery Hill Llamas

4. There are two types of alpaca: the huacaya, which comprises about 85–90% of all alpacas, and the suri, which comprises the remaining 10–15%

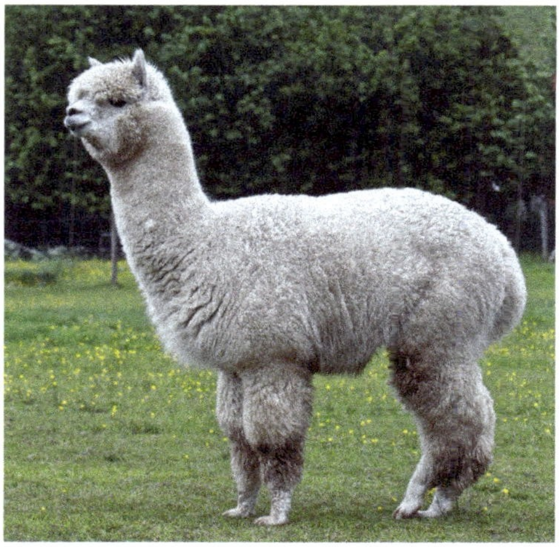

Figure 2. A huacaya type alpaca
Photo: Ken Whitehead

(*Figures 2 and 3*). The suri have long straight fibres organised in waves, falling in "pencils" from the top line. Breeders value lustre in suri fleece. In the huacaya, the emphasis is more on density. Regardless of the alpaca type, fineness is always valued.

5. Suris and huacayas can interbreed, but you wouldn't really want them to because it dilutes the qualities of each type of fleece. Llamas and alpacas can also interbreed, but again, you don't want them to. A llama/alpaca cross is called a "huariso" or a "wari."

6. Llamas are so much bigger than us, so if you're going to get them, handling them can be very challenging if you don't bother to handle them frequently and train them to walk on a halter. This is a responsibility you take on when you get llamas. You can get a handling system like a restraint chute, but if the llama

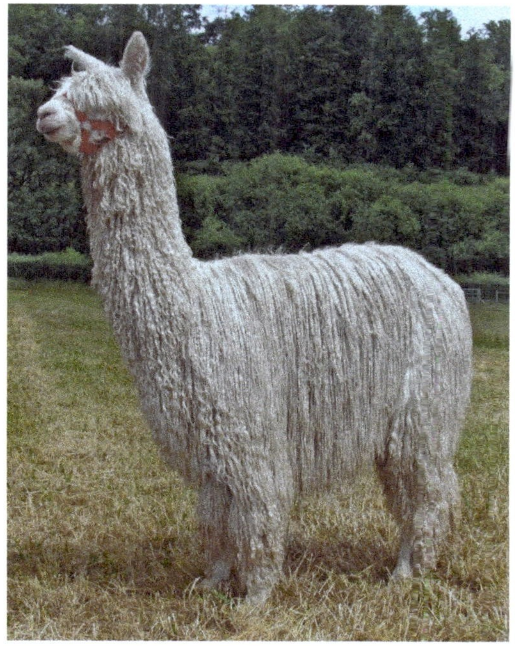

Figure 3. A suri-type alpaca
Photo: Ken Whitehead

isn't used to this and panics, either you or the llama could get injured. So be prepared to spend time with your animals – they're not just pasture ornaments. The same applies to alpacas, although since they're smaller, you won't get pushed around as much if your alpacas aren't handled often. However, if you don't handle them, doing husbandry tasks with them will be more challenging, and they will get more stressed. (And by the way, trust me when I tell you that I've ended up on my backside enough times with alpacas! I'm sure it's not just me!)

7. Some terminology:
   - Males can be called males, sires, studs, "machos" or geldings if castrated.

- Females can be called females, dams or "hembras."
- The babies are called crias. This term remains with them until weaning, generally around six months, when they become "weanlings" or "tuis." I rather like the word tui but never really hear anyone use it!
- Birthing has some alternative names: In North America, it tends to be called "criating/creation," while in Australia and New Zealand, it's "unpacking." People use various terms in the UK, but birthing is probably the most common.
- Collectively, the convention seems to refer to a group as a "herd" rather than a "flock." (I'd like to suggest an "assembly," or maybe an "addition" or "fluffle," as once suggested on a Facebook group!)
- The haircoat is called fleece or fibre (not wool!).

8. There are about 4 million alpacas globally. Compare this with 1.4 billion cattle and 1 billion sheep. You will need to get used to the idea that no medicines are licensed for use in camelids, nor will they ever be. Fortunately, these days, the public knows about both llamas and alpacas - although they don't know the difference and will still mix them up. Get used to explaining the difference...

9. Camelids have some unique anatomical and physiological adaptations:
   - They are adapted to arid climates, so they're good at absorbing most of the water they consume. They have a whole extra loop of intestine to deal with this, but they can still get dehydrated! Make sure they always have a source of fresh, clean water. Pond or marsh water does *not* count! (I once tried to help an owner who had thought it was acceptable for his alpacas to drink marsh water - it was their only source. They were dying from liver fluke infestations.)
   - They can tolerate low oxygen conditions due to small, elliptical-shaped red blood cells with a greater surface area for oxygen. These red blood cells pick up oxygen more easily in the lungs and release it more readily to the tissues. This also means that if they have a condition that reduces their oxygen availability, like anaemia or lung problems, the clinical situation might get serious before they notice.
   - They are used to colder climates rather than hot ones–no surprise there, given their thick fleece! As such, they are prone to heat stress because they are not adapted to it. So, if you live in a hot country or, worse, a hot and humid country, you must make special adaptations for them.

10. Camelids are susceptible to:
    - Parasites such as worms, coccidia and liver fluke. Camelids are not well adapted to these and appear to be very sensitive to them. If you have alpacas or llamas, be prepared to have an excellent parasite control strategy.
    - Vitamin D deficiency. In South America, camelids live at equatorial

latitudes and high altitudes, exposing them to high ultraviolet radiation. This helps them make vitamin D in their skin. Outside these zones, there is less UV radiation, and they struggle to make enough vitamin D. Supplementation with vitamin D is required to prevent rickets in growing crias and support their immune systems, foetal growth, and lactational performance, among other things.

- Skin problems. Camelids are prone to many skin problems, most commonly mange. Unresolved factors may contribute to their susceptibility to skin problems. Treating them can be a lot of work. Monitoring and catching symptoms early is a much better plan!

11. The digestive system of camelids is similar to that of cows or sheep, with a complex forestomach. However, unlike cattle and sheep, camelids have three stomachs. The first stomach acts like a big fermentation vat, containing millions of microbes that help them digest their food.

12. Camelids need to be shorn once a year. They do not shed their fleece naturally, and you must book a shearer well ahead of the summer to get a slot. Shearers are specialists with camelids, and they move around the country during the spring and summer. They need to plan their stops to be efficient. Don't leave it to the last minute because their diaries may be full, and your alpacas and llamas may become heat-stressed. If you can, aim to shear by the end of May before it gets hot (in the northern hemisphere, at least!).

13. Camelids normally have only one cria. Because their placentation is similar to that of a horse, they cannot carry twins to term, unlike cattle or sheep. There are exceptions, of course, but most twin pregnancies are aborted at around 5.5 months of gestation. If they do make it to term, the twins are usually delivered early and relatively small, needing a lot of extra attention.

14. The pregnancy length for alpacas and llamas is 343 days, give or take a few weeks. Pregnancies may be shorter in the autumn, when the days are shorter, and longer pregnancies are usual in the spring, when there's more time to enjoy the sunshine! The further away from the equator you are, the more you will notice this difference. The variability of pregnancy length does tend to cause some headaches for owners waiting for their newborns to arrive. However, camelids typically give birth during the day, making them much more considerate than horses, which usually give birth at night!

15. In terms of lifespan, camelids can live quite a long time. There are both alpacas and llamas living in their twenties that are even productive females, so be prepared for a substantial duration of your commitment. The average lifespan is 15 to 20 years. The problems affecting them later in life tend to be arthritis and worn down teeth, which makes it hard for them to eat sufficiently for their needs.

So, you've decided whether you want alpacas

or llamas (or both). What do you need to know now? Here are answers to some key questions, with more details covered in the following chapters.

"Can I have just one?"

No. Camelids are social animals and like the company of others. Keeping them singly would be contrary to good welfare as they need other camelids to engage in normal behaviour. We recommend having at least two alpacas or llamas. However, three is a better minimum number because if one dies, the other will be left alone, which can be incredibly stressful. Some people occasionally buy camelids as guard animals for sheep or poultry. In this situation, I would still recommend getting at least two camelids on welfare grounds.

"Can they go in my garden?"

No. Most people's gardens are way too small for camelids! Even if you have a stately home with massive gardens, a garden isn't the best place because it may be full of toxic plants (rhododendron, oleander, yew - to name a few). Additionally, gardens tend to have a monoculture of grass rather than the mixed species in pastures. When determining the best type of seed mix, it should be a mixed species of grass made for grazing animals like horses and cattle. Adding legumes like clover into the seed mix helps to fix nitrogen, and the grass grows better overall. With mixed species grazing, the soil biology improves, there is improved biodiversity, and the grasses are more pest-resistant. You can include grasses that confer parasite resistance, like sainfoin, too!

"How much space do they need?"

I usually recommend planning to have a maximum of an acre of pasture (0.4 hectares) per five alpacas—this is known as a maximum "stocking density." However, you should have twice this space available to rest the pasture, allowing the grass to recover and any parasites to die off.

If you have one big field, think about how you can divide this into smaller paddocks to allow you to rest areas of pasture. Also, consider where you can put a shelter (yes, you will need one of those, too) to use it from multiple paddocks. Set up fencing to allow access from different paddocks. Avoid long, thin paddocks that are more than twice the width length as they won't get grazed efficiently.

One thing to plan for is keeping males and females separate. If you intend to breed, you'll also need paddocks to wean crias away from their dams. Unless you're lucky, you'll end up with crias of both genders, which will also need separating—males and females can be precocious, so be warned! All of this increases the acreage you'll need, so ensure you have space to accommodate growth if you plan to expand. Many owners find themselves with far more animals than they originally intended!

"Do they need shelter?"

Yes, you will need to provide shelter. Hedgerows and trees will provide some shelter from inclement weather, depending on the direction of prevailing weather, and may also offer shade depending on the sun's position. However, you should at least have a field shelter that the animals can access to get out of horrid weather such as rain, wind or snow. In addition, you should think about how you will manage a sick animal – and *before* you have one on your hands. You will want to have a structure, ideally with light and power, that you can bring a sick animal in to treat it. A field shelter isn't always ideal, as containing the animal inside can be tricky while still giving the others access.

"What sort of fencing do they need?"

Avoid using barbed wire, as it can cause eye injuries. Sheep fencing usually works best for camelids. It has a large square mesh for two-thirds of the fence's height and two to three smooth wires above. Post-and-rail fencing will not be secure for crias. Badger-proof fencing is recommended for those where bovine TB is prevalent in the UK.

"Can I mix them with other species?"

If you intend to mix camelids with other animals, here are a few tips: Be cautious about cattle and horses due to their size difference and injury potential. However, some people manage to keep camelids with horses, and the camelids end up being the bosses! But since horses are large and have hooves, I urge caution. Also, horses carry *Streptococcus zooepidemicus* in their upper respiratory tract, which can cause severe infections in camelids.

While size issues aren't a concern with sheep, you must be careful about parasite control because camelids are much more susceptible to parasites than sheep.

"Can you train alpacas and llamas?"

Yes, you can. Like most domesticated animals, camelids are very adaptable to training. The first thing to do is to get them used to handling. Then, you can start to train them to accept a halter and to learn to walk with a halter and lead. This allows you to take them to shows, transport them to other farms or the vet, or complete obstacle courses – the latter more common at llama shows. You can also train them to walk comfortably on and off a trailer or van. Remember, they should never be tied during transportation.

You may have heard of clicker training for dogs, and you can use it on camelids, too, if you want to! I recommend getting some handling training from other breeders or owners. Breed societies and other providers in your country may offer courses. You will learn more about handling in Chapter 2.

"Do I need to research anything in advance?"

Yes, you do! Please don't stumble blindly into this! Getting alpacas or llamas is a big commitment. You need to look after them every day, 365 days a year, regardless of the weather. Do NOT buy animals from anyone who claims they're super easy to keep, downplays the effort required and leaves you to figure things out on your own. They are likely incompetent caregivers themselves.

There are lots of sources of information about looking after camelids. Breed societies are usually a great source of information, as well as existing owners of alpacas and llamas. Go and talk to them and learn from them, and you will learn all sorts of practical tips. If you buy from them, they should support you, but you need to do your part first, and that is *learning* so that you don't kill the animals they've entrusted into your care. While practical experience is a great teacher, proper research *now* will pay dividends. You need to know what you are doing, and the fact that you are reading this book already tells me that you are approaching this project responsibly. Read the whole book to learn all you need to know about keeping your animals healthy and productive, and the problems you need to watch for.

Find Your Veterinarian

Before you get your alpacas or llamas, look at the veterinary provision in your local area and find out if the vets are familiar with camelids and are happy to register you. Most vets do not learn much about camelids during vet school - much of what they know will be picked up after graduation. Some vets will be experienced and happy to work with camelids, others not.

If your vets are inexperienced but eager to help, invite them over on a mutually quiet day to meet your herd, listen to lung and gut sounds, and familiarise themselves with healthy camelids. If you develop a rapport with them, it will be much easier for them when you need them in an emergency - much better than throwing them in at the deep end when something's going wrong and expecting them to work miracles.

You can also encourage them to take some training. I offer training courses on camelid care for vets and owners, which can be taken online, so it doesn't matter where they are located. If necessary, offer to help them pay for training. Vets are usually keen to learn new things, but bear in mind that vets have a limited budget for continuing education. If their interests are in another species or discipline, they won't want to spend that precious budget on camelids just because it's important to you. However, you *can* get them interested just by helping them to learn! And frankly, what's not to love?

As veterinary patients, alpacas and llamas are fascinating and fun to work with. Since most camelid owners want to do everything they can for their animals, they tend to be a little more like small animal or horse owners than farmers and are keen to pay for diagnostics and other care. This makes being a vet much more interesting, as we do not have to guess as much. However, balancing this with practicality is also essential - particularly regarding costs. Always discuss your wishes with your vet so they know if you're willing to invest in extra tests when needed. They should be able to provide you with estimates for testing.

Calling for help is another option, particularly where a referral might not be possible. People like myself can provide remote consultations to your vet, assisting you and your vet in managing a complex case in the field. Visit www.ukalpacavet.com to get in touch with us.

Be Aware of Your Legal and Ethical Responsibilities

I explore this topic in greater detail in Chapter 15. At this point, though, I will say that you need to know the animal welfare laws in your country or state. Familiarise yourself with whether you need to register your animals with the authorities, their identification and what records you need to keep. Find out the legislation on the transport of live animals and if there are any restrictions over where you can travel and how long for. Check for disease testing requirements if travelling from country to country, state to state, or province to province. Your vet will know the answers to this one, although they may need to do some research for camelids specifically. Plan to give yourself plenty of time for testing if required.

Costs and Financial Planning

Having animals always carries a financial commitment, not just for the initial investment in the animals and the infrastructure required in fencing, field shelters, barns, water troughs and trailers, but feed and maintenance costs. You must consider routine veterinary fees, vaccinations, faecal testing and medicines such as wormers. There are also shearing, registration and rodent control costs to consider. Depending on the size of your holding, you should invest in farm equipment like tractors, trailers, a farm buggy (UTV) and something to help you clear faecal material from the pasture. On top of that are the unexpected costs that might pop up, like emergency veterinary visits due to animals being ill or injured. If you are thinking of showing, there are entry fees for the animals you wish to show. Also, think about who might look after your animals when you leave, as there may be added costs.

There may be some financial returns depending on what you intend to do with your animals. For example, if you are breeding, you can sell the progeny. However, you may be tempted to keep them at the start because you're trying to improve your herd, and it takes time before you are ready to part with any. Better quality animals with good conformation and fleece will fetch better prices, and this is proven if those animals are shown and doing well at the shows. Also, do not assume that all animals will sell for a certain price. Remember that most male offspring will not be of breeding quality, and they make up 50% of the cria crop. When you shear your animals, there is income if you sell the fleece, but you will get more for it if it's better quality and you put effort into sorting it first. If you process the products yourself, this will add value to the fleece but take time, effort and possibly added costs in equipment.

Camelids are also increasingly used in agritourism, which includes experiences, walking or trekking. They have been used alongside yoga sessions, as ring-bearers at weddings and for therapy. So, there are opportunities for revenue generation here that can be significant but must not become an animal welfare concern. Providing some of these activities can create potential conflicts for animal welfare, as what benefits people isn't always best for the animals. Unfortunately, there is no research to guide recommendations on what is acceptable or not. For instance, how many hours per day or week should animals be allowed to "work," such as being on a halter and going for a walk? At what point do these activities affect the animals' ability to consume enough nutrition or cause stress from being separated from their herd?

Finally, investigate how you structure your investment. It can all come from your finances if it's just a hobby. However, suppose you intend to be more serious and grow your animal population. In that case, setting up a business to offset costs against any profits may offer tax and liability advantages. Always seek advice from your accountant about these options' relative pros and cons, as the benefits will vary by country.

Time Commitment

Always remember that having animals that depend on you is a serious commitment and requires dedication every day of the year, regardless of the weather. It's wonderful wandering among them in the summertime when the sun is shining, and crias are bouncing around. But before you commit, think whether you would still enjoy having them if you need to be outside in torrential rain or snow, carrying buckets of water because the ground is frozen and you've had to turn off the mains water feed. Consider whether you'd still enjoy caring for these animals when you're sliding around in the mud as you carry hay out to the animals because you can't take your UTV on the muddy ground. Understand that you will need to schedule time to commit to husbandry tasks such as monthly body condition scoring, toenail trimming, vaccinations and more. More in Chapters 2 and 3 where I cover the 10 non-negotiable herd health activities.

Where Should You Buy From?

Take your time deciding where to buy your animals. Visit several breeders, ask plenty of questions and observe how they set up and manage their farms. This exposure helps you envision how you might structure your setup and provide valuable insights into animal care practices. Look for breeders who are open to questions, honest with their answers and genuinely invested in finding the right home for their animals. Sellers who prioritise their animals' well-being are also more likely to offer helpful after-sales support when you need it.

Be cautious if a seller claims they never have any issues with their animals or implies that camelids are easy to care for with minimal effort. Such statements suggest a stronger focus on making a sale than providing an honest picture of camelid ownership. Occasional problems are normal and can even be a positive sign, as they show the seller can recognise and address challenges responsibly. This demonstrates their knowledge and experience and gives you confidence that they can guide you if you encounter similar issues in the future.

In terms of making sure that you don't buy animals with disease risks, familiarise yourself with the biosecurity recommendations in Chapter 8.

Resources

Get in touch with the breeding society in your country as a first port of call. They usually have a lot of information freely available, and you can join the societies without actually needing to own animals. This gives you increased access to available resources, and most societies will offer training opportunities to help you learn how to care for camelids. In addition, you will meet loads of like-minded individuals who will massively enjoy sharing their passion and knowledge with you. There may also be regional groups you can contact to help you locate breeders in your area. Listed below are the societies for camelids in the English-speaking countries with the largest alpacas and llamas outside of South America. There are many countries around Europe with large and growing numbers of camelids, but there appear to be multiple societies in most of these countries. Therefore, I encourage you to get in touch with all of them and align yourself with the society you feel the most affinity with.

Australia: Australian Alpaca Association (alpaca.asn.au) and the Llama Association of Australasia Inc. (llama.asn.au).

Canada: The Canada Llama & Alpaca Association (claacanada.com) primarily covers the Registry. Under this umbrella, two divisions manage all other activities: Alpaca Canada (alpacainfo.ca) and Llama Canada (www.llamacanada.com).

New Zealand: The Alpaca Association of New Zealand (https://alpaca.org.nz) and New Zealand Llama Association (llamas.org.nz).

South Africa: South African Alpaca Breeders Society (www.alpacasociety.co.za)

United Kingdom: The British Alpaca Society (bas-uk.com) and the British Llama Society (britishllamasociety.co.uk). The BAS umbrella also includes 14 regional groups.

United States: Alpaca Owners Association Inc. (alpacainfo.com) and Llama Association of North America (LANA, lanainfo.org). Most states also have their own organisations.

Go to shows to meet with breeders and to learn what characteristics are valued by breeders. At the alpaca shows, the judges provide oral reasoning for their decisions that can be useful if you're trying to learn what makes a good alpaca and what makes one better than another in the show ring.

You must also take some training before you get your animals. Good breeders will help you learn the basics of animal husbandry, either through you volunteering to help them or offering courses for their buyers. You can also take advanced courses on husbandry, care, and alpaca evaluation, focusing on fleece and conformation.

I offer an online training course in camelid health management to accompany this book, *The Intensive Camelid Health Care Course for Owners*, available at camelidhealthukeu.thealpacavet.com. This course helps you apply your learning in practice and includes lifetime access to materials, my community and live Q&A sessions with me.

Key Takeaways

Camelids are fascinating creatures with many unique and appealing traits. They possess remarkable adaptations that help them thrive in the harsh conditions of the Andes mountains. However, when raising them outside their native environment, it's essential to remember that these adaptations may not offer the same benefits elsewhere, and you might need to adjust your management practices to help them adapt.

Have a clear understanding of why you want to keep camelids and keep these goals in mind as you begin your journey as a camelid owner. While you might initially plan to have a small herd of three, it's too easy for numbers to grow over time. So be sure this aligns with what's best for you and your animals. Look at the checklist at the end of this chapter to assess your readiness for taking the next step and purchasing your first alpacas or llamas.

Do your homework and ensure you're fully prepared before starting. These are important decisions, and you should take time to make them. If you've made it this far, you're already on the right track, so keep going - you've got this! In the next few chapters, we will cover everything you need to know about camelid husbandry and routine care that will get you well on your way.

Remember that learning is a lifelong journey. Particularly in camelid medicine, what we learn today may be out of date tomorrow. I will leave you with a quote that should comfort you as a new potential owner of alpacas or llamas, concerned that there is much to learn.

"Every expert was once a beginner. Embrace the journey."
- Robin Sharma

Self-Assessment Questions for Prospective Camelid Owners

<table>
<tr><th>Topic</th><th>Questions</th><th colspan="2">Answers</th></tr>
<tr><td rowspan="3">Lifestyle & Time Commitment</td><td>Do I have the time and energy for daily care and regular health checks?</td><td>Yes</td><td>No</td></tr>
<tr><td>Am I prepared for the long-term commitment of owning animals that can live 15-25 years?</td><td>Yes</td><td>No</td></tr>
<tr><td>Do I have a plan for handling the care of my animals when I'm away (e.g. holidays, emergencies)?</td><td>Yes</td><td>No</td></tr>
<tr><td rowspan="3">Space & Shelter</td><td>Do I have enough grazing land?</td><td>Yes</td><td>No</td></tr>
<tr><td>Is my property equipped with safe, sturdy fencing to prevent escapes and protect against wildlife where required?</td><td>Yes</td><td>No</td></tr>
<tr><td>Can I provide adequate shelter for weather protection?</td><td>Yes</td><td>No</td></tr>
</table>

Topic	Questions	Answers	
Financial Considerations	Have I budgeted for initial and ongoing costs (e.g. feed, routine veterinary bills, maintenance, shearing)?	Yes	No
	Am I financially prepared for unexpected expenses such as emergency veterinary care?	Yes	No
	Do I understand the potential income opportunities and limitations (e.g. fibre sales, breeding)?	Yes	No
	Have I looked into insurance options, especially if animals will be engaging with the public?	Yes	No
Knowledge & Preparation	Am I familiar with the behaviour, communication and social needs of alpacas/llamas?	Yes	No
	Have I researched their dietary needs and common health issues?	Yes	No
	Have I consulted with experienced camelid owners or attended workshops for hands-on learning?	Yes	No

Topic	Questions	Answers	
Veterinary & Health Care	Do I have access to a veterinarian with experience in treating camelids?	Yes	No
	Am I knowledgeable about necessary vaccinations, parasite control and common medical conditions?	Yes	No
	Do I know how to monitor their health, and can I recognise early signs of illness?	Yes	No
Legal & Ethical Responsibilities	Do I understand the animal welfare laws and regulations regarding camelid ownership in my country/region?	Yes	No
	Do I need any licenses?	Yes	No
	Am I prepared to meet identification, disease reporting and ethical care requirements?	Yes	No
	Do I know how to ensure my animals are not isolated and will have appropriate companionship?	Yes	No

Topic	Questions	Answers	
Personal & Family Considerations	Does my family or household support this decision and understand the commitment involved?	Yes	No
	Are there any safety concerns with other pets or children interacting with camelids?	Yes	No
	Have I considered how owning these animals might impact my daily life and schedule?	Yes	No
Sustainability & Future Planning	Do I have a plan of action if my circumstances change (e.g. moving, health, financial changes)?	Yes	No
	Do I have a plan for caring for my animals as they age, or if I can no longer care for them?	Yes	No
	Will I be able to cope with end-of-life care when a decision has to be made?	Yes	No
Experience & Support Network	Do I have access to a local community or organisation that supports camelid owners?	Yes	No
	Have I connected with a mentor or experienced breeder who can offer advice and assistance?	Yes	No
	Do I know where to find reputable sources for buying healthy animals?	Yes	No

2

General Camelid Management

In this chapter, I want to familiarise you with some unique aspects of working with camelids. It's helpful to understand their behaviour so that you can work with them rather than fight against them, and to understand the consequences of stress in camelids that can be significant. Learning how to handle your alpacas or llamas is the first part of your journey and will significantly facilitate any management tasks that you need to perform.

In the second part of this chapter, I will cover the basic husbandry requirements you will need to ensure are met to care for your animals, including fencing, shelter, pasture, water and feed.

Behavioural Considerations in Camelids

Camelids are generally curious animals and have excellent eyesight. They love investigating anything new, especially newcomers to the paddock – including humans and animals! They recognise if someone is a stranger to the paddock and will come over to inspect the newcomer. If a fox dares to enter their fields, once the alpacas spot the alien species, they gang up on the fox and drive him out of their territory. This characteristic makes them quite effective poultry guards, and people have used them precisely for this purpose. Alpacas can stamp a fox to death if they catch up with it! Once chased from the field in such a way, the fox will avoid repeating the conflict and skirt around the outside of the field without crossing it.

Camelids tend to greet each other by touching noses, and when meeting new humans, they attempt to do the same. This can seem a little intimidating for those not accustomed to llamas and alpacas! They will usually move away just as soon as they have made that initial contact. After that, you will notice that they prefer to maintain their space. The zone of personal space will increase or decrease depending on the available space around them. If you try to walk up close to an alpaca or llama in a large field, once you cross a certain threshold, they will start to move away. They may then stop to look at you until you once again try to cross that threshold, and then they will again move away from you. If you bring them into a smaller handling area, that threshold distance will be closer to the animal. In a handling pen of 12–14 ft^2 (3.5–4 m^2), you will most likely be able to get up to around

3–4 ft (1–1.2 m) away from them before they move away. Once they become accustomed to being handled, they may become more comfortable with you entering their personal space and permit you to approach them. There will be more on handling in the next section.

Camelids are very vocal and have quite an impressive repertoire of sounds. The most heard sound is their hum. If you sit out in a field near a group of grazing animals, you will often hear them hum to communicate with each other. Mothers and crias also hum to each other frequently. When you gather a group of alpacas or llamas together into a handling area, the amount of vocalisation increases. This vocalisation includes increased humming, and they will sometimes scream if you want to catch them or do something to them that worries them. They can elicit an alarm call if they are worried about something, such as when they spot a pasture invader like a fox. Usually, the animal making the alarm call will stand facing the object of the alarm, with their ears forward and their tails raised. Finally, the males have a very unique sound when breeding, known as "orgling."

It is worth being aware of some of the more negative behaviours that camelids may exhibit, such as kicking and spitting. If you learn to work sympathetically with your animals, you can certainly minimise these behaviours and avoid being in the kicking or spitting zone! Camelids can kick with their back legs in all directions, and the point at which they can kick you with maximum intensity is near full extension of the leg, around 150 degrees from their forward direction. Therefore, if you try to stand close to the animal rather than at its leg's length away, if they decide to kick, they will not be able to build up their full power, and the kick's intensity will be far lower. Happily, since alpacas are small, the worst injury you are likely to sustain is a big bruise. However, some llamas can push you around a bit due to their larger size, and accommodating them to handling is all the more important! Camelids rarely kick out with their front legs as they are not able to achieve a great deal with these, although they may stamp their feet – and stand on your toes if they get in the way! I suggest you always wear closed-toe shoes when working with camelids, as camelid toenails can be quite sharp; also, leather boots will protect your feet far better than flimsy trainers.

Camelids are often known negatively for their spitting behaviour; frustratingly, it is frequently the *only* thing that members of the public are aware of. They regurgitate small amounts of first stomach compartment contents (partially broken-down forages) and expel it with a blast of air from the lungs. The spit usually has a limited chance of reaching you if you are beyond six feet away – unless wind-assisted! More often than not, when the spit hits you, it's because you've been caught in the crossfire rather than being spat at on purpose! However, alpacas and llamas will also spit when threatened or as a response to a sudden insult, such as giving them an injection. Therefore, it should seem obvious not to stand directly in front of a camelid when it is being injected. Beware also of the "umbrella spit," where the spit is directed upwards and then seems to spray down on a relatively wide area!

Remember, spitting is normal behaviour

for camelids and often happens in small pens when animals bump into each other. They may turn and spit at the one that just bumped them. Spitting is also a reproductive behaviour, as females "spit off" when they are non-receptive to the male. It may also be used for asserting dominance over other animals in the herd, for example, at the feed trough, but it can also be a defensive behaviour. Once you have control of the animal, you are responsible for the direction in which the head points, and you should point the head away from other people if the animal chooses to spit. Spit does stink a bit – after all, it is partially digested food! The smell will stay with you all day unless you can wash it off effectively. So, don't wear your best clothes when handling camelids, and I would advise not handling them just before you are about to go out! But if you find yourself hit with a faceful of spit, all I'll say is, "It ain't gonna kill ya!"

Stress

Camelids are known to be quite susceptible to stress. It's important to understand what form that stress may take. Essentially, the source of stress may be anything that changes in their environment. A significant form of stress is relocation from one herd to another. Such relocation might seem innocuous to us, and as a buyer, there is a tendency always to think that you are giving them a "better home." From the alpaca's or llama's perspective, you've taken them away from their friends and family, transported them in a noisy trailer, and placed them in an unfamiliar environment with animals they don't know. Social interactions are very important with camelids, and they do become close to other animals. When you buy an animal and move them to a new farm, you need to be aware of the stress that creating those rifts causes. They will have to establish themselves within the social hierarchy of the new herd.

While less stressful, moving animals within the same herd to different paddocks still disrupts social structures. I remember one of our first alpacas, Totora, who would become incredibly upset at weaning time for her crias and whenever she was separated from her long-time friend, Palpa. She would pace up and down the fence for days. From her, we learned that while weaning is necessary, separating her from Palpa was not an option. Be mindful of these relationships when moving animals around your herd groups; it may be that certain animals have to stay together, and you'll have to figure out how to make that work.

Weaning is a period of significant stress for young animals, and changes in the weather add to this stress. Unlike us, outdoor-dwelling animals can't simply put on a jacket, wrap up in a scarf, or go inside and turn on the heating when it's cold and wet. Their bodies have to adapt to these changes without much external support. Camelids can tolerate gradual temperature changes well; however, when the weather becomes frosty in the autumn, this causes physiological stress that takes time to adapt to. Extra feeding of dry forages and some concentrates will assist camelids in dealing with the cold, but sudden changes are still hard to handle. Likewise, prolonged periods of wet, cold or hot weather will take their toll and constitute stress to the animal.

Finally, an animal can also be stressed by

disease, such as parasitism. Suffering from one disease weakens the animal's ability to cope with another if it occurs.

Signs of Stress

Stressed camelids exhibit some obvious signs of acute stress that may not be apparent to the untrained eye. For example, alpacas will develop a crease line below and parallel to the lower eyelid, and they may also tense their chins - although the latter is more evident in llamas. In addition, the lower eyelid may turn outwards such that you can see the redness of the conjunctiva inside the lower lid. When under severe stress, camelids will breathe open-mouthed (*Figure 1*) and flare their nostrils, breathing more deeply and rapidly to bring more air (oxygenation) into their lungs. You might see this if you try to force an animal to remain still for a procedure or chase it around a pen to catch it. Open-mouth breathing is also very commonly exhibited by males after fighting.

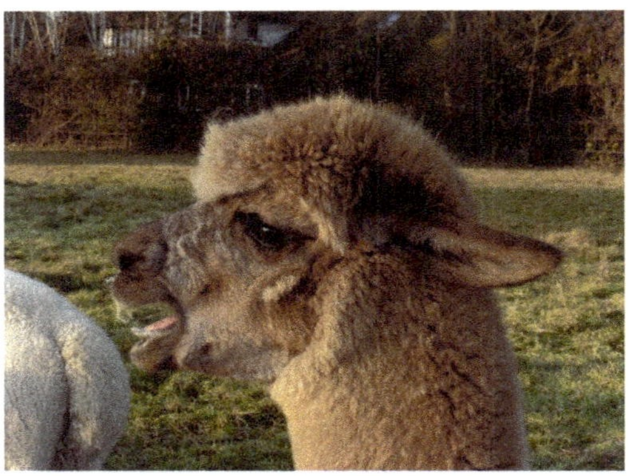

Figure 1. An alpaca shows signs of stress by open-mouthed breathing. If you look closely at the lower eyelid, you may also be able to recognise a wrinkle that also indicates stress.

Effects of Stress

We've talked about what causes stress, but what are the effects on the animals themselves? If a camelid has been under severe stress, you may expect:

Immunosuppression

Immunosuppression is the most significant aspect of prolonged periods of stress, commonly associated with situations such as weaning, relocation and abrupt weather changes as some examples. Stress causes suppression of the immune system that makes the body more susceptible to infections or parasites.

Third stomach compartment (C3) ulcers

It has been known for a while that stress can cause camelids to develop ulcers in their third stomach compartments. The ulcer is usually not the primary issue but is secondary to underlying stress, which may be caused by disease, relocation, or being hospitalised (particularly alone). They are likely the result of reduced blood flow to the mucosa that lines the stomach and/or alterations in the protective mechanisms of the mucosa to potential damage by the acid and digestive enzymes produced in C3. The use of non-steroidal anti-inflammatory medicines (e.g. flunixin meglumine) is also associated with the development of ulcers due to disruption of prostaglandin production. We will discuss ulcers in more detail in Chapter 13.

Pregnancy losses

Stress can cause pregnancy loss in many animals, including camelids. The stress hormone cortisol disrupts the function of the placenta, increasing the risk of pregnancy loss. In camelids, stress during the first and last 60 days of pregnancy is critical and should be avoided whenever possible.

Weight loss from prolonged stress

Camelids subjected to sustained stress levels over a prolonged period might experience weight loss by disrupting normal eating.

Handling

Regular handling of your animals makes management tasks much easier, including collecting faecal samples, weighing, assessing body condition, deworming (when necessary) and administering vaccinations. Not only will it make handling them a pleasure for yourself rather than a chore, but your alpacas or llamas will benefit from being more comfortable with the experience, too. They will be considerably less stressed if gathering them to carry out procedures is routine. Consequently, you can minimise the likelihood of associated problems. As mentioned, stress reduces the immune system's ability to ward off disease and also has the potential to cause pregnancy losses. Additionally, if you need to take your animal to another farm for breeding, to a show or to the vet, an animal trained to walk on a halter is much easier to handle and experiences far less stress.

Do everything you can to make the handling environment assist the process rather than hinder it. Think about constructing handling areas that enable you to catch the animals more easily without chasing them around. Construct the flow on the farm to minimise the amount of actual handling required to get animals to the handling areas. For example, you can install fencing to create pathways that let you move groups of animals easily between fields or to handling areas without needing to handle or halter them. Fencing also avoids dangerous situations, such as moving the animals on a road. If you have large groups of animals, consider creating staged handling areas. Start with a larger holding pen that accommodates the whole group, then use a smaller pen leading from this area to handle fewer animals at a time for procedures. The ideal size for a catch pen is around 8–10 ft^2. Camelids can be herded easily and calmly simply by following them. A few people walking behind the group can gently guide them toward open gates, and this process requires no physical contact – handlers should extend their arms to appear larger, encouraging the animals to move away. Avoid trying to split a group, as those ahead will likely turn back to rejoin those left behind.

A key first step when handling is to ensure that you do not put yourself or others into a dangerous situation. Always ensure that the immediate location for handling is safe and that you would not hit your head on the fencing if pushed over. Always be aware of your surroundings; if you are having trouble, back off and start again. For animals labelled as "difficult," a different strategy may sometimes be necessary. Sometimes, *less* handling is *more* effective: learning the techniques of Camelidynamics can be very helpful here and may result in considerably less stress, physical exertion and injury for both handler and camelid.

When catching a llama or alpaca, first begin by bringing them into a small pen as above. You want to avoid chasing them around a field! Chasing them will only increase their stress and potentially lead to exhaustion for you. Make it easier for yourself and the animals by approaching calmly from behind the head, holding your arms out to block their exit route, and then "catching" them by grasping firmly around the top of the neck. If using Camelidynamics handling, your hand position will be a thumb on one side of the neck, right under the ears, and fingers on the other side. Then, approach with the other hand to place under the jaw – this method is called the "bracelet hold".

When handling camelids, it is essential to learn how they move. Generally speaking, if you have control of the head, then you have control of the animal. If the head is free, they will use their long necks as a lever to try and wriggle themselves free. However, regardless of the handling method, you must always consider keeping them balanced. If you are pulling the head around to the side, this makes them unbalanced, and they will step around to put their head and neck back into straight alignment.

For most procedures that you might need to perform, you can hold them with an arm around the top of the neck, with or without a restraining hand on the withers. (Note that this is not the Camelidynamics style of handling.) The hand on the withers helps to stop them from jumping up. Be calm but firm so that they know that you are serious. If you are half-hearted about handling, they will sense this and easily throw you around. I also recommend talking gently to them during any handling, as they appear to find it calming. Say anything you like; it just needs to be done in a gentle tone! Always stand with feet apart for balance and your knees soft so that you are ready to respond if they move suddenly. Some animals do not appreciate this sort of close contact, and it is better to hold just the head with one hand below the mandible and the other behind the head (the Camelidynamics bracelet hold). Generally, it is not a good idea to touch the hindquarters as this worries them. Alpacas can seemingly move in virtually any direction, sometimes without warning, and they may try to pull away, twist around or spin. They may also rear up, possibly twisting simultaneously, or duck and spring back up! If you are ready for these behaviours, you are more likely to be successful in managing them. Sometimes, when they feel you relax, they *will* take advantage, so be ready for sudden, surprising movements.

If you need to move an animal from one area to another and it is not safe to herd the animal, put a halter with a long rope on it. Then, walk behind the animal using your arms to guide it. If you put your left arm out, it will tend to move to the right, and vice versa. Camelids are naturally curious so they will be happy to walk away from you to investigate where they are. I used to use this method to move alpacas around the hospital at Ohio State. Initially, I found that students had to drag the animals into stalls or to diagnostic and surgical locations – an exhausting process for both animals and handlers. But because the alpacas were curious and had to be on a halter, I would often just walk behind them, and they would naturally move. The key is to stay behind their shoulders. As soon as you get level with the shoulder, they will stop. Drop back and they will start to move forwards once again.

Chutes can help aid management, particularly for llamas, but be careful about the design of the chute you buy. Ideally, chutes should have solid sides so that the animals cannot get their legs stuck between bars and suffer from accidental fractures. If you buy one with bars, consider adapting it to line the side panels inside to prevent the animal from trapping its legs.

A chute should be designed to prevent the animal from twisting or turning around, but will not stop them from jumping up or cushing. You can't trap the head like you can with cattle because their head is no wider than their neck, so a head gate will not work for camelids. Instead, incorporate a shoulder brace at the front of the chute. The brace will stop the animal from pushing forward and out of the front of the chute; usually, they will exit the side through an opening side panel or reverse back out. However, the brace could cause shoulder injury if it lacks padding. Chutes don't necessarily *need* shoulder braces, but they are important for reproductive procedures where you want to minimise as much movement as possible to avoid soft tissue injury due to the instruments used at the back end.

Always use halters made especially for camelids. They should have two buckles for adjustment: one around the nose and the other that goes around the back of the head. Ensure the nose piece is loose enough before placing it onto the nose. It should be able to go all the way up the nose to just in front of the eyes. Then, secure and tighten the neck strap. If necessary, tighten the nose strap so that it can't fall over the nose.

Camelids have a short, bony nose section in front of the eyes where the nose strap can sit safely. When properly secured, halters on camelids should not be loose. If the strap slips down the nose, it may lie over the pliable cartilaginous section of the nose. If the handler pulls down on a rope hooked onto the halter, what may then happen is that the halter pulls down on the cartilage and squishes the nose so that the alpaca or llama cannot breathe. They will then potentially start jumping around to try to get away from you, and not because they don't want to be held, but because they simply want to be able to breathe! If this happens when your camelid is on a halter, quickly check that the strap isn't squashing their nose, readjust if necessary and then all should return to calm.

Camelidynamics

Camelidynamics is a particular approach to handling camelids using techniques developed by Marty McGee Bennett. The approach incorporates TTEAM and TTOUCH principles that Linda Tellington Jones developed, adapted for use with llamas and alpacas. The underlying principles are to respect the animal, use positive and less intrusive techniques for handling, and minimise stress caused by handling. The technique is based on an understanding of animal behaviours and teaches the importance of using balance and leverage in getting cooperation from the alpaca or llama. Handling is less about *restraint* and *force* than *containment* and *cooperation.*

It takes a little time and practice to learn these techniques and get your animals used to them, but those who take the time can work easily with their animals. A course in these methods is worth considering because it will enhance your understanding of how best to work with your animals. Although I don't use the techniques all the time, as I work both with clients who use them and those who don't, I do incorporate some of the techniques to enhance my handling. For example, the bracelet hold is surprisingly effective, particularly for those animals who only want to jump around when handled by other means.

You can also move your index finger around in clockwise circles around the occiput (the bony protrusion at the back of the skill) – this massage technique appears to be calming. Also, if I am trying to move an alpaca on a halter from point A to point B, I will use the ratchet technique to encourage them further along or through a doorway. Another important tip is to ensure that the animals are balanced when handling. If you pull their head around too far to the side, they will move their bodies around to keep themselves balanced. If you keep pulling, you will end up going around in circles! If picking up a foot to trim toenails, ensure that the animal is standing square and is balanced. When picking up a hind foot, resting the animal's stifle on your knee will help them balance all four points. With Camelidynamics, you are taught toenail trimming without picking up the feet at all.

Camelidynamics uses several handling aids to help with catching camelids. For example, a long wand can increase the length of your arms when herding, but the wand can also help place a catch rope around the top of the neck. There is also a "halter-helper" that helps with placing the halter.

I have been impressed with how much you can achieve using these techniques. I once visited the herd of a Camelidynamics instructor, primarily for teaching. However, while I was there she wanted me to remove the deciduous incisors from one of her alpacas. To do this, I needed to sedate the alpaca heavily. I knew that the owner would want to hold her animal using the Camelidynamics techniques, and I was doubtful that I'd be able to give an intravenous injection. However, I decided not to voice my concerns and just went with it to see what would happen – after all, she was a very experienced practitioner of the Camelidynamics techniques.

The owner held her alpaca at arm's length. I squatted down in front of the alpaca and proceeded to locate the jugular vein. I was ready for it to jump as soon as I placed the needle through the skin – but the alpaca didn't move! I managed to ensure I was in the vein by aspirating blood back into the syringe and then injecting the sedation. The alpaca didn't flinch for a moment, and the only thing stopping it from jumping around was its owner holding it with one hand below the jaws and the other on the back of the head. The job was done with no stress whatsoever.

General Husbandry Requirements

This section will discuss the basic requirements for caring for your animals, keeping them safe, and providing for their needs.

Fencing

Your pastures need to be fenced for two reasons. The first reason is to contain the animals and keep them safe from getting out onto a road where they could be hit by vehicles and cause accidents. Camelids can jump fences but tend not to most of the time. The exception would be for males trying to get into female paddocks. Expensive extra-high deer fencing is not usually needed to keep them from jumping out, but it can be used strategically.

The second reason for fencing is to keep groups of animals separated from each other, such as separating males, females and weanlings. Fencing is also there to keep other animals (and people) out of the fields where your animals are, and having decent fencing will help to keep stray dogs out of your pastures. Irresponsible dog owners, the numbers of whom appear to have increased in recent years, sometimes let their dogs wander. Groups of stray dogs can be hazardous, as they can attack and kill camelids. Well-constructed fencing will minimise this risk.

The type of fencing you choose can be particularly important if you need to restrict access to wild animals that may carry certain diseases. An additional use for fencing is to use it inside hedgerows to prevent animals from picking up vegetation in their fleeces when they rub against them.

Sheep fencing is considered the best type for camelids as it contains adults and crias and normally keeps dogs out. This type of fencing is a wire mesh type of fencing with large squares of about 10cm in size. Normally, to increase the total height of the fencing, you would put 2–3 lines of smooth wires above. You should not use barbed wire as it can damage fleeces and potentially cause eye damage since camelids sometimes rub themselves along fencing, and their large eyes are susceptible to trauma. Any wire fencing should be tensioned; loose fencing poses a risk to animals as they can get their legs or necks caught.

Post and rail-type fencing can work quite well, though be aware that crias are more likely to escape through the gaps between rails, so rails closer together can prevent this. However, be aware that post and rail-type fencing won't keep dogs out. Camelids will also occasionally graze through the fence. They may injure their necks if they move suddenly while their necks are between the rails. Cervical vertebral injuries (injuries affecting the vertebrae of the neck) are a relatively common injury in alpacas and are usually thought to be related to fencing.

Perimeter fencing can be used to restrict access from wildlife that could carry disease. For example, in the UK, in areas where there is bovine tuberculosis, badger-proof and deer-proof fencing can be used to keep potential carriers out. Badger-proof fencing must have wire mesh, and the wires should be no further than 7 cm apart. It also needs to be dug into the ground with the underground section angled at (ideally) 45° away from the vertical. (*Figure 2*) The dug-in portion prevents badgers from digging under the fence, as they will meet an underground portion of impenetrable fencing.

The alternative to dug-in fencing is to use electric wire around the outside of the fencing, though this can't be used on public footpaths. For this, use 2-3 strands of electrified wire, one near the ground to stop badgers from digging under the fence and one at the top of the fence to stop them from climbing over. Electric fencing requires a lot of maintenance as you must keep the grass and weeds from touching it, and the fence must be checked regularly to ensure it works properly. In the UK, deer-proof fencing must be at least 180 cm (6 ft) high to prevent deer from jumping over. In North America, if you wish to restrict access to white-tailed deer, go for 240 cm (8 ft).

Lastly, electric fencing alone isn't particularly effective for camelids, especially as their fleece insulates them from shocks.

Shelter

Camelids are well-suited to living outdoors year-round, as they are adapted to cold, arid climates. In Puno, Peru, at an altitude of 3,827 m, average annual temperatures between 1991 and 2022 ranged from 7°C to 11°C, with winter (May to September) temperatures between -3°C and 16°C and

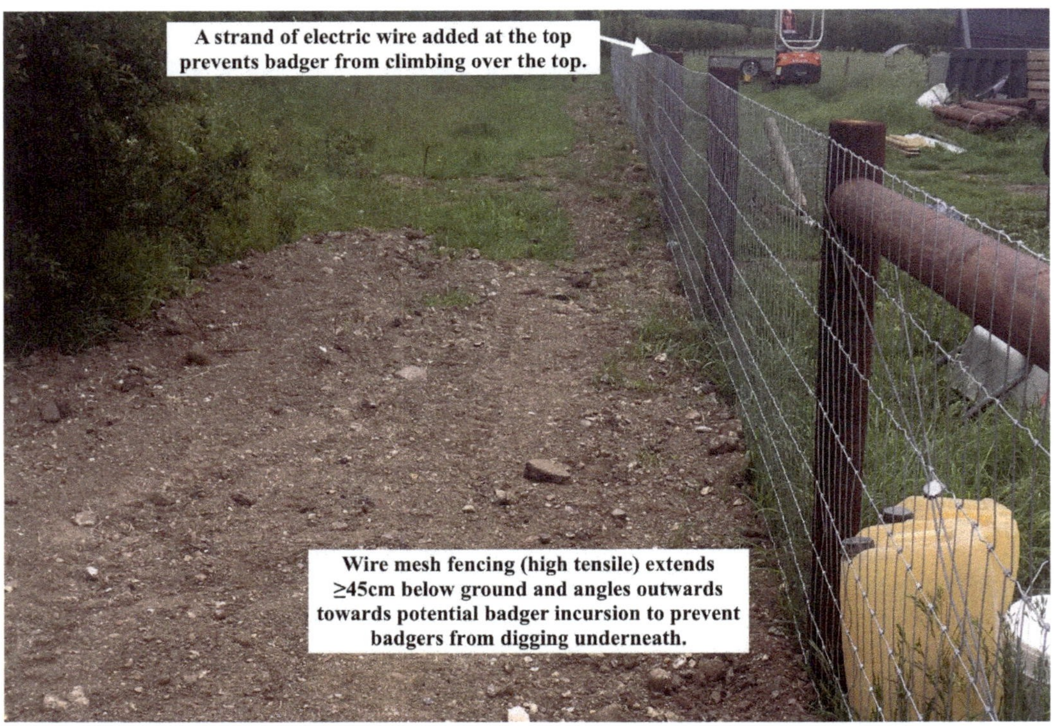
A strand of electric wire added at the top prevents badger from climbing over the top.
Wire mesh fencing (high tensile) extends ≥45cm below ground and angles outwards towards potential badger incursion to prevent badgers from digging underneath.

Figure 2. Badger-proof fencing with mesh dug in on the outside of the fence (unseen). Wires on this type of fence must be high tensile, properly tensioned and with wires no more than 7 cm apart. Electric fencing at the top deters climbing badgers.

summer (December to March) temperatures between 5°C and 18.5°C.[1] Precipitation is low in winter and higher in summer.

Outside South America, camelids face more variable climates. *Figures 3-7* illustrate these differences. In the United States, temperatures range widely - from an average minimum of -7°C in Ohio in winter to an average maximum of 29°C in summer. Florida's average temperatures are steadier, from 15°C to 28°C. In the UK, average temperatures range from 4°C in winter to 15°C in summer (1.5°C to 20°C overall), with higher rainfall in the colder winter months. While the south of the UK can get hot, heatwaves are usually short-lived. In New South Wales, Australia, average temperatures range from 10°C to 26°C, with extremes from 4°C to 33°C.

In particularly cold winter climates, such as those in northern parts of the US, Canada and Scandinavia, camelids may need to spend part of their time indoors. They should also have access to shelter to protect them from inclement weather, especially rain. Unlike sheep, which are well-adapted to cold and wet conditions due to the lanolin in their fleeces, camelids lack natural oils and can become soaked and chilled in cold, wet weather. They must have a way to get out of the rain.

While camelid fleeces provide good insulation against snow, temperatures below freezing require additional feeding to help them cope. If temperatures drop below -5°C (23°F), other problems can start to materialise due to the stress of dealing with the cold on the body. A three-sided shelter, positioned away from prevailing winds, is generally sufficient for most needs. However, having an enclosed space, like a stable or a pen in a barn, is also helpful for sick animals or newborn crias. Straw makes the best bedding for insulation.

Camelids don't like dark spaces inside shelters. They are more likely to use shelters with more light. For this, skylight panels on the roof may help improve the ambient lighting. Be sure to position shelters away from the prevailing weather and preferably at the periphery of the pasture. Avoid placing them where they block the view of grazing areas, as animals may avoid grazing behind shelters if they cannot see you approaching with feed.

Camelids also need shelter from hot weather as they are susceptible to heat stress, particularly during prolonged periods of heat and humidity. This vulnerability is due to their limited ability to lose heat, as most of their body is covered by fleece. Heat dissipation occurs only from less hairy areas such as the belly, inside the hind limbs, and armpits. If a camelid becomes recumbent from heat stress, its ability to cool down is further reduced.

The heat stress index (HSI) helps predict the likelihood of heat stress. To calculate for HSI, add the temperature (in °F) to the percentage humidity. A value over 150 indicates a high risk of heat stress. Camelids should be shorn early in the summer to reduce this risk, allowing their fleece to regrow before winter. Additionally, they must have access to shade on sunny days.

Camelids also need to be able to find shade when it is sunny. They love to "sunbathe" (I've lost count of how many times I ran out to check on an alpaca sprawled flat in the pasture!), but this behaviour can sometimes lead to heat exhaustion, particularly in darker-fleeced animals. In sweltering climates, fans, water sprayers, and water baths can aid evaporative cooling.

Not every pasture has to have permanent access to a shelter. Hedgerows and treelines make great windbreaks and can provide some shelter from rain. In summer, trees provide shade with excellent ventilation.

Barns provide valuable shelter for larger herds, but it's vital to ensure adequate ventilation to reduce the risk of respiratory disease. Barns can be made adaptable to facilitate various tasks, as movable posts and gates can accommodate various tasks throughout the year. For example, the space can be configured for animal handling, allowing procedures like pregnancy checks with ultrasound to be done out of daylight and rain. The space can then be repurposed for shearing, weighing, vaccinating animals or housing groups during winter. Additionally, sick pens can be set up to care for individual sick animals or crias.

Flooring in barns also requires careful consideration. While concrete is the easiest to clean and disinfect, it's a cold surface for

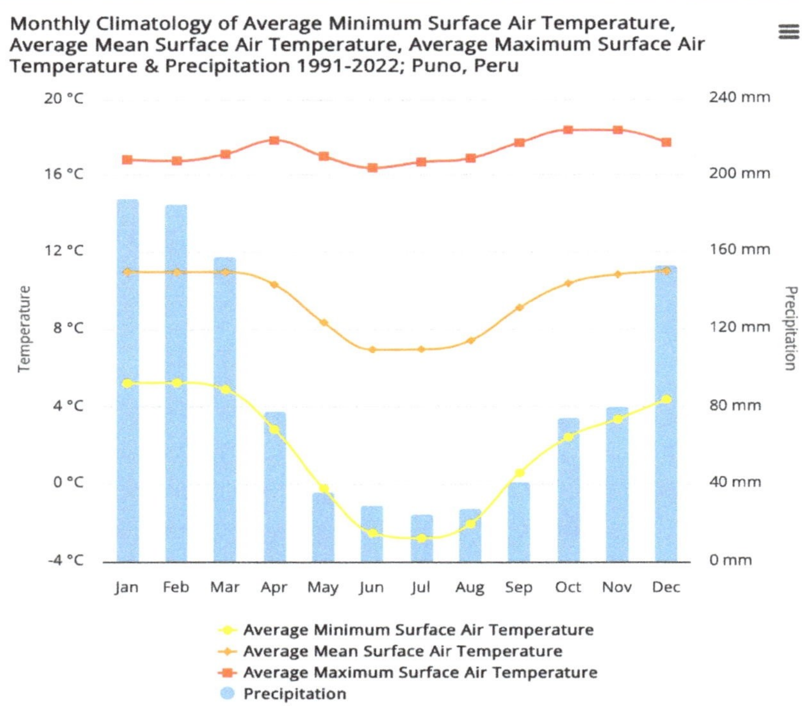

Figure 3.

Figures 3-7. These charts show the average monthly temperatures and rainfall in different parts of the world where camelids are farmed. Puno, Peru; United Kingdom; Ohio, USA; Florida, USA; New South Wales, Australia.[3]

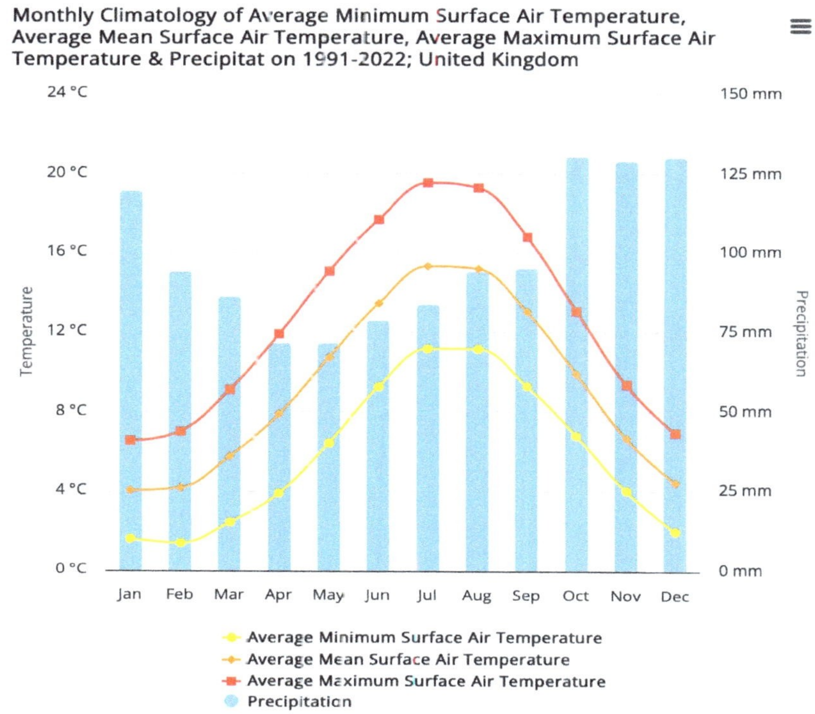

Figure 4.

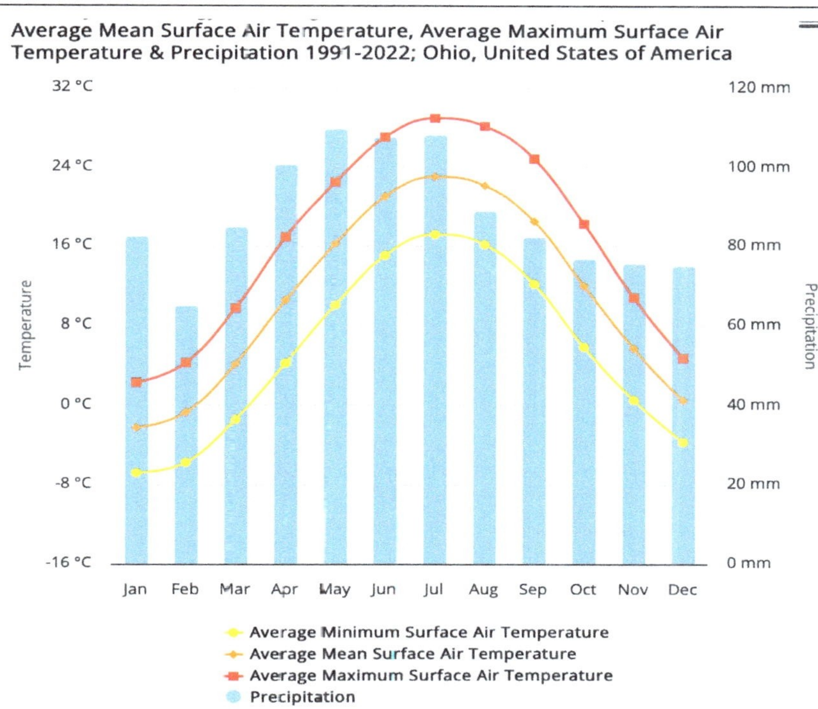

Figure 5.

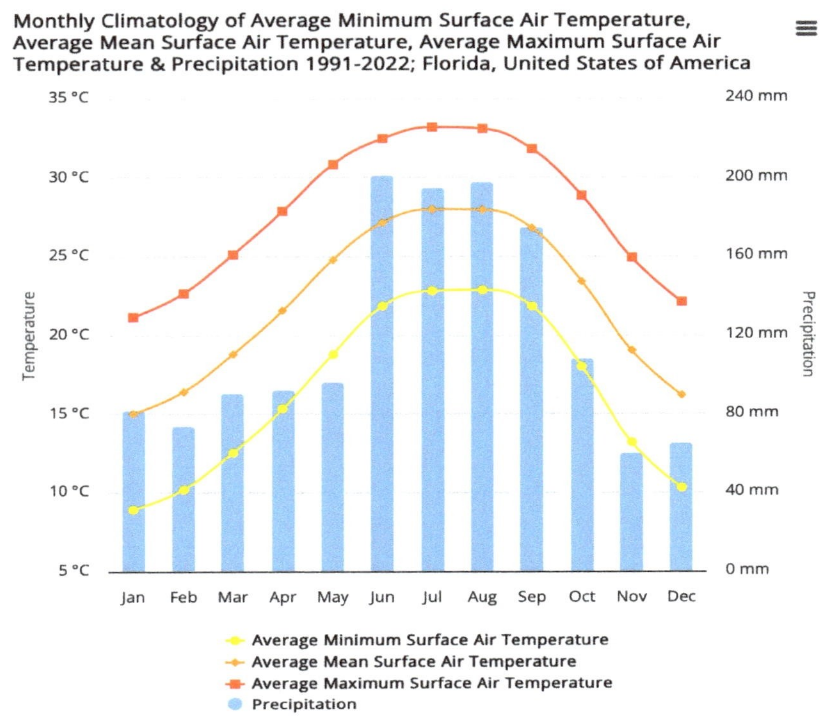

Figure 6.

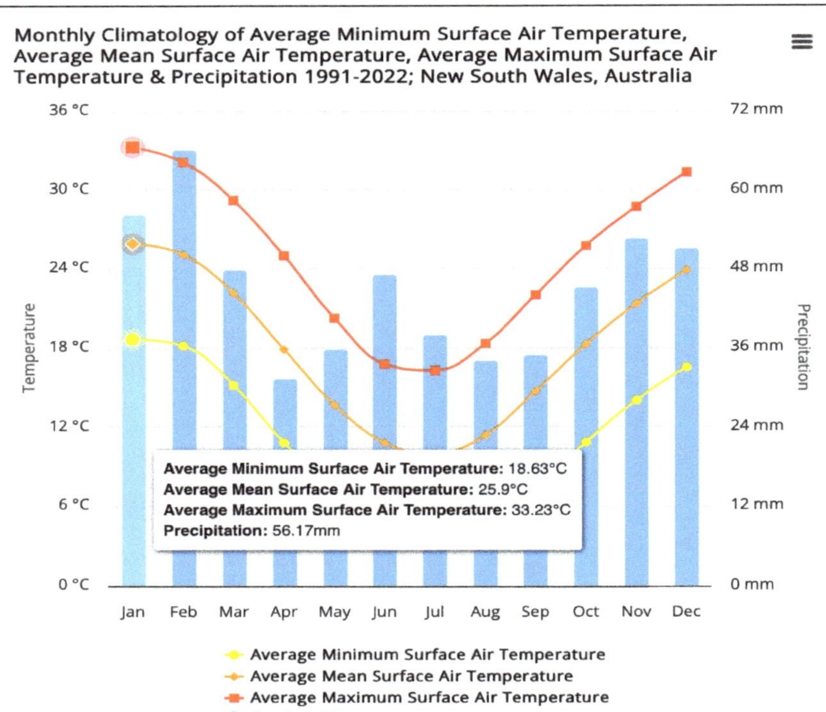

Figure 7.

sick pens and needs insulating with rubber matting and/or straw. Dirt floors or crushed limestone are difficult to clean or disinfect. Straw is the preferred substrate for sick pens due to its insulating properties, but some breeders avoid it because it can get into the fleece and reduce its quality. Similarly, wood shavings are rarely used as they also become embedded in the fleece.

Pasture

The amount of space needed for your alpacas or llamas will vary depending on the type of grazing that you have. On good quality grazing, stocking densities can be higher than those on poorer quality or more marginal types of land. For example, in the temperate UK climate, lowland pastures will be able to handle more animals than upland hilly areas in places like Scotland. Grazing in the northeastern USA will also be of much better quality than that found in places like Colorado or Montana.

There are two main types of pasture used for grazing animals: static or rotation grazing. Static grazing works best with larger areas and lower stocking densities, while rotational grazing allows pastures to rest and maximises the number of animals that smaller pastures can support. It should be noted that, over time, dung piles will accumulate, and camelids will avoid grazing near these areas, leaving the grass to grow lush but untouched, eventually reducing the available grazing space. Where minimal pasture is available, dung removal becomes more important for both parasite control *and* maintaining grass availability.

When resting pastures for parasite control, one frequently asked question is, how long should one rest the pastures? The goal is to rest it long enough for hatched larvae to die off due to a lack of a suitable host. The timescale depends entirely on environmental conditions, particularly moisture and temperature, because larval survival depends on this. Advice will therefore vary geographically. Hot weather increases the larvae's metabolic rate and shortens their lifespan, while cool, dry weather prolongs it. Moisture supports larval development, making wet conditions less ideal for parasite control. Overnight frosts are particularly effective at reducing parasite burdens, although *Nematodirus* presents a unique challenge. This parasite requires a cold period for larval development within the egg and then warmer temperatures of at least 10°C to hatch. If these conditions occur in quick succession, they can trigger the mass emergence of larvae, posing significant risks to spring lambs in the UK.

Coming back to the question of how long to rest pastures: In the UK, where conditions often favour parasite survival, a significant reduction in parasite larvae can be seen after four months. However, they may not be completely eradicated. It's also important to note that some parasites survive within the host. Although not yet clearly documented in camelids, it is known in small ruminants that some parasites can undergo a period of dormancy within the host. This dormancy allows them to wait for more favourable conditions and can be a problem during the summer. Specifically in camelids in the UK, when a hot and dry June or July is followed by wet weather in August, burdens can rapidly re-accumulate due to a sudden parasite "bloom," and we will often see a lot of *Haemonchus* cases at that time.

Generally, allow 1 acre of pasture per 5 animals on good quality grazing (equivalent to 0.4 hectares). Stocking density can be increased for short periods, but animals must be moved more regularly to allow the grass to recover. You never want to fill every spare piece of land with animals; you need to ensure that you always have spare ungrazed or rested pasture available to move animals onto. Doing this not only supports grass recovery but also helps manage parasites.

A common issue new camelid keepers face is that they have a single field available, allowing the animals to have access to the entire space all the time. When problems crop up later on – as they inevitably do – they have no capacity to move animals onto clean, rested pasture. This can make it very difficult to get on top of a worm infestation or a mange problem. If you only have one large pasture, consider dividing it into smaller paddocks. Since animals tend to graze unevenly in elongated paddocks, square paddocks are more efficient than long, narrow ones. Thoughtful placement of field shelters and fencing can allow shared access to the same shelter from multiple paddocks – for example, placing a shelter at the centre of four square paddocks.

In terms of the pasture itself, mixed species grasses are best. Stay away from single-species pastures such as ryegrass or garden mixes. If you have ryegrass in your pasture mix, use endophyte-free varieties to reduce the risk of ryegrass toxicity or staggers. Ryegrass staggers is a neurological problem caused by toxins produced by the endophyte fungus that infects perennial ryegrass. While ryegrass staggers are more common in the United States, Australia, New Zealand and southern Europe, it is less of an issue in the UK and northern Europe due to different environmental conditions.

Wet or poorly drained areas should be avoided or fenced off. Camelids are susceptible to liver fluke, which thrives in waterlogged pastures, particularly in regions like the UK and the Pacific Northwest of the USA. Wet ground can also lead to foot problems and make vehicle access more challenging.

Camelids are well-adapted to poor-quality grazing, reflecting their origins in the Andes, where mountainous pastures are variable and poor-quality. Research by Dulphy et al. showed that llamas are better than sheep at extracting nutrition from low-quality grazing. However, on good pasture, both species perform equally well.[2] That said, this does not mean keeping them on poor-quality grazing is compatible with optimum production or health!

Water

A fresh, clean source of water must always be available. Camelids appear to barely drink when grazing on lush, wet grass, but they drink noticeably more in hot weather or when grazing is dry.

Water can be provided in mains-water-fed troughs or buckets filled from a tank or bowser. Just make sure that *containers are stable and cannot be knocked over.* Keep the tanks or buckets clean, as algae and debris accumulate over time. The frequency of this is unpredictable and *will vary depending on location and environmental conditions.*

If you use on-farm water sources, such as boreholes or open rainwater storage dams, ensure the water is filtered before it reaches the troughs, and monitor filters during heavy rainfall to prevent them from becoming overwhelmed. I have seen giardia outbreaks in herds with overwhelmed water filters.

If you live in a region with freezing winters, you'll need to break the ice on water troughs or buckets so the animals can still drink. You may also need to turn off the main water supply to prevent pipes from freezing and bursting, and then you'll have to top up the water manually. In the northern parts of North America and Europe, you can get buckets with electrical heating elements to keep the water from freezing.

Camelids love water and will immerse themselves in it if at all possible! To prevent them from soaking themselves and potentially damaging their fleeces, it is a good idea to install bars across water tanks and fence off ponds. On the other hand, you may have a willing participant should bathing be required to treat skin problems! In particularly hot weather, children's paddling pools (not the inflatable ones) make quite effective areas for camelids to cool off, as they love sitting in the water to help keep themselves cool.

Feed

Camelids can thrive on good quality pasture, supplemented with stored forages such as hay, haylage or dried chopped grass during periods when the grass is sparse or of poor quality. Some animals, especially non-breeding females and non-working or gelded males, will gain weight on this diet. The same will be true in other parts of the world with temperate climates. One thing to be aware of is that lush spring grass can contain so much water that the nutritional content is lower than it would appear. Under these circumstances, to consume sufficient energy and protein to match their nutritional requirements, camelids may require supplementary stored forages and feed.

Supplementary feed will be necessary where grazing is of insufficient quality to meet their demands. This need may arise during cold or hot periods when the grass isn't growing, is of poor quality, or in locations where grazing is poor. Growing animals, as well as late-pregnant and lactating females, have the highest energy and protein requirements. Supplementation may also be necessary in cold weather, as camelids need extra energy to keep warm.

There are many feed manufacturers offering feeds marketed specifically for camelids, although not all will have researched camelid requirements specifically, so don't assume that if a feed is labelled for camelids, it is formulated with camelids in mind. Do your research! A pelleted ration is preferred to a coarse mix or muesli-type ration, as this ensures a more even spread of nutrients and discourages picky feeding.

Next, look at the ingredients on the label. These tend to be listed in order of priority in the bag. In other words, the first ingredient on the label will make up the highest percentage of the ration. Avoid feed that lists grains such as corn/maize, barley and wheat as the first three ingredients, as these can cause acidosis and third stomach compartment ulcers. Oats are the best of the grains as they are not ulcerogenic and

When I was working at the Royal Veterinary College, an owner brought in two alpacas on a Friday afternoon for evaluation of "not doing right." (When I was in the US, we would have called this "ADR" or "ain't doin' right!") One of the alpacas presented with a hunched-up appearance, grinding its teeth and exhibiting excessive salivation. I observed as the students asked the owners questions and performed their physical examination. It seemed to me that the students were not specific enough when asking the owners about the alpacas' diet. They had asked if the alpacas were eating, and the owners said no. I felt there was some missing information here, so when the students finished, I asked the owners to explain further. I started by confirming that they'd said the alpacas were not eating, then asked if they were eating concentrates. They replied that they were not. Next, I asked, "Are they eating forages, like hay?" They gave me a confused look.

Given that it had snowed on Monday night, stayed below freezing, and there were still three to four inches of snow on the ground, I asked, "You are feeding hay, right?" To my surprise, they replied that they had assumed the alpacas would move the snow and graze on the grass underneath. And there lay the problem: The alpacas had not eaten forage for nearly four days and were starving.

The clinical evaluation and diagnostic testing confirmed no underlying illnesses; the clinical signs being displayed were due to the effects of the stress of starvation. We gave the alpacas hay, which they tucked into gratefully, and treated the alpaca grinding its teeth and salivating excessively for third compartment ulcers. We then sent the owners home to source some hay for the remaining alpacas in their small herd so that they would not also succumb to starvation and ulcers!

The moral of this story is that alpacas and llamas need to be fed forages where none are available - not just concentrates! As owners, you need to ensure that you have stored enough forages ahead of winter and as feed in the event of drought or when the animals cannot get sufficient nutrition from the grass on their pastures.

are higher in fibre. Sugar beet is another excellent feed that provides energy without inducing ulcers. It is also recommended for weight gain and encouraging sick camelids to eat. Alfalfa or lucerne, which can come in hay, chopped hay or pellets, is great for added protein and promotes weight gain.

In terms of the micronutrients in the feed, the first thing to look for is that the feed has added vitamin D. Camelids are very sensitive to vitamin D deficiency when kept at low altitudes and non-equatorial latitudes (i.e. most places away from the Andes), because of the reduced ultraviolet radiation. However, those in the southern states of the US may see much more ultraviolet radiation year-round. A typical supplementation level would be between 8,000–18,000 IU of 25-hydroxyvitamin D per kilogram of feed.

The next micronutrient to look for on a feed label is zinc, which is important due to its involvement in skin health. Zinc deficiency can cause scaly, scurfy skin and increased susceptibility to skin problems such as mange. On the feed label, look for the form of zinc that is included. Zinc oxide or zinc sulphate is not well absorbed. Chelated zinc, such as zinc methionine, is absorbed far better. You should also watch out for high copper as camelids are sensitive to high copper levels, similar to sheep. Cattle rations should be avoided for this reason as copper supplementation tends to be much higher.

Key Takeaways

This chapter provides insights into camelid behaviour and helps you understand the very important issue of stress concerning camelids. If you understand how your animals behave and respond to events, you can minimise the stress experienced and help to keep them happy and healthy.

Handling is a key skill you must master to manage your herd effectively. Handling isn't something you can leave to someone else. There are different schools of thought concerning handling. You can learn both and practise one or the other, or incorporate techniques from both if this suits you better.

In this chapter, I have also outlined critical infrastructure - fencing, shelter, and pasture space - that you must consider when setting up your farm and highlighted the animals' absolute needs for fresh water and supplementary feed where required. We will discuss nutrition in much more detail in Chapters 5 and 6.

3

Routine Herd Health Activities: Part 1

There are several non-negotiable activities that must be scheduled and performed regularly to maintain your herd's health. Some activities are focused on monitoring your animals' well-being, while others aim to prevent diseases or other issues. All will help you keep your animals in the best health and help you stay ahead of the curve.

Monitoring is essential because it allows you to spot early signs of disease, and quick action can help minimise the potential impact on an animal's health while preventing the spread to other animals in the case of infectious problems.

Without a doubt, if you follow this list of non-negotiable activities and schedule them into your herd health plan, you will benefit from a more rewarding relationship with your animals. You will feel more confident as an owner because you'll know your animals' state rather than have to guess at it. You will also be less likely to find yourself in a herd health crisis.

You will find non-negotiables 1 to 5 detailed here in this chapter and non-negotiables 6 to 10 in the following chapter. We will look at each of them in turn.

The 10 Non-Negotiable Herd Health Activities

1. Observation
2. Body Condition Scoring
3. Checking the Mucous Membrane Colour
4. Faecal Testing as Part of a Parasite Control Strategy
5. Vaccinations
6. Toenail Trimming
7. Vitamin D Supplementation
8. Shearing
9. Dental Care
10. Plan Nutrition

1. Observation

Learning what is normal

Observation is a key tool in monitoring your animals' health. Clearly, if you are *not* watching your alpacas or llamas, you will *not* know if something is wrong. Understanding what is normal behaviour in your animals is key to recognising when something is off. This awareness comes from consistent observation and develops with experience. Part of your routine management is to spend time each day watching your herd. Daily observation allows you to notice important signs, such as an individual not approaching the feed trough, being bullied, or spending more time lying down than usual.

At the start, you may find that everything you observe raises a question about whether a particular behaviour is normal. But as you observe more and more, you will gradually become familiar with your herd's behaviour and learn to spot if something isn't quite right. Some individuals may exhibit odd behaviours that seem "normal" to them, and you will also learn the hierarchy of the animals in the herd.

You will also notice animals that have close relationships and realise that if you separate these animals, it can cause excessive stress. Closely related females often exhibit this bond and do not like being separated. These females are sometimes observed "helping out" and "reassuring" a young maiden female who's just given birth to a cria for the first time. They are also sometimes the designated babysitters. (I like to call them "aunties" when they're performing this role.) Recognising and learning these relationships can help you manage animals within your herd and groups, minimising stress-related concerns.

Once you have learned what is typical for your animals, you are more likely to spot if an individual behaves uncharacteristically. Most animals move together as a herd to eat and graze. Any animal that separates itself from the herd or spends more time lying down should raise alarm bells.

Behaviour at the feed trough

Observation at the feed trough will teach you quite a lot about the hierarchy within your herd, so you may miss useful information if you put the feed out and then just walk away. Dominant animals often go to the feed trough, push others aside or spit at them to clear space and secure more food. However, some spend so much time policing the trough and spitting at subordinates that they fail to eat enough to meet their own nutritional needs. On the other hand, recessive animals at the bottom of the hierarchy may hang back and wait for space, only to find that little feed remains by the time they approach. These animals also need adequate nutrition, and it may be necessary to feed them separately by coaxing them into a small pen with their own measured portion. Another way to resolve this is to adjust how the feed is provided. In small herds, using separate bowls spaced apart can reduce competition. Increasing the trough space may be sufficient in larger groups to ensure all animals have access to feed.

Camelid veterinarians recommend that alpacas require 3 ft (90 cm) of head space in a single-sided trough. By comparison, the Red Tractor Assurance Scheme recommends 40 cm of trough space per head for cattle weighing 200–299 kg, 70 cm for cattle weighing 700–799 kg (a typical dairy cow), and 45 cm for a medium-sized sheep. Given the size differences, alpacas need more space than other livestock to reduce competitive feeding! If the feed is accessible from both sides of the trough, one would imagine that trough space may be reduced. However, having the animals competing head-to-head adds further dimensions to competitive feeding within groups of camelids. Only by observing feeding behaviour within your herd will you learn how to manage groups effectively and select individuals that may require more sensitive management.

An owner in the United States recently shared a story about two alpacas with poor body condition: an adult alpaca that had become lethargic and a 10-month-old that wasn't growing. She took both alpacas to a referral centre, and they received a thorough diagnostic workup. The adult alpaca was known to be submissive in a hierarchy within the herd. She was found to have an ulcerated second stomach compartment, was not anaemic, had a normal total protein concentration, and had a faecal egg count that was in a range that didn't warrant treatment. The owner requested that she be treated for *Eimeria macusaniensis* in case a pre-patent burden caused weight loss. She was treated for the ulcer and started eating voraciously the day after treatment began. The 10-month-old alpaca was also quite submissive in attitude within the herd, but the referral centre could not find a reason for her failure to gain weight. When the owner returned the animals to the herd, she put out hay and feed and observed her alpacas for a full hour. She discovered that two adult females were intimidating the alpacas she'd evaluated, and they wouldn't eat. The owner had provided individual feed trays plus an extra two until then. She moved these so that there were 3 feet between each tray and moved the hay feeders (she provided one for every two alpacas) 10 feet apart. Ever since, these two alpacas have been gaining weight! Careful observation helped this owner find a simple solution to a serious and frustrating problem.

2. Body Condition Scoring

Body condition scoring is by far the single most important herd health monitoring tool that you should master when keeping alpacas and llamas – or any other type of livestock, for that matter. This is because it allows you to monitor the animals' health individually and in groups.

Weight loss in an individual animal may indicate dental problems, parasitism, or other diseases, prompting the owner to investigate these issues with their veterinarian. Diagnostic testing can detect parasites in faecal samples and identify changes in haematological or biochemical profiles, which can help diagnose other issues. A faecal sample should *always* be checked as a first port of call in any weight loss case.

Another common cause of weight loss is oral pain. Owners can palpate both jaws to check for evidence of tooth root abscesses. These will be evident as hard swellings on the mandible that are typically painful if pressure is applied. I advise against intra-oral examination without proper equipment because it is quite easy to get bitten (unintentionally) by an alpaca or llama, but this can be painful!

Faecal testing and checking for mandibular swellings are simple tasks owners can perform before they call their vet. However, if the weight loss is severe or the individual is inappetent, do not delay calling your vet to investigate further.

Weight loss consistent across most or all of a group is likely to suggest inadequate dietary provision. Since parasites tend to affect some individuals more than others, with 20% of individuals in a herd generally responsible for 80% of the parasite problems, parasitism is less likely to be the main cause of weight loss across a group. However, it may contribute to the problem in the herd. Poor nutrition will put the immune system under stress, and animals will be less likely to manage any parasite burdens they're exposed to.

Weight gain is more likely when the nutritional supply exceeds the animals' requirements. This may occur in individuals or across groups. It most often occurs with individuals when animals with lower nutritional requirements are fed with higher requirements. It occurs most commonly when non-pregnant or non-lactating females are fed alongside late pregnant or lactating females whose nutritional requirements are considerably higher than theirs. Strategic feeding can help manage this in smaller herds where keeping them in separate groups isn't feasible.

Body condition scoring should be done routinely, with the results recorded in each animal's records. I suggest checking animals monthly as a routine, but it can be done more frequently in animals that are either losing or gaining weight to assess the effectiveness of dietary changes.

Due to the presence of fleece, it can be difficult to judge the animals' condition from a distance, so hands-on body condition scoring is essential. Weighing your animals may provide a more accurate and immediate measure of dietary changes.

Body condition scoring is achieved using a scoring system. I prefer a 1–10 scale, with 1 being very thin and 10 being obese. Some people prefer a 1–5 scale, and others use a 1–9 scale. It doesn't matter which scoring system you use as long as you do your body condition scoring consistently. When speaking with your veterinarian or others about an animal and communicating their body condition, specify which scoring system you use. A score of 3 out of 10 is very different to a score of 3 out of 5 and will elicit a very different response if you're requesting advice. I use the 10-point scale because I have more pigeonholes to put animals into. With time, you will develop a particular sensitivity to the technique and find that you want to use half or even quarter scores. A body condition score (BCS) of 4–4.5 out of 10 could be termed 4.25/10, and this would be difficult to label on the 1 to 5 scoring system, as it would be a score of 2.125 – that would be hard to say and hard to write down!

On the scoring system of 10, I advise that you *aim* for a BCS of 5.5–6 out of 10 for females at all stages of gestation and lactation. Females may lose some body condition after giving birth, particularly 6–8 weeks into lactation when milk production peaks and the crias are growing at their fastest rate. If you notice females losing condition during lactation, you should try to increase their nutritional provision to match their demands. Suppose they get into a negative energy balance where their nutrition is insufficient for their needs. In that case, they can get into a dangerous situation metabolically due to mobilising fat as an alternative energy source.

Males should ideally have BCS of 6–7 at the start of the breeding season, as they can lose a little condition during this period. Aim for a BCS of 5.5–6 out of 10 if not working as a stud male.

The main area to palpate for body condition scoring is over the mid-back, but you will also need to drop your hand down to feel over the ribcage (*Figure 1*). You feel for the muscle and fat covering and supporting the spine and the fat covering over the last few ribs. Suris and Huacayas differ in how they store fat, which affects body condition scoring. Suris tend to store more fat along the topline for insulation, likely due to their distinct coat type. Because of this, in suris, the rib cover often can give a more accurate indication of body condition than feeling over the topline. In suris, the rib and spine can disagree, while in huacayas, the rib cover and back tend to agree.

Older animals also feel differently during scoring, as ageing makes them more concave along the spine. Thus, rib cover is a more reliable indicator of body condition. Males are also unique in that they tend to have more muscle around the spine, so again, it is important to feel for rib cover to get a proper idea of their condition.

Figure 2 illustrates a range of body condition scores, showing cross-sectional diagrams through the spine, a rear view and descriptions for clarity. For an animal with a BCS of 5/10, when laying your hand perpendicular to the spine and angled towards the ribs, your hand will feel as

While doing my residency at Ohio State, my mentor David Anderson and I occasionally discussed body condition scores. I liked to use half scores, and he would joke that it was because I couldn't make up my mind! I would argue, "But it's between a 4 and a 5 out of 10!"

When I returned to the UK, I was amused to see quarter scores listed on my family's farm faecal submission forms. I thought to myself, maybe *here* was a person who couldn't make their mind up! Was it even possible to differentiate a quarter score?

One day, while checking alpacas on the farm, I decided to test the theory. I found an alpaca whose body condition score I couldn't quite decide – was it a 4 or a 4.5 out of 10? So I asked Iain, my cousin's husband, what BCS he would give that alpaca. He palpated her for a few seconds before confidently declaring, "Four and a quarter!" Touché, my friend!

Sites for Body Condition Scoring

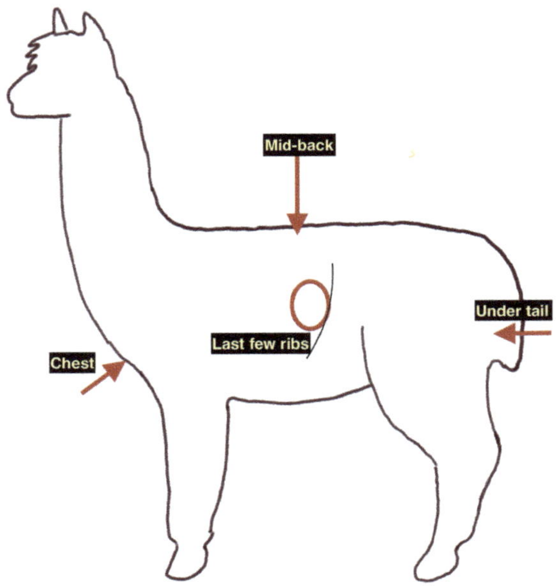

Figure 1. This diagram shows the main sites for performing body condition scoring in camelids.

though it's sitting flat, neither concave nor convex. Below a 5/10, it will become progressively more concave until there is very little muscle or fat, and the animal is literally a bag of bones. Above a 5/10, the fat and muscle will fill out progressively until there is a flat surface over the back, which would be a 10/10. For a 6/10, the topline should feel slightly rounded on either side of the spine, and the ribs should be palpable, but they should feel as though they have healthy muscle coverage and a little fat. When animals become skinnier, you can fit your fingers between the ribs. As they become fatter, the ribs become harder to palpate.

Fatter animals can be hard to BCS using just the topline and the ribcage. If an animal is overweight, the next place to look is under the tail. Animals start to store fat in the perineal area (under the tail) when they have a BCS of 7.5/10. This will be evident as fat pads on either side of the anus, just above the bony protuberance there (the tuber ischium of the pelvic bones). Typically, this area is dished and hollow in females. Once there is fat there, the area becomes more flat in profile, and you can tap the fat, and it will wobble a little. Males tend to be a little flatter in profile in this area already, but you can still appreciate the fat deposition from 7.5/10. As they get fatter, they start depositing fat at the

BCS (/10)		Spine	Rear View	Description
BCS 1	Emaciated	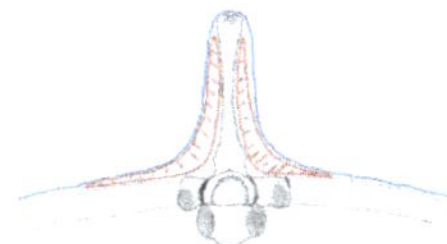	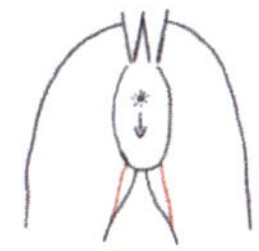	The spine will feel like a knife-edge and ribs are very prominent (you can fit your fingers between them). Very slim legs – no muscle.
BCS 3	Poor / thin	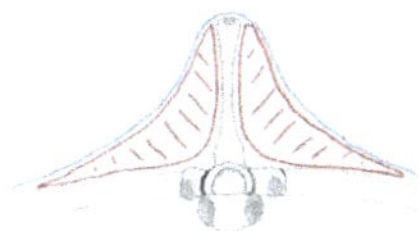	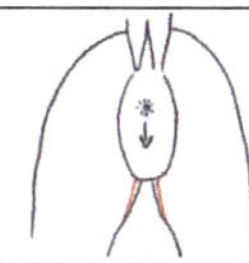	The alpaca is thin, and the muscles are concave either side of the spine: ribs are prominent. Slim legs.
BCS 5	Borderline	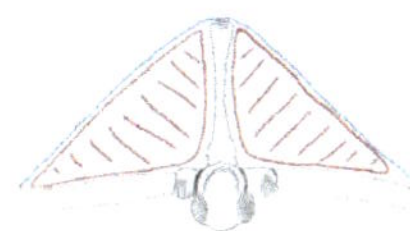	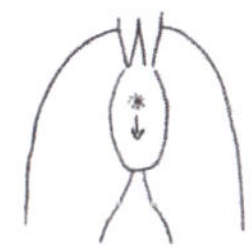	A straight line from the top of the spine to the rib – hand lays flat. No rounding, no concavity. Legs have a healthy profile.
BCS 6	Good / Ideal	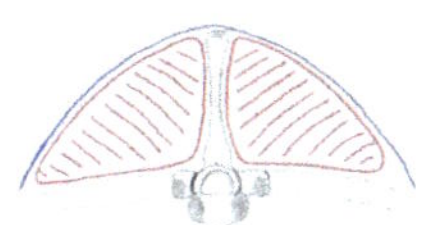	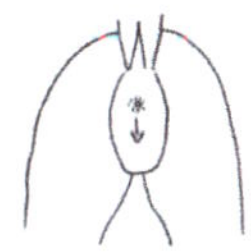	A BCS of 5.5-6 is IDEAL. The muscle cover around the spine is slightly rounded and you can feel the ribs (but not fit your fingers between). Legs have a healthy profile.
BCS 7.5	Overweight	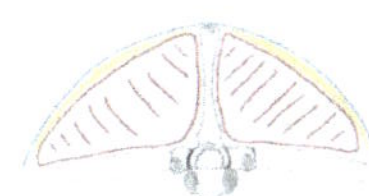	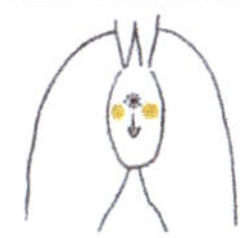	The ribs are palpable but not obvious. Rounded over spine. At BCS 7.5 and above it is possible to feel fat padding either side of the anus above the pelvic bones.
BCS 9	Obese	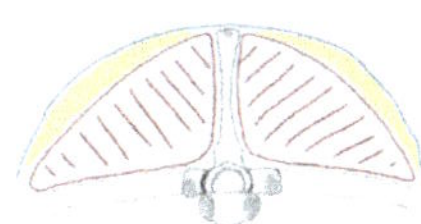	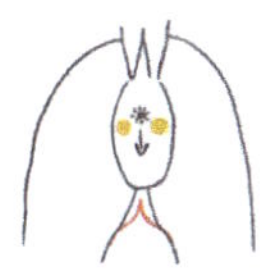	More rounded over back. Cannot feel ribs at all. Fat around anus and on chest. Also present: fat padding either side of the anus, upper leg and chest area.

Figure 2. Guide to body condition scoring showing cross sections through the spine and rear view diagrams to illustrate the findings at different body condition scores

tops of their thighs. When females become even fatter, the anatomy of the vulva begins to become distorted. If you want to check if they are fatter than a 7.5/10, the next place to look is on their chests, above the front legs. Fat will start to be deposited here from BCS 8/10.

Look at the pictures below for guidance on how to condition score your camelids. You will also find a video resource in the resources that accompany this book.

3. Mucous Membrane Colour Checking

Every time you perform a body condition score on an alpaca or llama, take the opportunity also to check the colour of their mucous membranes. The mucous membranes are the areas inside the mouth and under the eyelids. These tissues are kept moist by the body's secretions.

Looking under the eyelids is the best place to understand whether an animal might be anaemic. Anaemia is a common problem associated with parasitism, mainly due to the roundworm *Haemonchus*, also known as the Barber Pole Worm. This is an issue in camelids worldwide. Checking for anaemia should be a routine part of parasite monitoring in conjunction with body condition scoring and faecal testing. Each of the three tests tells you something about the state of individuals in the herd, and you need all three together to interpret your herd's health.

When checking for anaemia, you need to push the upper eyelid down over the eye while gently pressing. Simultaneously, you evert the lower eyelid to show the mucous membranes underneath (*Figure 3*). You want to see a nice, healthy red-pink colour. As an animal becomes anaemic, the colour will become paler. You will likely notice a difference when the packed cell volume (PCV) drops below 15%, although some people may detect anaemia below 20%. Severely anaemic animals can appear completely white (*Figure 4*). These animals are likely to have a packed cell volume of <5% and are likely to be very lethargic and weak.

If you practise mucous membrane colour checking regularly, you will soon learn to spot when an animal is anaemic. The FAMACHA© colour chart provides a visual guide for assessing anaemia and guides

> ***What is a PCV?***
>
> PCV is an abbreviation for packed cell volume and is the proportion of red cells in the blood. The red cells collect oxygen in the lungs and carry it to the tissues. When an animal becomes anaemic, its PCV reduces, meaning that the proportion of red cells in the blood decreases, and its ability to provide oxygen to the tissues is correspondingly reduced. Having fewer red cells in the blood makes your animals appear paler. We can measure the PCV by filling a narrow tube with whole blood and then centrifuging it down so that the red cells are packed into the bottom of the tube - we can then measure the proportion of red cells on a scale. A normal PCV for an adult alpaca near sea level is around 24-28%. We would normally recommend a blood transfusion for an animal with a PCV of <12%, but definitely for an animal with a PCV of <10%. At this level, reduced oxygen delivery can cause organ failure.

when a wormer should be given. You will find a video resource showing you how to check mucous membrane colour in the resources that accompany this book.

How often should you check the mucous membrane colour of the animals in your herd?

Do this routinely every time you catch an animal for any procedure. It's quick and easy and makes sense since it can be such a sensitive indicator of *Haemonchus*. I suggest doing this alongside your routine body condition scoring, which should be done monthly.

However, at high-risk times of the year or where conditions are optimal for *Haemonchus*, you should increase the frequency of checking mucous membranes to every two weeks. If you notice an animal that might be anaemic, collect a faecal sample and have it analysed for worm eggs, and if the anaemia is significant, call out your vet to evaluate the animal, check its PCV and total protein (at the very least) and determine what further actions need to be taken (e.g. anthelmintic treatment, blood transfusion, etc.)

If parasites are suspected, initiate a herd parasite investigation, starting with body condition scoring, membrane checking of the entire herd and faecal testing of a representative selection of animals from each group and the herd.

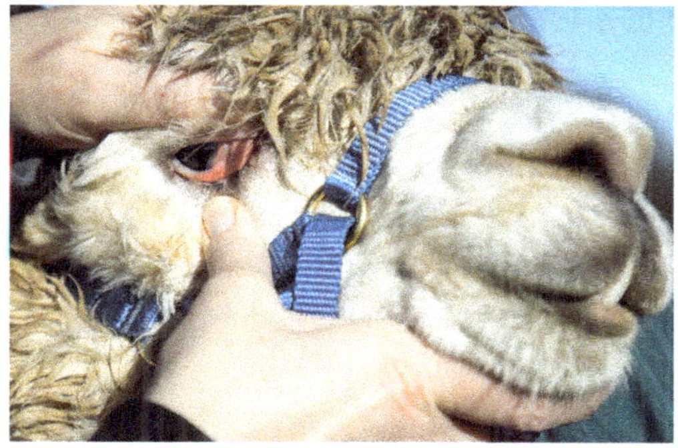

Figure 3. This image shows how to evaluate an alpaca's mucous membrane colour, which indicates whether the animal is anaemic.

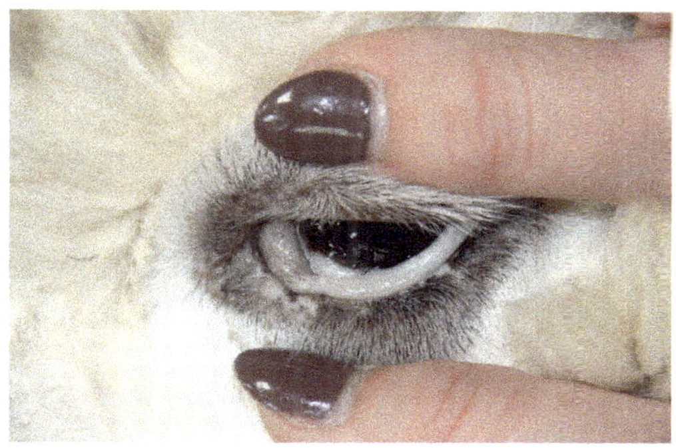

Figure 4. This alpaca exhibits extremely pale mucous membranes and has a PCV of 5%. She will need a blood transfusion.

Haemonchus can be present in animals in high numbers and this can result in high egg counts. However, it's important to note that anaemic animals may still have good body condition scores (BCS) and normal faecal egg counts. This can occur when the *Haemonchus* population in the third stomach compartment consists mostly of larvae, and egg production has not yet increased. However, not all anaemia is due to *Haemonchus*, so looking at each animal individually and as part of the herd is important. What's going on in one individual doesn't necessarily tell you the whole story. If you identify an anaemic animal with severe anaemia, you can treat it empirically for *Haemonchus* while awaiting individual lab test results. At the same time, submit faecal samples from a representative selection of the group for a broader assessment. Use the finding of anaemia as a warning that tells you that *Haemonchus* may be present in the herd. It may be symptomatic of conditions on the farm. This parasite is promoted when conditions have been wet and the temperatures mild. Use this warning to investigate the herd and find animals that might have increasing egg counts that you can deal with before further animals become severely anaemic.

4. Faecal Testing as Part of a Parasite Control Strategy

Faecal testing is an essential component of any parasite control strategy. Here are the key components of your parasite control strategy:

1. Pasture management
2. Body condition scoring and mucous membrane checking
3. Faecal screening
4. Use of anthelmintics (wormers) and anticoccidials where appropriate
5. Quarantine of new/travelling stock

Chapters 9 and 10 discuss parasite control in great detail. Here, we will focus on faecal testing as a non-negotiable activity for monitoring and maintaining your herd's health.

What is faecal testing all about? Examining faecal samples allows for detecting gastrointestinal parasites, such as worms and coccidia, by identifying parasite eggs and oocysts. Routine screening gives you a snapshot of the parasites present in your animals at the point of collection and the magnitude of any problem. You can also test a faecal sample from any animal that is losing or not gaining weight, isn't eating well, or seems off-colour. I recommend routinely testing a faecal sample for any of these complaints because parasitism is so common as an underlying or contributory problem. Determining which parasites are present in your animals allows for appropriate treatment, as different parasites have varying susceptibilities to different drugs. Using a random wormer without knowing what you're treating leaves you uncertain if parasites are present or even what type they are. As a result, you cannot determine if the treatment was effective or if the issue lies elsewhere, ultimately delaying an accurate diagnosis.

In the past, people used a wormer every six months or every year as a blanket treatment for every animal in a group or herd. This type of practice has not been recommended for many years now because parasites have started to develop resistance to wormers, and we have learned how this occurs and how to prevent it. Blanket worming kills all susceptible worms in a population but leaves the resistant ones to pass on their resistance genes to the next generation. This hastens the development of resistance in a population of worms, so more strategic control methods must be developed. We will discuss this in more detail in Chapter 10. The key thing is that faecal testing allows us to monitor the amount of worms and coccidia in a herd to manage them more strategically and with targeted worming.

Ideally, you should check 10% of the herd or 10 animals, whichever is the highest number. If you have fewer than 10 animals, then test all of them. You will be in an ideal situation because you can treat each animal individually. These numbers are the minimum numbers to test. However, you must remember that the greater the proportion of the herd that is tested, the less likely it is that any problems will be missed, and you are leaving less of your parasite control strategy to chance. In addition, targeted treatment can be employed if most or all of the herd are tested. This helps reduce the use of anthelmintics and reduces the risk of developing resistance.

When choosing which animals to test, consider which animals you are most concerned about and which are likely to have the most problems. Select animals in poor body condition, have lost weight or condition recently, or have any paleness of the mucous membranes. Older animals can be good to include as their immunity wanes, and they become more susceptible to parasites once again. Young stock up to two years old are more likely to carry higher burdens of worm eggs and coccidia, making them good candidates for testing. In contrast, crias under two months are unlikely to have worm eggs but may show coccidia starting around three weeks of age. Ensure you include animals from each group in your herd and select a representative sample from each. Testing one sample from a group of five provides limited information while testing only 10% of a group of 50 animals (five samples) offers too superficial a representation.

Samples must be as fresh as possible when they arrive at the lab to avoid any hatching of eggs that will result in an underestimation of egg counts. If you need to collect them on a weekend, the ideal day would be Sunday, so the samples can be kept in a refrigerator overnight for posting on Monday. Refrigeration is important as it will slow the development of the larvae. Samples must be taken from individual animals and not from a communal pooping area, and the samples should be labelled with the individual animal's name or number. Labelling is vital as it allows you to identify specific animals with problems requiring treatment and can reveal patterns indicating a herd parasite issue. Some individuals are more susceptible to parasites, so identifying them allows for closer monitoring and ensures they can be kept away from vulnerable animals, such as youngsters or those under stress.

Avoid pooling samples, as this method can miss heavily parasitised animals due to dilution by others with very low parasite burdens. You also will have no idea who any "problem" animals are on the farm and which individuals require treatment. Pooling samples is done primarily on sheep farms where profit margins are low, and parasite control is practised as a flock rather than per individual. Farmers accept that losses may be associated with less rigorous screening, but most camelid owners I have worked with would not be prepared to accept those losses.

There are two ways to collect samples. Both require disposable gloves and collection pots to put the samples in. A permanent marker is handy for labelling.

1. Watch and wait for animals to defecate and then collect their sample from the ground. Tip: If you bring your alpacas or llamas into a small area for feeding or to gather them for body condition scoring, let them out in batches. They often poop as they leave the enclosure and return to the field. Just be ready to collect the samples with pre-labelled pots because they will often go to the toilet *en masse*. You'll know who you want to sample based on BCS and mucous membrane scores.

2. Collect samples directly from the anus (*Figure 5*). You will need disposable gloves and a tube of lubrication for this. You will also need a second person to hold the animal for you. Put a blob of lubricant jelly on your index and middle fingers on your dominant hand. Hold the base of the tail with your non-dominant hand and then pop your two lubricated fingers gently in through the anus. There is typically enough faecal material sitting right inside the anus to collect a sample.

How much sample is enough? Eight to ten faecal beans are typically enough for most faecal methods. However, you may need more if you want to test for fluke.

The use of wormers, called anthelmintics, and anticoccidials will be recommended based on faecal testing results alongside results from your body condition scoring and mucous membrane checks.

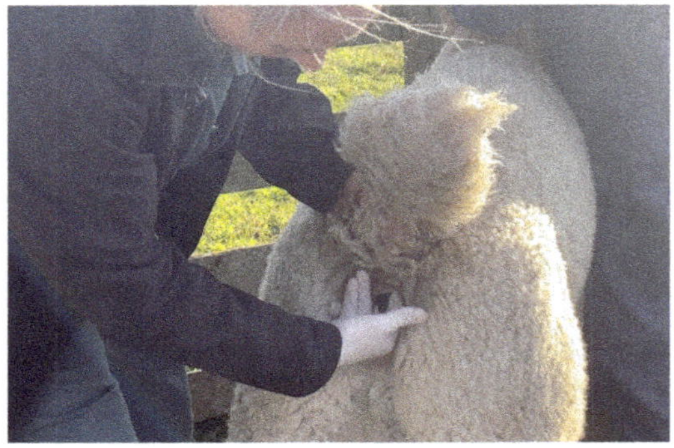

Figure 5. Collection of a faecal sample directly from the anus of an alpaca.

5. Vaccinations

Currently, clostridial diseases are the primary diseases we need to vaccinate against in camelids globally. However, outside of the UK, Australia and New Zealand, which are rabies-free, it might be recommended to vaccinate against rabies.

If leptospirosis is a concern, usually in the face of an outbreak, consider vaccinating against leptospirosis. However, the leptospirosis vaccines' effects are very short-lived, necessitating frequent vaccination (every 3–6 months) to be effective. It is rarely necessary if adequate rodent control is in place.

Vaccination against the bluetongue virus is sometimes recommended in the UK and northern Europe, depending on the risk of disease incursion from the south. Previously, BTV-8 was the most common strain, but more recently, BTV-3 has become more prevalent. Bluetongue generally poses a risk to UK livestock industries late in the summer (late August to September) as the virus spreads northward through France.

Southeastern and eastern parts of the UK are at the highest risk due to their proximity to mainland Europe. Once the virus reaches the British Isles, it can spread within livestock populations through the local midge vector. Different strains of the bluetongue virus are prevalent in other parts of the world, and vaccination may also be advised there. Consult your veterinarian about bluetongue and its prevalence in your area.

It should be stressed that, as for other medications in alpacas, there are no products licensed for use in camelids. Therefore, our recommendations for using vaccines are extrapolated from using these medicines in other species and from small-scale studies and personal experience. For some vaccines, studies are available to show which protocols initiate an appropriate antibody response, but few studies include experimental infection studies that would show whether the vaccines are effective in the face of exposure. These vaccines should be killed vaccines; live vaccines must never be used in camelids as these carry the risk that the virus recovers its virulence and causes disease in the recipient.

Remember that vaccines should be stored and used according to the label directions. This usually means a bottle cannot be used after opening it, and vaccines typically require refrigeration.

Never vaccinate sick or stressed animals because their immune response may be insufficient to ensure the vaccine provides effective protection. A commonly deployed "time-saving" method is to vaccinate at shearing because it's easy to do so. However, this is best avoided since shearing is stressful for camelids and could significantly impair the immune system's response to vaccination.

Clostridial Diseases

Multiple vaccines are available for clostridial diseases, offered by different manufacturers, and a range of options for the number of clostridial diseases (or antigens) covered. The specific vaccines available vary by country; all are licensed for use in sheep, cattle or both. Clostridial diseases include tetanus, enterotoxaemia, blackleg, bighead, malignant oedema and bacillary haemoglobinuria.

In crias, we are particularly concerned about enterotoxaemia caused by *Clostridium perfringens* (often shortened to *C perfringens*). However, since all clostridial diseases can affect alpacas, it's important to vaccinate against a broad range of them.

Lambivac (MSD; Europe, UK) covers Clostridium perfringens types B, C, and D, as well as tetanus. CD&T is available in North America but it does not include type B protection. The 7-, 8-, and 10-way vaccines (the multivalents) cover a broader spectrum of clostridial diseases, including tetanus. The 10-way vaccines are the only ones that protect against type A clostridial enterotoxaemia and *C sordellii.*

Most clostridial enterotoxaemia cases I have encountered were type A, diagnosed before 10-way vaccines became available. If offered in your country, the 10-way vaccine may be a good choice. In the US, a separate type A vaccine is now also available if needed.

There are two main strategies for vaccination against clostridial diseases, with arguments for and against both. Neither of these strategies has been proven to be best in camelids to date. It is, therefore, suggested that you discuss your vaccination strategy with your veterinarian. Together, consider the relative risks and benefits to determine the most appropriate for your herd. The following notes provide two strategies for where multivalent vaccines are available in the UK and Europe. There are notes later in this chapter for those in the US.

Strategy #1: Vaccinate pregnant dams 3–8 weeks prior to parturition

- In this first strategy, you will vaccinate pregnant dams 3-8 weeks before parturition. Please check the recommendations on the vaccine label for specific advice on timing. This is the more traditional approach to vaccination, which aims to "boost" colonic immunity and improve the passive transfer of vaccine-specific antibodies to the newborn cria
- Crias are not vaccinated until they reach about 12 weeks of age (but at least 10 weeks), at which time they receive a farm-chosen multivalent vaccine and begin the full primary course. A primary course consists of two doses, usually 4-6 weeks apart. The second vaccination dose is necessary to produce an anamnestic response so that the body will recognise the disease and produce antibodies more quickly in the face of infection.
- The crias will then be re-vaccinated a year later or the following spring as appropriate, depending on the date of birth. Aim to vaccinate most animals in spring as the highest risk period for clostridial diseases is during the warmer months. This may mean shortening the inter-vaccination interval so that this booster may be given 6 months after the primary course.
- Animals are then boosted once annually, again ideally in the spring. This should be pre-breeding for maiden females.
- It should be noted that pregnancy loss may be associated with vaccination using multivalent vaccines during pregnancy. It is possible that some of these pregnancy losses may be due to handling stress during a potentially vulnerable stage of pregnancy. Pregnancy loss is much more likely if you provide a primary vaccination course during pregnancy - this is the two-dose course given the first time you give a vaccine. This is because the body is more likely to produce an inflammatory response to a vaccine on first exposure than a booster vaccine. Therefore, I would recommend only *boosting* vaccination during late-stage pregnancy. In other words, do not complete a primary course of vaccination during pregnancy. Animals handled more frequently may be better suited to this strategy in case of stress losses.

Strategy #2: Vaccinate young crias; avoid vaccinating pregnant dams

- Option 1: Give a primary course of Lambivac, with the first dose at 3 days old and the second 3 weeks later. Do not use a multivalent vaccine at this age!

- Option 2: At one month of age, start vaccinating using a more multivalent vaccine (e.g. 10-way). Give a primary course of two doses.
- Only vaccinate healthy crias. Sick crias will not mount an appropriate immune response, and vaccination will fail.
- Vaccinate at 4–6 months using a multivalent vaccine that includes tetanus (full primary course again), then repeat in the spring or at pre-breeding for females.
- Dams are vaccinated between pregnancies, avoiding potential stress effects that may induce preterm labour

When I first returned to the UK, my family's farm was quite large at that time. The farm had some females birthing in March due to recent imports from South America. Several crias died from those early births. Postmortem examination revealed clostridial enterotoxaemia, specifically from type A C perfringens was involved. That year, the farm was expecting around 300 crias, and an outbreak of clostridial enterotoxaemia could have been devastating. Raul Rosadio, a veterinarian in Peru, reported that outbreaks in alpaca farms in Peru had caused mortality rates of up to 70% among crias aged 3-9 weeks old1. I was very alarmed. Fortunately, a 10-way clostridial vaccine had just become available in the UK, and we decided to pre-emptively vaccinate the pregnant dams to prevent a devastating outbreak. This required a two-dose primary course of vaccine. We estimated that 9 or 10 females aborted their crias following the use of the vaccine, but the losses could have been worse. No further crias were lost to enterotoxaemia.

I have worked with another large farm in the UK that regularly dosed pregnant females prepartum with the 10-way vaccine. Generally, they vaccinated the dams once at shearing and then again prepartum, but they did not report any abortions as a result of using the vaccine. Since this was a large farm, these animals were unlikely to be habituated sufficiently to handle and not be stressed. Therefore, the stress of handling shearing and vaccinations did not cause pregnancy loss, and the vaccine didn't appear to be causing noticeable problems.

I know one other farmer who contacted me asking about the use of vaccines. This owner had decided to upgrade his clostridial vaccine to the 10-way vaccine and completed a primary vaccination course in his pregnant females. He reported seeing several abortions associated with the use of the vaccine.

Based on this information, using multivalent vaccines in pregnant animals is likely to be safe if they receive their initial exposure before pregnancy. However, administering the vaccine for the first time during pregnancy may trigger a fever or other immune responses that could lead to pregnancy loss. This may be the case for any vaccine.

or abortions. Vaccinate dams with your choice of vaccine, preferably one of the multivalents, as these offer more coverage.

- This strategy was tested in unpublished studies in which the crias were shown to have developed appropriate antibody responses following the second dose. However, the effectiveness of this strategy versus exposure has yet to be discovered. In the US, many thousands of crias have been vaccinated using this approach, but using CD&T (which contains slightly less protection) and have shown promising results, meaning that "not much clostridial disease is observed." However, I have seen clostridial enterotoxaemia from type A *C perfringens* in crias in both the US and the UK. This is not prevented with Lambivac or CD&T vaccination in neonatal crias, and this strategy will not provide as much passive immunity versus clostridial diseases either. I have personally moved more towards recommending the first strategy in the UK, where we can use 10-way vaccines that confer protection against type A *C perfringens.*

Consider both options carefully, weigh the relative risks and discuss with your vet which is best for you and your farm.

Regardless of the strategy employed, a primary course of two doses is required to properly "prime" the immune system. If you ever "upgrade" vaccination to cover more antigens, from Lambivac to a 7- or 10-way vaccine, for example, it will be necessary to do a primary course again. Annual re-vaccination of adults is recommended, ideally in the spring to early summer, which ensures coverage over the highest risk time of year. Twice-yearly vaccination against clostridial diseases does not appear to be necessary. Use the label dose for sheep.

For owners based in North America

As with everywhere else in the world, vaccines are used "off-label" because nothing is licensed for use in camelids. Always discuss your vaccination strategy with your regular veterinarian to determine which products to use and the most appropriate plan for the diseases present in your area.

The following vaccines are available for use in North America.

CD/T (3-way vaccine)	Confers protection against *C perfringens* types C and D and tetanus
7- or 8- way vaccines ultivalent vaccines)	Confers protection against *C perfringens* types C and D, tetanus and 4 or 5 other clostridial diseases
C perfringens Type A Toxoid	Recommended on farms that have had problems with *C perfringens* type A enterotoxaemia. This vaccine was evaluated in alpacas at Washington State University and showed a measurable antibody response. However, its efficacy was not tested in challenge studies. There were no adverse reactions, but it was not tested in pregnant animals.

Options for Clostridial Vaccination in North America

Strategy #1: Vaccinate pregnant dams 3-8 weeks prior to parturition

- Vaccinate pregnant dams 3-8 weeks before parturition using a clostridial vaccine. Note that the dam should have received a full primary course of vaccine prior to pregnancy for this booster to be effective. This boosts the antibodies transferred to the cria in the mother's colostrum. The "maternal antibodies" protect the cria during the first few weeks of life.
- Crias are not vaccinated until 3 months old when they are vaccinated using a clostridial vaccine (based on farm choice). A full primary course is also required. Revaccinate as above annually (pre-breeding for maiden females). It doesn't matter if you give a booster vaccine earlier than a year after the primary course.
- If the dam has been vaccinated prepartum, you must not provide neonatal vaccination because the circulating maternal antibodies from colostrum will cancel out the effect of any vaccine given to the cria. This will leave the cria susceptible to clostridial organisms and may even harm the immune system. Maternal antibody wanes over the first few months of life and is virtually gone by 3 months of age.
- This is the traditional approach to vaccination. It should be noted that the use of multivalent vaccines prepartum in camelids has occasionally resulted in early birthing or pregnancy loss. This may be associated with handling stress or using a new vaccine in a pregnant animal, which may result in fever. It is best to avoid giving a primary course of a new vaccine during pregnancy. Animals that are accustomed to handling *may* be less likely to experience problems due to stress.

Strategy #2: Vaccinate young crias; avoid vaccinating pregnant dams

- Give a primary course of CD/T, with the first dose at 3 days old and the second 3 weeks later. Do not use a multivalent vaccine at this age!
- Only vaccinate healthy crias. Sick crias will not mount an appropriate immune response, and vaccination will fail.
- Crias can be revaccinated in spring with CD/T or upgraded to a more multivalent vaccine that includes tetanus at 4–6 months of age. This requires completing a full primary course and then revaccinating annually (pre-breeding for maiden females). When increasing valency (e.g. switching from CD/T to a 7- or 8-way vaccine), you must complete the full primary course to ensure the body is fully primed for future exposures.
- In this strategy, the dams are vaccinated between pregnancies to avoid potential stress effects that may induce preterm labour or pregnancy loss. Vaccinate dams with your choice of vaccine.

Depending on your preference, you can use either CD/T or 7-/8-way vaccines in your herd. Discuss with your vet what is most appropriate for your area. Never use the 7-/8-way vaccines in young crias; stick to CD/T instead. Additionally, some people have reported more soft tissue reactions at the injection site for the more multivalent vaccines.

Rabies

Rabies has been reported in camelids, and vaccination should be considered in areas where the disease is endemic. Only veterinarians can administer rabies vaccines, such as IMRAB-3®.[2] This can be given to crias from 3–6 months of age.

Leptospirosis

Vaccination against leptospirosis is only necessary when the problem has been confirmed on a farm and the serovar(s) causing the disease have been identified to ensure the vaccination will be worthwhile. Leptospirosis antibodies are short-lived, so vaccination may need to be repeated three to four times yearly. Since leptospirosis usually spreads via rodents and some wildlife species, other environmental controls, particularly rodent control measures, can also be employed.

West Nile Virus (WNV)

Camelids can be affected by West Nile Virus. The clinical signs tend to be neurological, and cases are difficult to treat when they occur. Initially, WNV was found only in the Eastern US but has since spread west. Check with your veterinarian to discover the disease status in your area. Vaccination will be timed to occur prior to the mosquito season.

There are two vaccines licensed for use in horses that have been evaluated in camelids:

- Ft. Dodge West Nile-Innovator→: 3 doses, 3 weeks apart. Only one dose is required in subsequent years [3]
- Merial Recombitek Equine WNV vaccine→: 2 doses, 2-3 weeks apart. Only one dose is required in subsequent years. There are no published studies, but this product has been evaluated in camelids.[4]

Key Takeaways

This chapter covers the first five non-negotiable herd health activities: Observation, body condition scoring, checking mucous membrane colour, faecal testing and vaccinations. Here are some key takeaways:

- Observation is a key tool in monitoring your animals' health. Do this regularly and familiarise yourself with what is normal for your animals as a group and as individuals. If anything seems out of the ordinary, investigate.
- Body condition scoring is the most important herd health monitoring tool. You should master it, practise it regularly (at least monthly) and always record your findings. Body condition scoring helps identify issues within the herd and in individual animals.
- Check the mucous membrane colour whenever you score body condition. Your observations from these two key tools will inform your parasite control strategy.
- Faecal testing is an important component of any parasite control strategy. Make sure you test a minimum of 10 animals or 10% of the herd (whichever is the highest number) at least twice a year and in between as necessary, depending on the problems you experience and changing conditions. Understand that the more significant the proportion of the herd that is tested, the less likely it is that any problems will be missed, and you leave less of your parasite control strategy to chance. Always do follow-up faecal tests to check that any wormers/anticoccidials used were effective.
- Check with your regular veterinarian to determine the prevalent diseases in your area. Consider the various vaccination options, and plan to ensure you don't miss any vaccination dates.

We will move onto the next chapter, covering the final five non-negotiable herd health activities.

4

Routine Herd Health Activities: Part 2

In Chapter 3, we looked at the first five non-negotiable herd health activities: observation, body condition scoring, checking mucous membrane colour, faecal testing as part of a parasite control strategy and vaccinations. We will now discuss five more, no less important than the first five, and these include toenail trimming, vitamin D supplementation, shearing, dental care, and nutrition planning.

6. Toenail Trimming

Toenails on alpacas and llamas grow continuously in the same way that our fingernails do. They will wear down on hard ground, but the toenails may overgrow when the animals are kept on soft ground. If this overgrowth becomes excessive, it can tilt the toe upwards and alter how the animal bears weight. As a result, the animal's comfort may be affected, potentially leading to foot lesions. Later on, the toenail will be forced to tilt sideways, which may result in the nail altering its growth direction, which may cause problems later. Occasionally, the nail may grow all the way around and start growing into the pad itself, which will cause pain and may result in infection within the foot.

Toenail trimming should be done on a routine basis to prevent these issues. The frequency with which it needs to be carried out will depend on your land and your individual animals. Areas of hard standing will increase the wear of toenails and reduce the frequency of toenail trimming, but this rarely makes a difference in UK pastures! Animals with dark toenails require less trimming than those with clear toenails. Get into the habit of noticing the toenails on your animals, especially when gathering them in for other routine husbandry such as body condition scoring. Trim them when required – you will start to see a pattern of how regularly this is needed. It is most likely to be every 3–4 months.

The toenail trimmers I prefer have sharp, straight and non-serrated blades. If you're in the US, you can purchase this type of toenail trimmer on the Camelidynamics website. If you're in the UK, you can find these trimmers on our products page at www.ukalpacavet.com. These toenail trimmers are easy to hold and have sharp blades that make trimming toenails easy.

Camelid feet have soft pads on two digits, overlain with a nail. It is the nail that overgrows, and it should be trimmed back so that the nail is level with the soft pad. When standing, the toenails should sit above the ground rather than on it (*Figure 1*). You will need to pick the feet up to trim them, although Camelidynamics has a method where the foot stays on the ground during toenail trimming.

Make sure you have a handler holding the animal squarely, and always aim to keep the animal balanced. Start with a front foot on either side. Standing beside the shoulder and looking towards the tail, bend down and run your hand down the leg to the fetlock. Then, pick the foot up. You might need to gently push the animal slightly away from you to get them to transfer their weight to the other front leg. The foot will now be upside down, and you can examine the nails and pads (*Figure 2*).

When picking up a hindfoot, stand beside the hip and stabilise the animal by placing a hand on the opposite hip. Then, run your hand down the back leg to just above the hock. Pick up the leg from the hock, reach down with the hand stabilising the hip, and hold the lower limb so that the foot again faces upwards. When picking up a hind foot, alpacas and llamas may try to kick your hand away. I advise you to just hold on to the leg, and usually, after one or two kicks, they settle down and let you examine the foot.

Ensure that the animal remains balanced because if you pull their leg out to the side or unbalance them in any way, they will not be comfortable and will continue to fight you. I position myself so that the animal's stifle (knee) rests on my leg (*Figure 3*). This position allows them to remain squarely balanced, as some of their weight will pass through your holding leg. While this works well with alpacas, it's not as effective with llamas because of their height! Always put the feet down gently once you've finished.

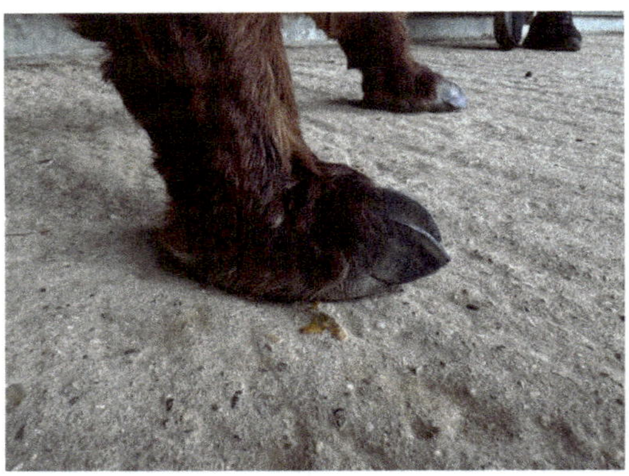

Figure 1. These toenails are the correct length. They are resting above the ground when the animal is standing normally.

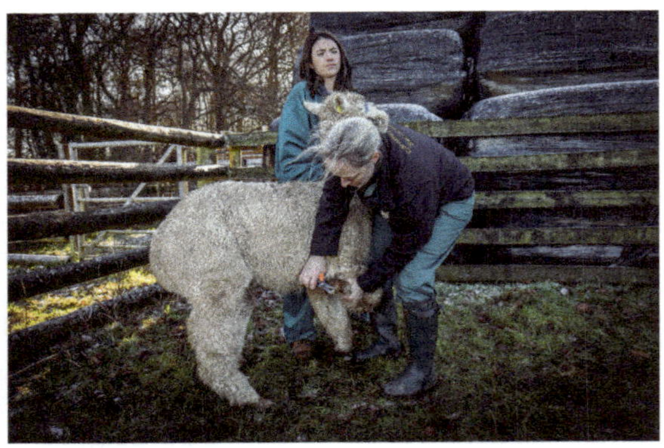

Figure 2. This image shows the author picking up a front foot for toenail trimming.

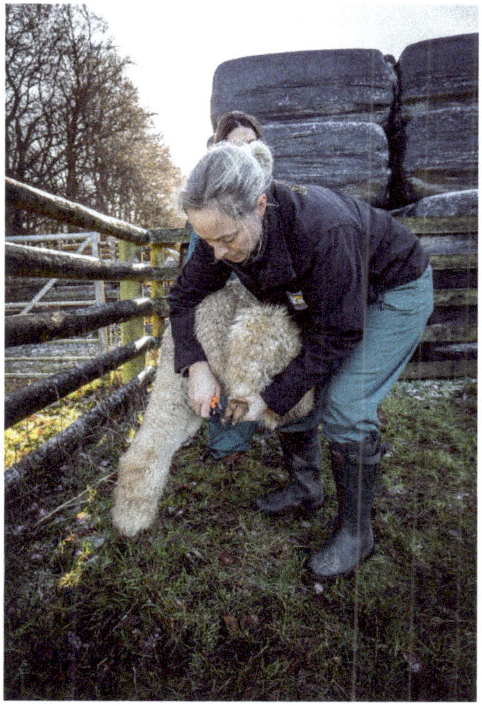

Figure 3. In this image, the author shows how to pick up a hind foot. Note that the alpaca's stifle is positioned on the handler's knee to support the body's left side.

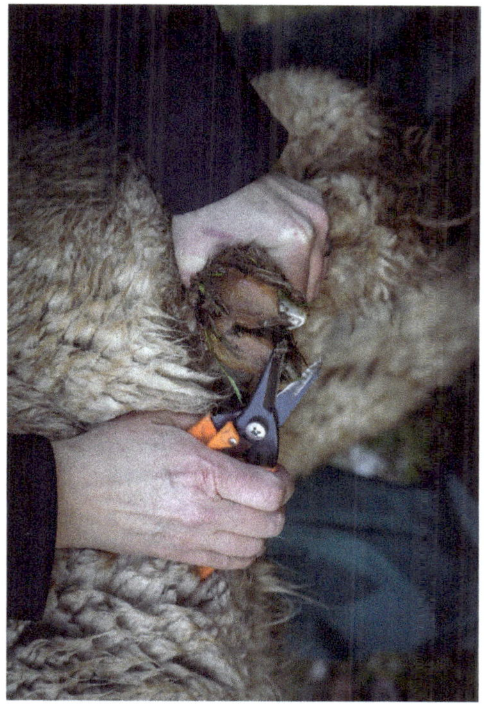

Figure 4. This image shows the author removing the excess nail length from the toenail, with the clipper blades angled perpendicular to the toe, to avoid squeezing the sensitive nailbed.

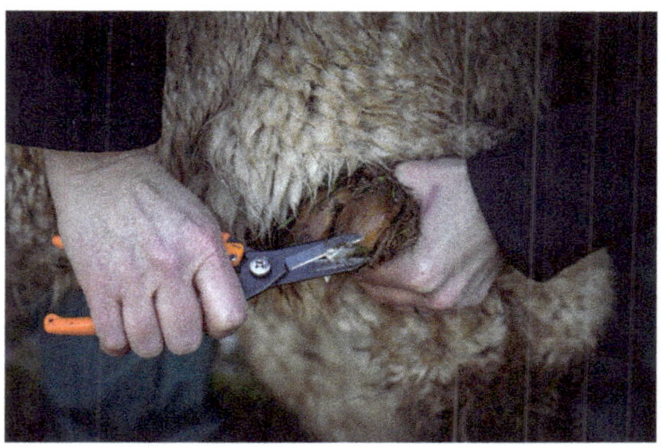

Figure 5. This image shows how to angle the toenail clippers to reduce the excess nail along one side of the toenail. This needs to be repeated for the other side.

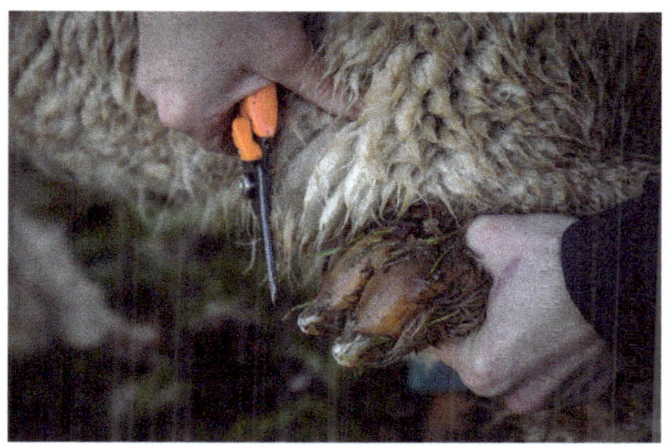

Figure 6. In this image, the toenails have been trimmed down to level with the pad. A small section of the nail has also been clipped from the very tip of the toenail.

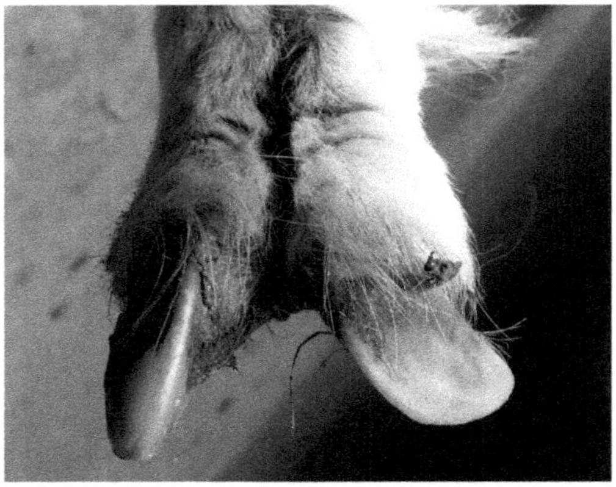

Figure 7. The left hind foot of a white alpaca with lateral deviation of the lateral toe.

When trimming the toenail, I will initially brush any mud off the foot and use the tips of the toenail trimmers to pick any mud out from the tip of the toenail, the part from the toe pad to the tip of the nail. Once I can clearly see where the toe finishes, I usually remove the excess toenail by cutting perpendicular to the toe pads (*Figure 4*). In this way, I'm not squeezing the nail bed, which might cause the animal pain. I then trim down each side of the nail separately until the toenail is trimmed level with the pad itself (*Figure 5*). If you do it this way, don't apply pressure to the nailbed, as this can be painful. Finally, I take a little nip off the front edge of the nail. I do this because I feel as though this helps to slow the regrowth. You can see this in *Figure 6*.

Some animals have "twisted toenails" where the outside (normally) digit on the hind feet will deviate laterally (*Figure 7*). These nails are more challenging to maintain and are related to the rotation of the 3rd phalanx (equivalent to the last section of your fingers or toes) of the affected toes, as evident on radiographs. Limited research based on examination of the feet of 861 alpacas suggests that this is a heritable problem.[1] They do not appear to be associated with any other issues but will not wear properly, necessitating frequent and difficult toenail trimming.

7. Vitamin D Supplementation

South American Camelids are susceptible to Vitamin D deficiency. In growing animals, this manifests clinically as rickets. Affected animals exhibit stunted growth, angular limb deformities and lameness. They may also be lethargic, have depressed appetites, may walk with a hunched back due to pain and are typically smaller than age-matched herd mates. Vitamin D deficiency also causes reduced immunity, which may affect camelids of any age. Vitamin D supplementation is provided to prevent rickets in crias, support the immune system at any age of camelid, and improve foetal development and lactational performance in pregnant and lactating females.

There are two sources of vitamin D for herbivorous animals, including camelids. These are dietary vitamin D2 (ergocalciferol), available from plants, and vitamin D3 (cholecalciferol), made in the skin by the action of U-V light on pro-vitamin D3. Dietary vitamin D2 is more abundant in mature grass and hay, while spring grass contains relatively little vitamin D. As a result, spring can be a high-risk period for summer- or autumn-born crias. These young animals, weaned over the winter and turned onto fresh spring pastures without supplementary feeding, may not receive enough vitamin D if it's assumed that spring grass alone will suffice.

A seasonal variation in vitamin D3 has been described in llamas, alpacas[2] and sheep[3], where blood concentrations drop during winter due to reduced ultraviolet light availability. It is believed that reduced exposure to U-V radiation at reduced altitudes and non-equatorial latitudes (i.e. outside the South American Andes) causes reduced vitamin D activation in the skin. It has also been suggested in sheep that increased pigmentation and amount of fleece result in reduced vitamin D photobiosynthesis and that darker, unsheared animals are more susceptible to rickets.[3] Similar findings were found in alpacas by Smith and van Saun[2] and Judson and Feakes.[4] Having tested alpacas and llamas of all colours for vitamin D concentrations and tested clinical cases of rickets, I can personally corroborate that camelids with darker fleece colours are more prone to vitamin D deficiency. Vitamin D may also be passed transplacentally or via the dam's milk to neonates.[5]

Camels kept in locations away from the Equator and low altitudes (e.g., Europe, North America, and Australasia) receive significantly less UV light. As a result, most animals become deficient in vitamin D, which has the most obvious effect on growing animals. Therefore, vitamin D supplementation during the winter months is vital.

Dosing Recommendations

You can use injectable or oral products to supplement your alpacas or llamas with vitamin D. The product you choose comes down to personal preference and the availability of products in your country. The following dosing regime is recommended to prevent rickets in growing alpacas and llamas.

Using Injectable Vitamin D Products

These products are usually more regulated than oral formulations. In the UK, for example, they are prescription-only products, meaning they must be prescribed by and purchased from a vet. However, they are not licensed in the UK, meaning vets must complete a Special Import Certificate to purchase them. They are available in the UK but require this extra step to comply with regulations. There may be different rules in your own country.

- Dose 1000-2000 IU of vitamin D per kg of body weight, given subcutaneously (SQ). Darker animals may benefit from a higher 1500-2000 IU/kg dose, particularly at the first dose, to get them up to a good concentration since they will start from a lower point.
- Injectable vitamin D lasts 6–8 weeks at this dose, so repeat this dosing every 2 months.
- Start in October and continue until April in the Northern Hemisphere, where conditions are dull and there is little UV radiation. If August has been dull, start dosing in September, especially for darker animals.
- The ideal injectable product contains 100,000 IU of vitamin D per ml: This concentration means that the dose for 10kg is 0.1 ml.

- 10 kg x 1000 IU = 10,000 IU
- If the product contains 100,000 IU/ml, the volume of product to be administered is given by the formula:

$$\frac{\text{Required dose}}{\text{concentration of product}} = 10{,}000 / 100{,}000 = 0.1 \text{ ml}$$

More concentrated products, such as those containing 500,000 IU/ml, can be dangerous because it is easier to overdose and cause toxicity. An adult weighing 80kg would require a dose of 0.16-0.32ml while a cria of 10kg would only require 0.02-0.04ml, which is rather difficult to measure and administer. Cases of death due to toxicity have been reported at doses of just over 6000 IU/kg.

Using Oral Vitamin D Products

Oral supplements are usually regarded as nutritional products and, therefore, fall outside the realm of prescription products (again, check the rules in your own country). Thus, less regulation governs the production of these products, making them easier to acquire. However, their contents may also be less reliable as they are not subjected to the same levels of scrutiny.

- Dose 1000-2000 IU of vitamin D per kg of body weight, as above, but provide this orally, using oral formulations typically provided as paste in syringes. These doses provide the same effect as the injectable products but don't last as long, so they must be supplemented more frequently - every 4-6 weeks.
- Take care to dose based on body weight rather *than* per cria, as crias have a wide weight range!
- These products sometimes come in large tubes; typically, these may contain 100,000 IU of vitamin D per 10ml, but you must check the ingredients of any products purchased. The label dosing may be per cria or adult, but I recommend calculating the correct and safe dose for crias due to wide weight ranges. At a concentration of 100,000 IU per 10 ml, each 1 ml contains 10,000 IU. A 1 ml dose suits animals weighing 5-10 kg, and a 5 ml dose suits animals weighing 25-50 kg, depending on whether you target 1,000 or 2,000 IU/kg of body weight.

For Treatment of Rickets or Vitamin D Deficiency

If you are treating a clinical case of rickets or vitamin D deficiency, I tend to use the higher dose of vitamin D because these animals are starting from a lower point. I also repeat the dose one month later, regardless of whether I use oral or injectable products. The dose should be 2,000 IU of vitamin D per kg of body weight using either oral or injectable products.

It is important to note that dosing above these recommendations can induce vitamin D toxicity and is not advisable. Vitamin D toxicity results in the mineralisation of soft tissues such as the kidneys, liver, gastrointestinal tract wall and blood vessels. This results in organ failure and potentially death from ruptured major vessels and is irreversible.

8. Shearing

Shearing needs to be done on an annual basis for most animals. It is best done in the spring or early summer to prevent heat stress in hot weather and also so that they can regrow their fleece in time for the following winter. Specialist camelid shearers are available in most countries where camelids are kept. Do not leave it until the last minute to book. Shearers travel the country on a schedule determined by bookings, and it's best to get yours scheduled in advance so that the animals aren't left waiting until they're back in the area again!

After booking your shearing date, there are some other preparations to help you get prepared and ensure shearing day happens smoothly and efficiently. Prepare the area in advance of the shearer's arrival. Ideally, the area will be indoors, in a barn, to protect against the rain. You should also have a concreted area to use. This area should be thoroughly cleaned, preferably power-hosed some time ahead, and swept and cleared of all dust right before shearing starts. If you use a dirt floor, there will be a much higher chance of contamination of the fleece. You will also need space to put fleece, check them before skirting, and decide whether to bag them for show or sale. If it's going to rain during shearing, you'll need somewhere to lay out the fleeces to dry.

Next, you'll need to ensure that your alpacas are clean and dry before the shearer arrives. If it's raining, this can be difficult, but chances are that rescheduling isn't going to be possible. If you can get at least some animals inside overnight, that will help get you started. You can use fans to assist in drying any wet animals.

Make sure you also have toenail trimmers available to trim toenails, bags and weighing scales for fleece, and boards for shearing on and collecting the fleece. Another helpful tip is to get some knee pads to use as you might be kneeling at times, particularly if you have the job of holding the head! Lastly, have a first aid kit handy in case of any shearing injuries. On shearing day itself, you should create a calm and stress-free environment by minimising noise and distractions. This will help keep your alpacas relaxed during the shearing process and ensure a positive experience for everyone involved.

For alpacas, shearing is usually performed with them positioned in recumbency. Thick, soft ropes secure their front and back feet to fixed points. The alpaca is manoeuvred into position, the ropes are looped over the fetlock of all feet, and a pulley system pulls the feet outwards while the handler guides the alpaca down to the ground. The ropes are pulled just enough to prevent the animal from struggling without causing ligament injury. A handler always remains with the alpaca while it is recumbent and holds the head in position.

During shearing, the alpaca is rotated from one side to the other, and the head and neck are shorn, with the animal sitting upright. Usually, the blanket part of the fleece over the body is collected separately from the fleece of the head, neck and legs because it is of superior quality and may be processed for fleece showing. At the end of shearing, the ropes are loosened, and the alpaca hops up of its own volition and is released. A professional alpaca shearer can shear an alpaca using this method in 3.5 to 4 minutes.

An alternative way to shear alpacas is by use of a shearing table. There are different models of these tables with slightly different working methods. But essentially, when using a shearing table, the table is rotated into a vertical position, and the alpaca is then walked in alongside the table. The alpaca is secured to the table using either a padded belly band or a padded restraining arm that levers into place, holding it firmly between the table and the padded arm. The table is then rotated horizontally, and the alpaca's legs are extended and secured.

Having alpacas restrained using either the rope or table method helps to minimise the risk of shearing injuries from the clipper blades. These occur when the skin rolls and gets caught by the blade, and are most common on the flank close to the hind legs and at the top of the hind legs. Most of these will be little nicks that can be cleaned with antiseptic spray. When cleaning wounds, use iodine solution diluted in water or just salt water. You can also use chlorhexidine solution (the pink stuff), but if you are using chlorhexidine or iodine, ensure that it is a solution rather than a scrub, as the scrubs contain soaps that can damage exposed subcutaneous tissues. Avoid using cotton wool to clean wounds, as this can leave little fibres in the wound. Gauze swabs are better to have on hand for this purpose. Larger wounds might need to be sutured by your veterinarian.

Llamas may be sheared in the same way but are often shorn standing up. In the US, many llamas are shorn with a barrel cut that removes the fleece from the trunk, leaving the fleece on the neck and legs. Please note that this *can* leave the animals more susceptible to heat stress because less of the body is accessible for cooling. Instead, owners will have to provide shade, ventilation and perhaps water to assist in cooling so that the animals remain comfortable. If shearing llamas with the barrel cut, it is important to groom the fleece so that it doesn't become matted. Matted fleece will make it even harder for the llama to keep cool and increase the potential for dermatological issues. If you have no patience or time for grooming, just shear the entire animal in the same way as an alpaca.

Activities That Can Be Done During Shearing

Some activities can be done during shearing, while others should not be done during shearing. For example, when an animal is restrained for shearing, it becomes a perfect opportunity to do toenail trimming. This will save time for you and stress for the animals, as you won't have to gather them in on another occasion.

While toenail trimming is acceptable, I do not recommend providing vaccinations at shearing. The reason for this is that although it may seem a short and relatively innocuous event, studies have shown increased faecal cortisol metabolites 33 hours afterwards, indicating a longer-lasting stress response. Their stress levels may remain increased for longer, but this still needs to be studied.[6] Why is this important? Well, stress reduces the immune system's ability to respond to stimuli. When you administer a vaccine to an alpaca or llama, you are relying on the body's immune response to recognise the vaccine antigens as foreign and to mount an antibody response so that, if faced with the infection you're trying to prevent at a later date, the immune system recognises it and reacts more quickly to prevent the illness. If the immune system is compromised by stress, the body's response to the vaccine will be reduced, so the effects of the vaccine are likely to be reduced.

Therefore, if you want to ensure your animals can mount the optimal response to a vaccine you administer (trust me, you want to increase the chances that it works!), separate vaccines from stressful events such as shearing! If you don't know how to give a vaccine, get your veterinarian to do a batch and ask them to show you how. I also recommend that you practise handling needles and syringes. You can vaccinate under the skin of a whole chicken before roasting it (although I would suggest using honey and soy rather than the vaccine so that you can still eat it afterwards), or if your dietary preferences are more vegetarian, practice on fruit!

Another practice that I hear about is shearers providing worming at shearing time. As I've discussed elsewhere in this chapter, blanket worming without consideration of faecal egg counts, body condition scoring and mucous membrane colour checking will often result in unnecessary resistance developing to your available wormers. If you need help with worming individuals that you have decided need worming based on the above, then get your appropriate medication ready ahead of shearing to be administered to selected individuals only on that day. However, in my experience, wormers are more likely to be needed at times other than shearing, and you should not rely on this single date on the calendar.

Shearers sometimes offer other services, such as incisor trimming or castrations. It may be legal in some countries and illegal in others. Hence, it's important to be aware of the legislation in your own country but also consider what is good versus bad for the welfare of the animals concerned. In the UK, castration is considered an act of veterinary surgery, and it is an offence for anyone other than a veterinarian to perform castration on camelids. While there are many levels of anaesthesia for castration, from local anaesthetic only to sedation with local or full general anaesthesia, your decision on how castration is performed must consider legal requirements, budget and preference. Local anaesthetic must *always* be used as a minimum standard for prevention and relief of pain. I would also recommend the use of a non-steroidal anti-inflammatory medicine.

I have seen cases where shearers have applied elastrator bands to the testicles of adult male alpacas to castrate them. Elastrator band castration is extremely painful. It is a technique in which a thick elastic band is placed over the base of the scrotum to cut off the blood supply to the testicles and scrotal skin. The lack of blood supply causes the tissues to die and the dead tissues then fall off. In the UK, this technique is only permitted in lambs less than seven days old and is permitted purely for cost-saving in economics-bound livestock farming. It is highly inappropriate to use this technique in an adult male due to the pain it would cause the animal. Furthermore, it has also been shown to be an ineffective method of castration in adult alpacas, primarily because of anatomical differences.[7]

Shearers may also offer to trim incisor

teeth. It is often done, quite unnecessarily, for cosmetic reasons. Trimming is only necessary if the incisors are overgrown and causing problems for the animal. In the UK, it is illegal for anyone other than a veterinarian to perform dental procedures of any kind on animals.

9. Dental Care

Camelids have a pair of incisor teeth present at birth, normally just poking up above the gum margin. If they are not present, this can indicate prematurity of a minimum of about 2–3 weeks. The first pair of permanent incisors will erupt at 2–2.5 years of age. At this time, the deciduous incisors are pushed outwards and will be lost while the permanent incisors come in behind them. During this period, the front of the mouth can look quite messy, and owners often think they've broken their teeth (*Figure 8*). However, this is entirely normal! The second pair of permanent incisors erupt at 3–3.3 years, and the third pair between 3–6 years of age. Camelids are also born with one or two deciduous premolar teeth on each arcade, and these are replaced between 3.5–5 years of age. The molar teeth erupt as follows: the first molars soon after weaning at 6–9 months, the second pair at 1.5–2 years and the third pair at 2.75–3.75 years.[8]

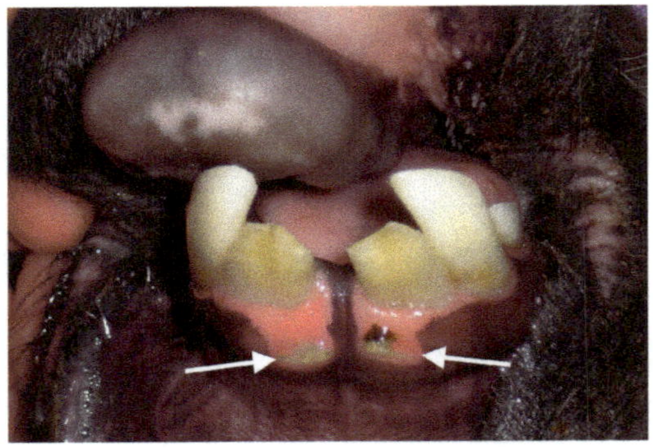

Figure 8. The changing dentition of a young camelid, aged between 2 and 2.5 years. You can see the broken stumps of the deciduous incisors (arrows) with the permanent incisors partially erupted.

Retained Incisors

Occasionally, the deciduous incisors may be retained when the permanent teeth erupt. When this happens, the deciduous incisors are pushed to the outside but not lost. They are smaller than the permanent incisors (*Figure 9*). Most of the time, these teeth will shed naturally in their own time. They do not normally cause any problems, but sometimes feed becomes impacted around them, and removal becomes necessary. If necessary, these teeth may be removed under sedation - but it is essential that none of the roots remain as they may become infected.

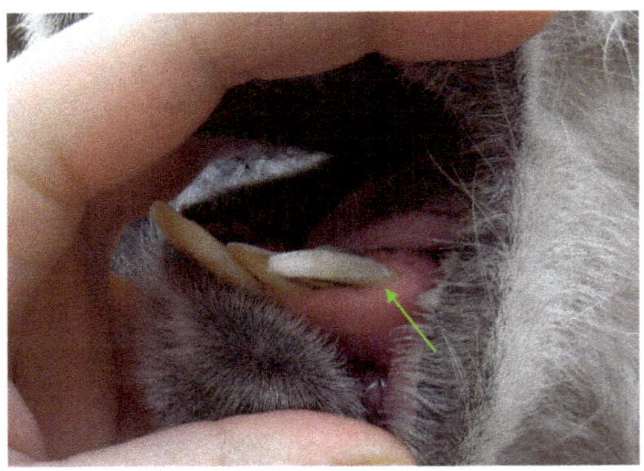

Figure 9. Retained 3rd incisor tooth (green arrow). This tooth is not causing any problems and can be left to fall out on its own.

Tooth Root Abscesses

Tooth root abscesses sometimes occur in camelids, usually associated with the mandibular molar teeth. They are palpable as firm, sometimes painful, swellings on the jawline. Some animals with lots of fleece around the face can be difficult to see, so it is helpful to feel the line of each mandible when you catch your alpacas or llamas for any reason. Early treatment inevitably results in a better outcome for the patient while also being more cost-effective.

Dental Trimming (Incisors)

Tooth trimming is only necessary for animals with poor dental conformation or for adult males to prevent fighting injuries. Sometimes, the incisors will overgrow if they are not level with the hard palate. This overgrowth occasionally results in feed material getting stuck around the incisors or causes difficulty with grazing such that the animals lose weight. In severe cases, the overgrown incisors may restrict lateral chewing motions. To address this, your vet can trim the incisors back to an appropriate length, and level with the hard plate. Make sure to sedate the animal and use a mouth gag and a rotary tool with a diamond cutting disc (*Figure 10*). Your veterinarian can do this for you, and should involve sedation and pain management as required.

In the UK, only veterinarians are permitted to trim teeth or perform any sort of dental manipulations. This is because your veterinarian is best placed to judge whether dental trimming is actually required and because you can cause quite a lot of harm in trimming teeth yourself if you don't know what you are doing. The incisor teeth grow continually, but there are nerves and blood vessels within the tooth under the enamel. If too much of the tooth is trimmed, the pulp cavity that contains the nerves and blood vessels may be entered. Excessive trimming can result in pain and infection getting into the tooth roots. Vets are trained to know what to do if this occurs.

Additionally, never trim teeth by clipping them using something like dog toenail clippers, as this carries a high risk of fracturing the teeth. This will not only be acutely painful but will allow infection to enter the sensitive parts inside the tooth and may cause abscesses that require surgery.

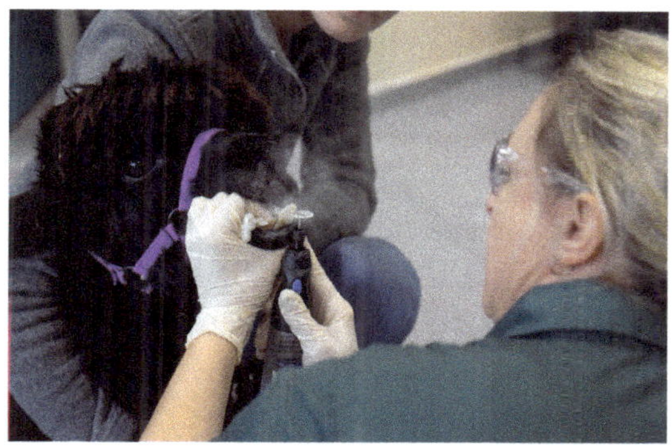

Figure 10. The author performed incisor trimming on a male alpaca with overgrown incisors who was experiencing weight loss. The alpaca is sedated.

There is a tool called the Tooth-a-Matic that is marketed to alpaca owners. This is essentially an angle-grinder with an attachment that the operator slots the teeth into, grinding them off. The problem with this tool is that it is extremely crude – the operator cannot visualise where the tooth is in the attachment or where the blade will cut. The incisor teeth often grow at different angles, and a one-size-fits-all attachment just doesn't make sense. In addition, the tool leaves sharp edges and makes a horrific noise from the alpaca's head. The availability of this tool makes it highly likely that owners worldwide are trimming alpacas' teeth unnecessarily. Again, I emphasise that owners are not legally permitted to trim teeth in the UK, and I do not recommend that anyone use this device.

Dental Trimming (Fighting Teeth)

Camelids have some teeth known as fighting teeth, prominent in males (*Figure 10*). Females sometimes have them, but they are usually much smaller and positioned below the gum line or only just emerging from it. They are more evident in female llamas than female alpacas.

The "fighting teeth" comprise two teeth on the upper arcade (one canine and one incisor) and one canine tooth on the lower arcade. The teeth are positioned on the side of the jaw, in the space between the incisors and premolars. The fighting teeth erupt between 2–7 years, with an average of 2.5 years, but they may not be ready to trim for a little while. They are sharp and point backwards, and in males, they can be used as weapons to inflict injury on their competition. In fact, it has been known for males to slit open the scrotum of another male.

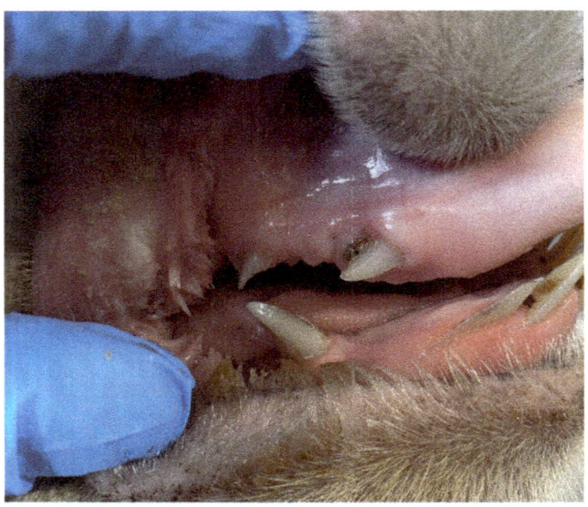

Figure 11. Fighting teeth in a male alpaca.

Fighting is more prevalent among males who are kept close to females, but males will fight even without females present. Therefore, to prevent injury, the fighting teeth can be trimmed to remove the sharp points. How close to the gum margin is safe depends on the animal's age at the time of trimming. Older males will have larger teeth, and the pulp canal will extend further above the gum margin.

Again, clippers must not be used as they may fracture the tooth and cause mandibular abscessation. In the UK, this procedure must be done by a veterinarian and with the animal under sedation. A rotary tool is the best for this as it is quick and can be guided accurately. In addition, any sharp edges can be smoothed off to prevent tongue laceration. Obstetrical wire is sometimes used, but I prefer the use of the rotary tool to the obstetrical wire for a couple of reasons. Firstly, when using wire, the operator has to pull the head to the side to see the wire over the tooth. Secondly, it is difficult to be accurate when placing the wire. It's one go, and that's it. Not to mention, the edges will still need to be smoothed off with another tool.

The Cheek Teeth

The cheek teeth (premolars and molars) of camelids are sharp and pointy. They are supposed to be that way due to their figure-eight chewing pattern. The teeth are positioned with the teeth of the jaw sitting inside the teeth of the upper jaws. The cheek teeth are sharp, adjacent to the tongue on the lower jaw and adjacent to the cheeks on the upper jaw (*Figure 12*). "Floating" of teeth, as in horses, is not necessary in camelids. Floating the teeth will age the animal by simulating what happens as camelids age, and their dental grinding surface may become flatter. It can also result in fractures of the teeth and jaws. The tools used by equine dentists on most horses are too big, and the grinding profile creates too much vibration. Very occasionally, camelids may develop sharp points on their cheek teeth, which may result in lesions on the tongue or cheeks. These animals may pack feed material around such teeth that may be visible as a bulge on the side of the face. If these lesions occur, they may cause reduced appetite due to oral pain.

An oral examination can help determine whether this is a problem, though it is quite challenging to do effectively without the right tools due to the very narrow opening of a long mouth. I use a head torch with a laryngoscope slid down inside the cheek. Vets use the laryngoscope to intubate animals for anaesthesia, providing excellent illumination inside the mouth.

Protecting one's hands and fingers is also imperative for oral examinations. I use a cut-resistant glove inside a latex or nitrile glove on my non-dominant hand to open the mouth. Llamas may require a mouth gag for a proper oral examination. This is because it is harder to keep their larger, stronger mouths open with just fingers, as they will constantly chew while doing this. Very rarely, it is necessary to smooth a sharp molar tooth if it is causing lesions on the tongue or cheeks, mostly in older animals.

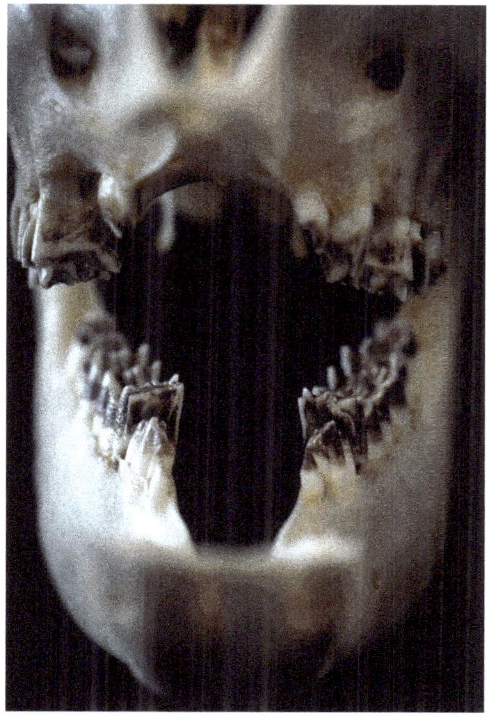

Figure 12. This picture shows the normal angulation of the cheek teeth in alpacas and llamas. The profile is meant to be angled.

10. Plan Nutrition

Nutrition planning for your herd is the last non-negotiable herd health activity. Nutrition is fundamental in ensuring that your animals are healthy and productive. A critical fact to acknowledge is that camelids have unique gastrointestinal anatomy and physiology; understanding this will aid you in planning the nutrition for your herd. Different groups of animals have different requirements, so you cannot manage all animals the same way and hope to get the best out of them. The next two chapters are dedicated to nutrition.

Key Takeaways

This chapter covers the second group of non-negotiable herd health activities: toenail trimming, vitamin D supplementation, shearing, dental care and nutrition planning. Here are some key takeaways:

- Camelid toenails will need trimming from time to time to stop them from overgrowing and causing abnormalities of weight-bearing. The frequency of trimming depends on whether the toenails are pigmented or not and also on the hardness of the ground on which they are kept. Check the feet monthly and trim as necessary.
- Camelids are susceptible to vitamin D deficiency when kept at low altitudes and latitudes away from the equator. Growing animals develop the most apparent signs of deficiency, manifesting as rickets. Supplementation will be required.
- Camelids do not shed their fleece naturally and will need to be sheared. For most animals, this will need to be done annually. It is best done in spring before the weather gets too hot, as camelids are very susceptible to heat stress.
- Monitor your animals' teeth for abnormalities. The most common are incisor overgrowth and tooth root abscesses.
- Nutrition planning is fundamental in ensuring that your animals are healthy and productive. Make sure that your nutrition matches your animals' requirements.

Over the following two chapters, we will cover nutrition in a lot more detail so that you can get to grips with this key component of camelid care.

5

Nutritional Management of Camelids: Part 1

Nutrition is one of the most fundamental features of any herd health plan and is crucial to understand. It forms the foundation for keeping your animals fit and healthy, helping them develop sufficient immunity, ensuring crias grow to their full potential and enabling alpacas to produce fleece of high quality and adequate quantity. Sounds like quite a lot! To do this, you must give your animals the building blocks to help them achieve it. Putting them into a paddock and chucking any old camelid feed at them will not be adequate. It may provide too much or too little nutrition or have an incorrect nutrient balance. Different animals have different needs depending on whether they are growing, pregnant or lactating, or are just wandering around in a field. So, you have to think about their needs as individuals and as groups, figure out what they might be getting from pasture and stored forages such as hay and haylage, and then supplement as necessary with concentrates and minerals.

In this chapter, we will cover the gastrointestinal anatomy and physiology of camelids and explain what makes them unique. We'll also discuss the terminology you should understand to help you manage your herd's nutrition and the nutritional requirements of individual camelids.

In the next chapter, we will discuss how to feed them and monitor the effectiveness of your feeding strategy. We will also discuss the importance of forage analysis in nutritional planning. The information in this book should be more than adequate for most people, but if you want to learn more, I recommend joining the Advanced Camelid Nutrition Masterclass with Dr. Bob Van Saun. For more details, visit www.thealpacavet.com.

The Basics

Gastrointestinal Anatomy & Physiology

Camelids have a complex forestomach comprised of three compartments, imaginatively named compartments 1, 2 and 3. *Figure 1* is a photograph of the stomachs, liver and intestines from a post-mortem specimen showing what the stomachs and intestines look like.

Compartment 1 (C1). This is essentially a large fermentation vat, occupying most of the left side of the abdomen and loaded with microbes (bacteria and protozoa). What do these microbes do?

The microbes break down otherwise indigestible forages to produce volatile fatty acids (VFAs) that are absorbed and used to provide energy.

- Camels provide a source of high-quality protein as they can make all the "essential" amino acids, the so-called building blocks of protein, that camelids need to live. They make the proteins from urea, a by-product of nitrogen metabolism. The proteins then act as a source of protein themselves when they flow downstream and are digested.
- They synthesise B vitamins. Mammals can only synthesise two of the B vitamins themselves. Fermentative microbes found in camelids (and ruminants) can make all of them. Deficiencies only occur when the fragile ruminal or C3 environment is disrupted, and this may occur if too much carbohydrate is suddenly ingested or the microbes aren't given time to adapt to a new diet. An example of this is thiamine (vitamin B1) deficiency.
- The microbes live in a symbiotic relationship with their host. The host feeds the microbes with what they ingest, and the microbes do their part to digest forages and provide proteins and vitamins. Keep the microbes happy, and you'll keep the animal itself happy. As my large animal mentors repeatedly told students during my residency on the farm animal rotation: "If you have a happy rumen, you have a happy cow." The same is true for C1 with alpacas and llamas.

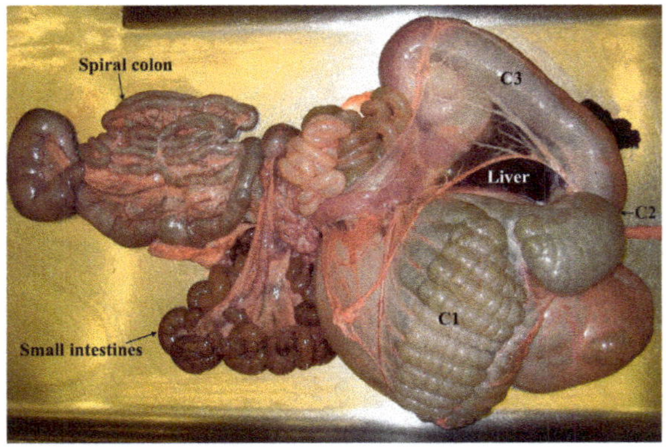

Figure 1. Photograph showing how the stomachs, liver and intestines relate to one another. C3 is reflected upwards to show the medial surface of C1 and its saccules – C3 normally lies over this area.

Compartment 2 (C2). This is a connecting tube between C1 and C3, where most of the action occurs. Some fermentation occurs in C2, along with the absorption of water, VFAs and other solutes.

Compartment 3 (C3). This is the "true" stomach. The first 80% is where further absorption of water, VFAs and solutes occurs. The terminal 20% is glandular; these glands secrete digestive enzymes and acid, resulting in a very much-reduced pH in this portion of the stomach. Camelids are susceptible to C3 ulcers because of the differing pH of these adjacent and physiologically distinct areas. Ulcers tend to form at the boundary between these two zones.

The **small intestine** terminates at a small caecum from where the ascending **colon** arises. Camelids have a long spiral colon relative to other ruminants, making them extremely efficient at re-absorbing water from intestinal content. Their relatively dehydrated pellets are produced here. This adaptation helps them survive in arid climates like the Altiplano. The adaptation also means that when camelids develop diarrhoea, it is much more likely to be significant because it takes a fair amount to overcome this water-absorbing capacity. While sheep will often develop diarrhoea if they have worm burdens, it is rare for camelids to present with soft stool. In fact, based on our having performed thousands of faecal tests in our lab, it is impossible to predict the animals that will have high burdens from the consistency of their stool samples.

The **omentum** is a vascular fatty lace-like structure overlying the intestines within the abdominal cavity. It is not nearly as well developed in camelids as in ruminants. In ruminants, the omentum can wall off pockets of infection in the abdominal cavity, such as stomach ulcers, abscesses or accidental contamination of the abdominal cavity during surgery. However, the camelid omentum is so poorly developed that it has limited ability to deal with any such insults. This means that any abdominal surgery in camelids, including C-sections, needs to be approached with greater attention to sterility than is often taken with ruminants in the field. Generalised peritonitis and post-operative adhesions between loops of bowel, the body wall and other organs may occur more readily. I recommend using sterile surgical drapes, sterile gowns, gloves and masks. Ideally, abdominal surgery should also be performed in a veterinary surgery rather than in a dusty barn.

Adaptations of Camelids

Apart from the anatomical and physiological differences discussed above, camelids are known to be very efficient at surviving on poor-quality forages. When you put camelids and sheep on poor-quality grazing, the camelids will do much better than the sheep. Why is this?

- There is rapid absorption of volatile fatty acids or VFAs. This helps stabilise forestomach pH, which is good for the microbes that are sensitive to changes in pH. VFAs are absorbed 2–3 times faster than in the rumen of ruminants. Camelids also have a high buffering capacity due to the secretion of alkaline bicarbonate, which provides a higher pH in C1. The higher pH improves the ability of cellulolytic bacteria to break down forages.
- Camelids exhibit enhanced recycling of urea. Camelids can consume forage that is low in nitrogen because they can achieve greater nitrogen recycling through the stomach wall. This means that the ammonia-nitrogen content in C1 and C2 remains higher, thereby supporting microbial protein synthesis. This is because nitrogen is a component of amino acids that are the building blocks for protein.
- Large particles of food are retained for longer in the forestomach, resulting in improved breakdown of plant cell walls.
- Liquids flow faster through C1 and C2. This means that microbial growth needs to be more efficient, and only a minimal amount of energy is required to maintain the microbes.

Camelids have developed these adaptations to cope with poorer quality forages in their native habitats in the Andes. Does this mean you can put camelids on poor grazing and they'll do just fine? Well, those with only maintenance energy demands will most likely manage. But it is important to realise that most *productive* animals have higher energy demands, including growing animals, pregnant and lactating females and working males. If you want to optimise the growth of youngsters and have females produce and raise healthy crias annually with excellent fleece, it is necessary to match the level of nutrition to energy demands. This might be difficult on marginal land, which is land with poor-quality grazing.

Another important consideration is that animals with lower energy demands will quickly become fat if fed too much forage or grazed on too-high-quality grass.

Nutrition Terminology & Explanations

The terms in the tables on these pages are used in nutritional analyses, including forage analyses, and they are also found on feed bag labels. Understanding what these terms mean can help you determine the relative nutritional value of the feed you are providing your animals.

Abbreviation	Term	Description
MER	Maintenance Energy Requirements	The amount of energy needed to maintain body weight and for basal metabolic functions. Most animals have energy requirements higher than "maintenance" due to merely walking around.
DM	Dry Matter	The proportion of a feedstuff that is not water. It is expressed as a percentage. Dry Matter is determined by weighing the feedstuff "as fed," drying it out overnight, and re-weighing it to determine the weight of the dried portion.
DMI	Dry Matter Intake	The amount of feed an animal consumes, excluding its water content.
DDM	Digestible Dry Matter	The proportion of dry matter in feed that is actually digested and absorbed. This is an important measure of forage quality since higher digestibility means more nutrients are available for maintenance, growth and production.

Terms Relating to Nutritional Content of Forages

Abbreviation	Term	Description
ADIN	Acid Detergent Insoluble Nitrogen	Important in determining forage quality and can be used as an index of heat damage
	Proteins	
CP	Crude Protein	Positively correlated with quality
RDP	Rumen Degradable Protein	Protein that can be broken down by microbes
UDP	Undegradable Protein	Protein that can't be broken down by microbes
	Fibre Analyses (Used to estimate available energy in feed analyses)	
ADF	Acid Detergent Fibre	Includes lignin and cellulose; used to determine how digestible forages are
NDF	Neutral Detergent Fibre	Includes lignin, cellulose and hemicellulose
	Energy	
TDN	Total Digestible Nutrients	An estimate of the energy content of a feed. Based on the digestible portion of the nutrients that can supply energy, carbohydrates, protein and fat
ME	Metabolisable Energy	The amount of energy available from food after energy lost in faeces, urine and gases has been subtracted

Some key interpretations to have in mind when evaluating rations:

- The more immature a forage is at the time of harvesting, the higher the quality and the lower the ADF value. The more mature the forage, the lower the quality and the higher the ADF.
- Higher-quality forages have lower

NDF, and poorer-quality forages have higher NDF.

- Lower-quality forage results in lower DMI; higher-quality forage results in higher DMI.

Alpacas or llamas with maintenance energy requirements consume 1–1.5 % of their body weight in dry matter. Growing, lactating and pregnant animals will require more than those at maintenance. Alpacas with only maintenance energy requirements may consume more than they need!

Nutritional Requirements

The main nutritional requirements for camelids are water, energy, protein, fibre, and vitamins and minerals. We'll talk about each of these in turn.

Water

Water is the most essential nutrient. It is necessary for maintaining blood volume, normal cellular functions, gut activity, milk production and more. Water makes up around two-thirds of the body weight of adult animals and up to 90% of newborns. Fresh, clean water always needs to be available for camelids to drink. Camelids need 5–8% of their body weight in water daily, depending on activity and production levels. This equals 3.75–6 L per day for a 75-kg alpaca. Some of this water is obtained through grazing, so their requirements are lower when grazing on pasture, especially when it is very wet, compared to eating hay. However, if you are keeping an alpaca or llama indoors or in a dry lot with access only to stored forages, this is a good estimate of the water requirement that they will have. Requirements for water will increase in hot weather and during growth, late pregnancy and lactation. Each litre of milk will require one litre of water intake.

Dehydration results in organ failure, reduced milk production, weakness and, ultimately, death. Neonates are more sensitive to the effects of dehydration since a more significant proportion of their body weight is water. It is important to know when young crias aren't drinking or are losing water in the form of diarrhoea, as they may need to receive intravenous fluid support much earlier to prevent organ failure.

Energy

Carbohydrates are the primary source of energy for camelids. They may be sugars, starches, cellulose or hemicellulose. Unlike humans, camelids can use cellulose and hemicellulose as energy sources because of the microbial populations present within their forestomach. Carbohydrates are fermented to produce volatile fatty acids that are used as energy.

Generally, we calculate energy requirements as "maintenance" (M) and then use a multiplier to account for different activity levels or add on a calculation to account for growth, milk and/or fleece production. This is usually called metabolisable energy (ME). The following calculations are from Van Saun, 2006.[1]

- ME for maintenance (kcal/day) = 72.85 kcal/kg $BW^{0.75}$
  - 1.25 x M: for light work or grazing on moderate to good quality pasture

  - 1.75 x M: for heavy work or grazing on sparse/mountainous grassland
- For growth, we add 7.25 kcal per g of weight gain
- For lactation, add 946.2 kcal per kg of milk produced
- For fleece production, add 30 kcal per kilogram of fleece (annual yield)
- Pregnant females have only maintenance energy requirements (+ those for fleece production) until the 8th month of pregnancy:
  - 8th – 9th month: Add 65.34 x Birth weight (kg) – 33.50
  - 9th – 10th month: Add 131.68 x Birth weight (kg) – 39.74
  - 10th – 11th month: Add 203.51 x Birth weight (kg) + 86.12

These calculations look somewhat complicated and require quite a lot of work in nutrition planning, but please don't feel overwhelmed! Instead, you can make things a little easier by considering an easier model:

Camelids consume about 1.0–1.5% of their body weight daily as dry matter (DM) to *maintain* body weight. Growing alpacas need 1.8–2.0%, late gestation females need 2%, and lactating females need 2.5%. In the next chapter, I will provide more information on how to ensure each group receives the right nutritional balance.

Protein

Protein is required for several functions, including normal cellular functions, growth, pregnancy, lactation, etc. The "building blocks" of proteins are called amino acids. The microbes present in C1 break down proteins (rumen degradable protein or RDP) into amino acids and ammonia. Consequently, camelids get their protein from the microbial production of protein, from the microbes themselves as they are flushed down from the stomachs, and also from protein that isn't broken down by the microbes (undegradable dietary protein or UDP).

Protein requirements vary according to physiological state, as shown in *Table 1*.

It is only possible to use these numbers if you know what your feed is providing. This holds true for stored forages such as hay, haylage, silage and concentrate feeds. Stored forages will vary greatly in quality depending on soil, rainfall, time of harvest, conditions during harvest and storage factors. Therefore, analysing their content is worthwhile if you want to know what you are feeding your animals. This will help you figure out what supplements they need to make up for any deficit. Spring grass generally has higher protein and lower fibre, making it higher in quality and providing more energy to grazing animals. Hay harvested later contains more mature grasses with less protein and higher fibre.

The crude protein content of common feedstuffs is shown in *Table 2*. Note that actual values will vary – this table is for use only as a guide.

If the protein content of the forage being provided is not enough to suit the physiological state of the animal, then you can supplement it with feeds rich in protein, such as alfalfa, peas or soybeans. Feeding higher-quality forage is generally

Physiological Status	Crude Protein Requirement (%)
Maintenance • Over 1.5 years old and not working • Working males, increase the percentage by a bit	8-10
Pregnant (1-8 months)	8-10
Pregnant (9-11 months)	10-14
Lactating	12-14
Growing (weanlings up to 1.5yrs)	14-16

Table 1. Crude protein requirements for different groups of camelids are based on their physiological state.

cheaper than adding expensive protein supplements. Avoid overfeeding as well because animals will excrete any excess nitrogen (which is 16% of all amino acids) into the urine at an energy cost to the animal. In addition, excessive nitrogen causes an increase in blood urea nitrogen that can be detrimental to fertility. It has been shown to cause increased embryonic loss, resulting in reduced pregnancy rates as well as increasing the incidence of endometritis (inflammation in the uterine lining).[2]

Fibre

Fibre is related to Energy. It is required to maintain microbial populations, as they need the structural components of plants, cellulose and hemicellulose, to break down into volatile fatty acids, which are used as an energy source. Forages higher in **crude fibre (CF)** have lower energy content, while forages lower in CF have higher energy content. Hay is higher in fibre but lower in energy, while spring grass is lower in fibre but higher in energy.

Fibre should ideally be long-stemmed (at least 4 cm long) to stimulate salivation, rumination and forestomach motility.

Ideally, a minimum of 25% crude fibre should be included in the diet. Looking at forage analysis, using the ADF value, this would be equivalent to 25% of dietary dry matter intake. Using NDF, this would be 30-35% of dietary DMI.[1]

Table 2 shows the crude fibre content of some common feedstuffs. Please note that actual values will vary; use this only as a guide. Examine the values for oats and sugar beet. These feeds have a higher crude fibre content than other cereal grains such as wheat, barley or corn while having similar energy densities. Therefore, they are favoured for energy supplements over other grains.

Feedstuff	Crude Fibre (% DM)	Crude Protein (% DM)	Energy Density (MJ ME per kg DM)
Spring grass	25 - 30	12 - 15	10 - 11
Clovery pasture hay	28 - 32	10 - 20	6 - 8
Grassy pasture hay	30 - 35	10	7.5 - 9
Straw	45 - 60	3 - 4	6
Alfalfa hay	28 - 40	13 - 20	7.5 - 9
Leafy pasture silage	30	20 - 25	8.5 - 9
Mature pasture silage	35	7	7.2
Oats	11	13	11 – 13.5
Wheat	3	12 - 14	13
Barley	5	12	12.5 - 14
Corn	2	9 - 10	13 - 14
Peas	7	25	13
Soybeans (whole, extruded or roasted)	9	40	14
Soybean meal	3 - 6	45 - 55	12.5 – 13
Soybean hulls	38	13	11.5
Sugar beet pulp	16	9	12
Wheat feed (a byproduct of flour milling)	9	15	11.5

Table 2. Nutrient composition of common feedstuffs. Adapted from Nutrient Requirements of Small Ruminants, NRC 2007.[3]

Vitamins & Minerals

When animals are grazing, most vitamins and minerals will be there in adequate supply. However, under certain circumstances, there may be deficiencies related to soil type or physiological conditions. For example, most soils in the UK are known to be deficient in selenium. This is also true for many parts of the world. There is very little information that defines the requirements of camelids for vitamins and minerals. Most information is extrapolated from known values for beef cattle, sheep and goats and adjusted for differences in the intake of camelids.

Van Saun has summarised the recommendations for minerals for llamas and alpacas based on a model shown in Table 3 below. He suggests that these should be viewed as providing the lower end of requirements and may need to be adjusted upwards under specific circumstances. These values do not consider the impact of any mineral interactions that may be inhibitory, and this may mean adjustments need to be made according to the presence of these in the forages and rations consumed. You can check mineral status by getting your vet to blood sample a selection of your animals.

Vitamin C deficiency is not usually a problem in camelids because this vitamin is made in the liver. Vitamin D, on the other hand, is the primary vitamin in camelids for which the possibility of serious deficiencies must be considered. However, it must alsobe noted that there is a risk of potential toxicities as well due to overzealous supplementation.

For this vitamin, it is definitely a case of "more is definitely *not* always better."

Camelids are susceptible to vitamin D deficiency when kept away from their native environments. In South America, they are exposed to higher levels of UV radiation at high altitudes and equatorial latitudes. Therefore, supplementation is required in most parts of the world where camelids have been exported.

The other fat-soluble vitamins (A, E and K) are generally present in adequate quantities in green grass. However, newborns are deficient at birth and will acquire these in colostrum if the dam has sufficient concentrations in late pregnancy. Since the fat-soluble vitamins are involved in helping the body's immune system function, this can impact their susceptibility to disease.

The B vitamins are all made by the gut microbes or found in milk for nursing crias. Therefore, if you look after the gut microbes by feeding sufficient forage to your animals and not overfeeding concentrates (or introducing them too rapidly), these should be present in sufficient supply. Disrupting the gut flora by introducing a rapidly fermentable carbohydrate too quickly, such as apples or a concentrate feed, may result in clinical signs of vitamin B1 or thiamine deficiency. The most consistent sign associated with B1 deficiency, and the clinical sign that is virtually pathognomic for it (except in cases where animals have access to lead sources such as old car batteries or paint), is sudden onset blindness. Affected animals may also become depressed and inappetent, and they will die without urgent treatment to protect the brain and replace the missing vitamin.

Mineral deficiencies and toxicities may occur. In addition, interactions between minerals mean that oversupplementation of one mineral may result in deficiency in another. Accurate mineral requirements for camelids are not known, and they have largely been extrapolated from other species.

Camelids are known to be sensitive to copper, although possibly not quite so much as sheep. Rations formulated for cattle

Nutrient	Averaged Requirement[1]	Extrapolated Requirement		
		Intake, mg/day[2]	Diet (ppm)[3]	Group[4]
Cobalt	1.76 μg/kg BW	0.11 – 0.28	0.12 – 0.15	M, G, P, L
Copper	0.12 mg/kg BW	7.2 – 19.2	8 - 12	M, G
	0.15 – 0.18mg/kg BW	9 – 27.2	9 – 12	P, L
Iodine	8.8 μg/kg BW	0.5 – 1.4	0.55 – 0.65	M, G, P
	15.7 μg/kg BW	0.9 – 2.5	0.65 – 0.75	L
Iron	0.6 mg/kg BW	36 - 96	35 - 40	M, G, P, L
Manganese	0.33 mg/kg	19.8 – 52.8	22 - 25	M, G, L
	0.52 mg/kg	31.2 – 83.2	28 - 30	P
Selenium	6.5 – 6.8 μg/kg BW	0.4 – 1.07	0.42 – 0.45	M, G
	7.0 – 7.5 μg/kg BW	0.44 – 1.2	0.46 – 0.5	P, L
Zinc	0.56 mg/kg BW	33.6 – 89.6	45	M, G
	0.8 – 1.3 mg/kg BW	60 - 160	55 - 60	P, L

μg/kg BW, microgram per kilogram of body weight: *mg/kg BW*, milligram per kilogram of body weight.
[1]Extrapolated from nutrient requirements for beef cattle (National Research Council: *Nutrient requirements of beef cattle*, ed 7, Washington DC, 1996, National Academy Press), sheep and goats (National Research Council: *Nutrient requirements of small ruminants: sheep, goats, cervids and New World Camelids*, Washington DC, 2007, National Academic Press).
[2]Estimated daily requirement based on a range of adult body weights from 60 to 160kg.
[3]Dietary concentration (mg/kg) on dry matter (DM) basis. Nutrient density calculations based on an assumed range of DM intake between 1.25 and 1.5% of body weight.
[4]Physiologic states of maintenance (M), growth (G), lactation (L) and pregnancy (P) for which the requirement is defined.

Table 3. Suggested dietary concentrations for the essential microminerals in llamas and alpacas for various physiological states. Reproduced with permission from Van Saun. [4]

are, therefore, likely to oversupply copper. Molybdenum interferes with copper absorption, so the suggested ratio of Cu:Mo is 6–10:1. Camelids tend to be zinc-deficient in most management systems outside of South America. Zinc is required for optimal skin health; therefore, zinc supplementation may help manage skin problems. Camelid rations are better if the zinc is provided in a more bioavailable form. Chelated zinc (e.g. zinc methionine) is far more bioavailable than zinc oxide or zinc sulphate.

Notes on Grains and Ingredients in Feeds

It can be confusing looking at the labels of different feeds and trying to figure out what is best to feed your alpacas. Not only are the contents very different, but there are also different ways of processing the grains to improve their digestibility. Some terms may be unfamiliar or leave you wondering what makes them different. Here's a quick guide to help:

Mechanical processing involves rolling or grinding, breaking the grains into smaller pieces. Grinding is required before grains can be included in pelleted rations.

Thermal processing involves roasting or micronising. It uses heat to help break down the complex carbohydrates of starch and increase the availability of nutrients.

Micronising is a specific type of thermal processing in which the grains are heated with infrared heat until all moisture has evaporated. This ruptures the grain's endosperm, breaking down the starch and making the grain more soft and pliable. Immediate flaking thereafter further breaks down the starches, resulting in improved digestibility. In case you are now wondering what the endosperm is, this is the largest part of a whole grain and is the food supply to the "germ," which is the embryo part of the grain that can sprout into a new plant. The endosperm contains carbohydrates, proteins and small amounts of vitamins and minerals.

Thermo-mechanical processing involves flaking or extruding. When rations are made into a pellet formulation, the ingredients are ground and then heated using steam to 80–90°C for around 20 seconds. They are then formed into pellet shapes, cooled and dried. For forage pellets, the forage is dried out before processing. During extrusion**,** the ingredients are ground and mixed. The mixture is then steam-cooked at high temperature and pressure. Pellets are formed that expand and pop like corn kernels. This process results in greater starch breakdown than pelleting.

The labelling convention means that ingredients are usually listed in descending order of importance within the ration. It is best to avoid feeds that list corn, maise or barley as one of the top two or three ingredients. Their fibre content is low compared to oats or sugar beet pulp, but they have similar energy densities. Additionally, oats and sugar beet are less likely to result in the development of C3 ulcers. Corn's protein content is also lower than that of other grains.

Key Takeaways

You should now clearly understand camelid gastrointestinal anatomy and physiology, their unique adaptations for processing the food you provide and their specific nutritional requirements. Key takeaway points:

- Camelids have unique gastrointestinal anatomy and physiology. Their biology is similar but superior to that of ruminants.
- Nutritional planning requires some thought. Don't just toss camelids into a field, throw them some hay and rely on a supplement just because the bag says it's for camelids.
- Animals' physiological states determine their needs for energy and protein. Therefore, it is important to be aware of which groups need more and which need less.
- Think forage first. Supplements make up any deficit.

We now need to consider how to approach feeding your alpacas and llamas. We will do this in the next chapter.

Group	Physiologic State	Feeding Plan	Dietary Guidelines
Nursing Dams with crias	Lactation	Highest nutrient requirements, feed best-quality forages, with energy/protein supplements	60 to 70% TDN, 12-14% Crude protein, 0.9% BW NDF, 0.45-0.62% Ca, 0.32-0.45% P, **
Weanlings up to 1.5 years	Growth	Highest nutrient requirements, feed best-quality forages, with energy/protein supplements	55 to 65% TDN, 14-16% Crude protein, 0.6-0.8% BW NDF, 0.53-0.73% Ca, 0.27-0.38% P, **
Males >1 year	Maintenance	Low requirements unless working, then adjust accordingly, low-to-moderate quality forage	55 to 60% TDN, 8-10% Crude protein, 0.8-1.0% BW NDF, 0.3-0.48% Ca, 0.21-0.28% P, **
Pregnant females 1-8 months	Maintenance	Low requirements, but ensure no loss of body condition, adequate protein, minerals, and vitamins	50 to 55% TDN, 8-10% Crude protein, 0.8-0.9% BW NDF, 0.2-0.24% Ca, 0.12-0.2% P
Pregnant females 9-11 months	Pregnancy	Moderate to high forage quality with supplement for additional mineral and vitamin needs	55 to 70% TDN, 10-14% Crude protein, 0.6-0.8% BW NDF, 0.45-0.56% Ca, 0.28-0.33% P, **, †
Breeding females	Maintenance	Low to moderate; ensure do not become fat or lose condition	50 to 55% TDN, 8-10% Crude protein, 0.8-1% NDF, 0.2-0.24% Ca, 0.12-0.2% P
Obese females	Sub-Maintenance	Low; low-quality forages with mineral/vitamin supplement unless pregnant	45 to 53% TDN, 8-9% Crude protein, 0.8-1% BW NDF, 0.2-0.24% Ca, 0.12-0.2% P

*Ensure adequate available water and free choice salt. White salt should be used when trace minerals are included in a supplement. Otherwise, trace mineral salt should be available.

** These feeding groups require higher amounts of trace minerals and vitamins preferably delivered by a supplement (refer to text for details).

† Dietary energy and crude protein content may need to be increased further in late pregnancy if dry matter intake drops below 1.5 percent of body weight

Table 4. Suggested feeding groups based on physiologic state and nutrient requirements. More precise dietary needs will be determined by the level of production (milk, rate of growth), environmental conditions and desired changes in body condition. Reproduced with permission from Dr Robert Van Saun. Published in: Van Saun, R.J., 2009. Nutritional requirements and assessing nutritional status in camelids. Vet Clinics: Food Animal Practice, 25(2), 265-279.

6

Nutritional Management of Camelids: Part 2

In Chapter 5, you learned all about the way camelids consume their food, digest it and turn it into useful components. You also learned about the main nutritional requirements of camelids: water, energy, protein, fibre, vitamins and minerals. In this chapter, you will learn how to approach feeding your animals and how to assess its effectiveness.

Feeding Alpacas and Llamas

Feeding alpacas and llamas is about more than asking, "How many scoops do I give my animals?" or "How many grams or ounces should I give them?" Although numbers can be helpful – and we will use them in some calculations in the next section – feeding also involves providing the right food with the correct composition and food that the animals can physically consume and digest.

Where supplementary feed is provided, feeding systems need to be designed to allow all animals in a group to feed. Therefore, the provision of adequate hayrack and trough space is vital. All animals must be able to come in and feed at the same time. Generally, allow 3 ft of space (90 cm) per head for single-sided access. Theoretically, half of this should be used for two-sided access. However, you may need to increase the allowance for two-sided access because having the animals competing head-to-head adds further dimensions to that competitive feeding within groups of camelids. Interestingly, camelids need quite a lot more space per head than other livestock to reduce competitive feeding. Thus, observation at feeding time is key to ensure that you get the balance right. Also, ensure that feed is provided in a space that encourages feeding. If the paddock is exposed to frequent windy conditions, site your hay feeders and troughs in a sheltered spot. Hay feeders with lids will help keep hay dry and make it more palatable.

Monitor the behaviour of your animals. Camelids have very unique personalities, and as you work with your animals, you will learn which animals are dominant feeders and which are recessive and stand back to allow others to feed first. Observation will allow you to identify potential problems within each group.

The dominant feeders may spend so much time fending off the others that they don't actually eat (although these are generally the farm fatties!). On the other hand, the recessive animals may struggle to eat enough

I once visited an alpaca farm at a winery in France. The owner had purchased 31 females and a stud male that arrived in spring and asked his winery staff to manage the herd. Fortunately, the chap in charge of the winery had a lovely wife who was very taken with the alpacas, and she stepped in to manage them.

They had no prior knowledge of working with any type of livestock, and the seller appeared now and again to worm the alpacas (blanket worming with injectable ivermectin - see my comments on this in Chapter 4!) and administer vitamin D injections. The seller had told them, "Alpacas are hardy and don't need much extra care." They were not advised to do any training on how to manage alpacas. All went well until October, when the animals started dying. A complicating factor was that the alpacas had been imported from the southern hemisphere and were due to give birth beginning in October. The owner had not planned for additional nutrition to support late gestation and lactation, nor had they planned to provide shelter.

I met them in December when they attended my Camelid Reproduction & Cria Care Course, and they discussed their problems with me. We arranged a herd health visit soon after. When I arrived on the farm in January, they had lost 6 adult alpacas and 10 crias. They also had to bottle feed 12 crias, and another adult died shortly after my arrival. They did have a lot of parasite problems in the herd, but it's the nutritional provision that I will focus on here.

The average body condition score across the herd was 3.5 out of 10 (ranging from 2 to 6 out of 10). The pasture quality was very poor. Parts were marshy with inedible reeds (*Figure 1*), while other parts were mossy with very little grass (*Figure 2*).

Only one small shelter was available and it was used by 10 females and 12 crias, who only just fit inside at night when they were closed in. Two bales of hay were being placed in the shelter daily, but only in one corner of the shelter so that only four or five alpacas could eat at the same time. A dog kennel was in use at the bottom of the paddock, but the alpacas could only access this through the dog access opening. Concentrates were being fed out of a single bucket, and the carer moved among the herd to try to ensure that all the alpacas could get some.

My recommendations regarding their nutritional provisional was to start feeding hay-free choice, with hay racks fixed to the inside walls of the shelter all the way around and mobile hay feeders out in the paddocks, allowing 3 ft per alpaca. I recommended they buy troughs for concentrate provision, again allowing sufficient trough space. They were already feeding a standard camelid pellet plus a protein source, so I added sugar beet. We also discussed the quality of the grazing, managing the moss and reseeding to provide better grass. They also planned to fence some additional grazing areas for the alpacas. There were many other recommendations in different areas, and I showed them how to do toenail trimming and how to body condition score their alpacas, which I asked them to do every other week.

When I revisited the farm four months later, the change had been nothing short of outstanding! The average body condition score had increased to 5.5/10 10. They had instituted all the management changes I suggested, got the parasite problems under control and moved the animals to much better-quality grazing. Finally, they felt so much more comfortable and confident with their alpacas.

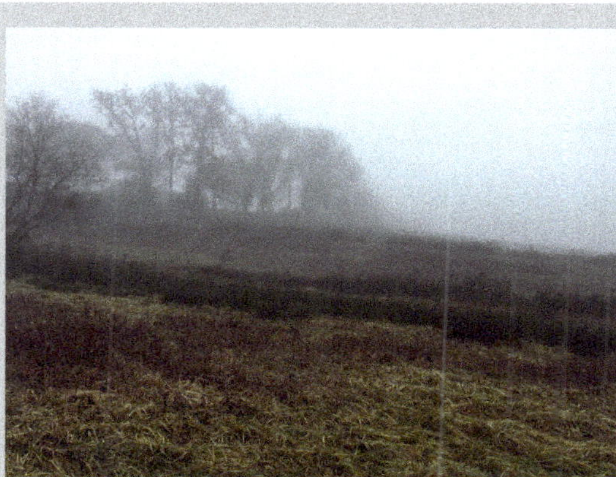

Figure 1. Poor quality pasture with marshy areas.

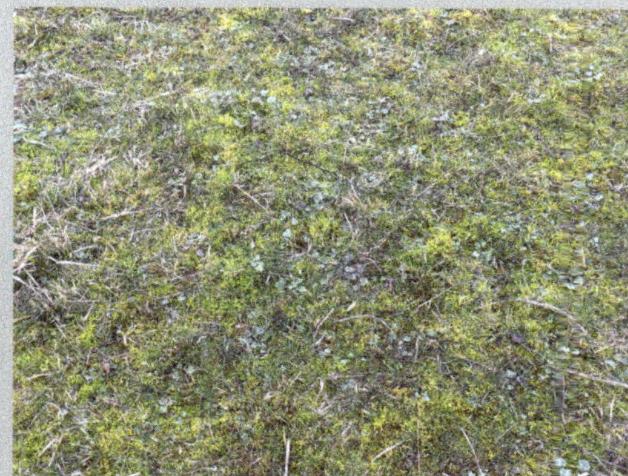

Figure 2. The pasture quality was very poor. Here, I estimated 80% moss, 10% weeds and 10% grass.

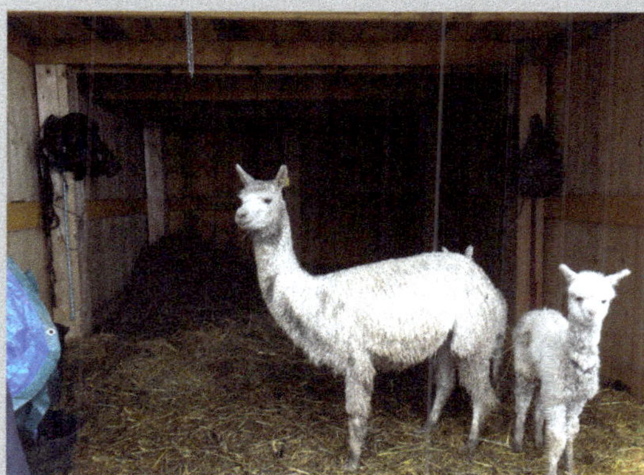

Figure 3. Inside view of the single shelter on the farm. Note the pile of hay stacked in one corner and the poor condition of the alpaca in the foreground.

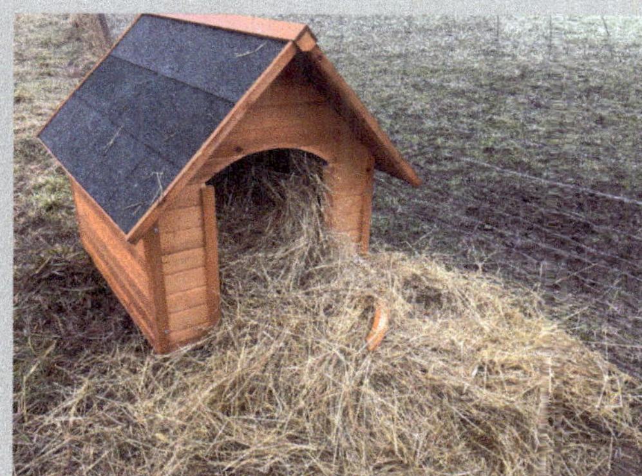

Figure 4. The only other place where hay was being provided in the paddock.

to meet the energy requirements of growth, gestation and lactation. Watch out for this sort of issue and consider separating these animals or at least feeding them separately to ensure that all get sufficient feed.

Animals with differing physiological states will also have differing energy, protein and nutrient requirements. *Table 1*, put together by Dr Bob Van Saun[1], shows suggested feeding groups based on physiologic state and nutrient requirements. This gives you a good idea of how to divide your animals based purely on nutritional needs. This might not always be possible on a small holding because you simply can't have that many groups, but you *can* manage their feeding in groups.

If you feed the same amount and quality of feed to those with only maintenance needs, as well as lactating females, the

Group	Physiologic State	Feeding Plan	Dietary Guidelines
Nursing Dams with crias	Lactation	Highest nutrient requirements, feed best-quality forages, with energy/protein supplements	60 to 70% TDN, 12-14% Crude protein, 0.9% BW NDF, 0.45-0.62% Ca, 0.32-0.45% P, **
Weanlings up to 1.5 years	Growth	Highest nutrient requirements, feed best-quality forages, with energy/protein supplements	55 to 65% TDN, 14-16% Crude protein, 0.6-0.8% BW NDF, 0.53-0.73% Ca, 0.27-0.38% P, **
Males >1 year	Maintenance	Low requirements unless working, then adjust accordingly, low-to-moderate quality forage	55 to 60% TDN, 8-10% Crude protein, 0.8-1.0% BW NDF, 0.3-0.48% Ca, 0.21-0.28% P, **
Pregnant females 1-8 months	Maintenance	Low requirements, but ensure no loss of body condition, adequate protein, minerals, and vitamins	50 to 55% TDN, 8-10% Crude protein, 0.8-0.9% BW NDF, 0.2-0.24% Ca, 0.12-0.2% P
Pregnant females 9-11 months	Pregnancy	Moderate to high forage quality with supplement for additional mineral and vitamin needs	55 to 70% TDN, 10-14% Crude protein, 0.6-0.8% BW NDF, 0.45-0.56% Ca, 0.28-0.33% P, **, †
Breeding females	Maintenance	Low to moderate; ensure do not become fat or lose condition	50 to 55% TDN, 8-10% Crude protein, 0.8-1% NDF, 0.2-0.24% Ca, 0.12-0.2% P
Obese females	Sub-Maintenance	Low; low-quality forages with mineral/vitamin supplement unless pregnant	45 to 53% TDN, 8-9% Crude protein, 0.8-1% BW NDF, 0.2-0.24% Ca, 0.12-0.2% P

*Ensure adequate available water and free choice salt. White salt should be used when trace minerals are included in a supplement. Otherwise, trace mineral salt should be available.
** These feeding groups require higher amounts of trace minerals and vitamins preferably delivered by a supplement (refer to text for details).
† Dietary energy and crude protein content may need to be increased further in late pregnancy if dry matter intake drops below 1.5 percent of body weight

Table 1. Suggested feeding groups based on physiologic state and nutrient requirements. More precise dietary needs will be determined by the level of production (milk, rate of growth), environmental conditions and desired changes in body condition. Reproduced with permission from Dr Robert Van Saun.[1]

"pasture ornaments" will quickly get fat. In particular, consider the maiden female who has reached maturity but may be floating around in the same group as pregnant and/or lactating females. In an ideal world, these animals will be split into different groups based on physiological state (growth, stage of pregnancy, lactation), but this can be difficult to manage on small farms. In this situation, you will need to come up with ways to make it work. For example, animals with higher energy demands can be fed supplements in a separate area, and they will quickly learn to come into a different location for extra food. This may require careful thought when designing your farm and handling area layouts. For those owners having animals that fall in the maintenance-only physiologic state, such as most males, geldings and non-pregnant non-lactating females over 1.5 years of age, it should be noted that these groups may require little supplementation - if at all - if they are receiving forage of good to average quality.

One group of animals deserves special consideration in terms of feeding management, and that is the pregnant females. Pregnant females have restricted stomach capacity owing to the presence and expanding size of the developing foetus, particularly in the last few months of gestation. Therefore, this group's feed *quality* must increase to compensate for their reduced intake volume. They simply cannot eat enough to supply their increasing energy demands if the quality of food they are presented with is poor. One potential problem to consider for this group is that if they get into a negative energy balance situation, they will start mobilising fats from storage sites in the body as an alternative energy source. If this process becomes excessive, it can overwhelm the liver's capacity to deal with it, and that can result in metabolic syndrome.

You should also minimise the accumulation of any rain in troughs by turning them over once they're empty. This will also minimise rodent contamination and potential disease transmission. Leptospirosis, for example, is spread via rodent urine. In TB-endemic zones of the UK, sitting troughs out of reach of badgers will make your troughs less of an attraction. Ideally, they need to be at least 90 cm above the ground, and the troughs should be sprayed so badgers can't climb up adjacent structures to access them. For example, if troughs are hung at an adequate height on stock fencing but a badger can climb up and access the trough, it won't be out of reach.

Determining How Much to Feed

As a general rule, you should aim to feed camelids about 1.5% of their body weight daily as **dry matter (DM)** to *maintain* body weight. Growing alpacas will need 1.8–2.0%, late gestation females will need 2%, and lactating females will need 2.5%.

If we consider a 70 kg alpaca, they will need 1.05 kg of dry matter per day (70 x 0.015) to maintain body weight.

- If this alpaca is on grass with 20% DM content, this alpaca will need to eat 5.25 kg of grass to satisfy this requirement.
- If the same alpaca is only receiving hay with 90% DM content, this alpaca will only need to eat 1.17 kg of hay. Use the formula below to calculate these amounts:

$$\text{Amount of subtrate to feed (kg)} = \text{Total DM requirement (kg)} \times \frac{100}{\text{\% DM of feed}}$$

You should aim to feed *at least* the maintenance energy requirement as forage. Forages (fibre) are required to maintain the function of C1 in maintaining the microbial populations and stimulate salivation, rumination and stomach motility. The rest could be made up with supplements or concentrates if necessary. Use this as a rough guide only. Depending on the actual energy content of the provided forage, this may either under or over-supply requirements. Therefore, I suggest using this as a starting point and then monitoring the effectiveness of what you supply by monitoring body condition and/or weight. If your animals are gaining and you don't want them to, feed a little less. If they are losing weight and you want them to maintain, feed them a little more. In addition, if they eat every blade of hay within a few hours, they probably need more hay. If they are wasting it, feed a little less, and you will waste less forage that gets trampled into the ground.

When adding concentrates, always introduce them gradually, starting with a small amount and increasing gradually over 10–14 days. Concentrates in this context include any feed that comes in a bag or contains grains of any sort. The rule of slowly introducing feed also applies when changing to a substantially different ration or adding different feeds to supplement a ration. This allows those all-important microbes to adapt to the changes.

So, once you've got your forage provision sorted as above, the next step is to calculate how much concentrate or supplement you might need to add to the forage provision to make up for any deficit. If you know the relative content of different feedstuffs at your disposal, you can determine how much to feed. Let us look at some examples using the Pearson Square tool to illustrate this.

The Pearson Square tool is a useful tool that allows you to calculate an appropriate blend of two feed ingredients to meet a desired level. The number in the centre of the square is the nutrient requirement - that is, what you aim to provide. For example, you want to supply a diet that contains 12% CP (crude protein) for a late pregnant female. First, list the nutrient composition of the two different feeds at the square's top and bottom left-hand corners. Then, subtract the nutrient requirement (middle of the square) from the nutrient concentration (on the left-hand side, top and bottom) across the diagonal. This gives the "parts" of the two feeds you need to feed. Any negative numbers are considered positive. Then, add these together to give the total number of parts to feed and divide each of the figures on the right-hand side of the square by the total. This will give the relative proportions as a percentage.

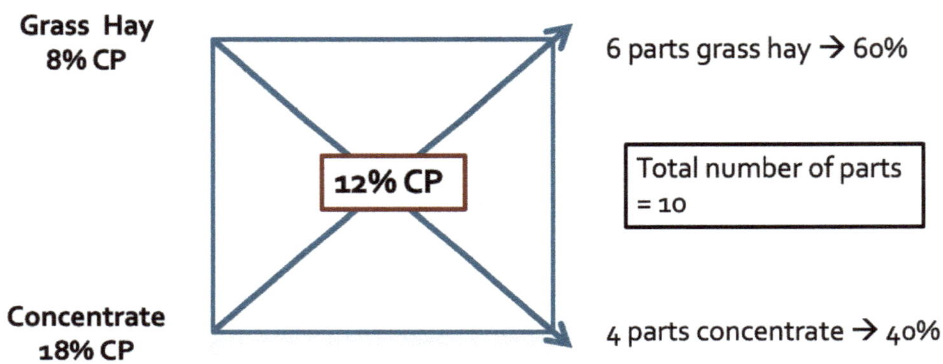

Figure 5. Pearson Square completed using poor-quality hay, trying to reach a target crude protein of 12% overall

Example: You want to mix some grass hay with a concentrate ration to make a diet with 12% crude protein. The grass hay is quite poor at 8% crude protein, and the concentrate is 18% CP. Follow the diagonals to give the equivalent parts of both grass hay and concentrate. Add the total number of parts, and then determine the proportions of each component you need to feed. In this

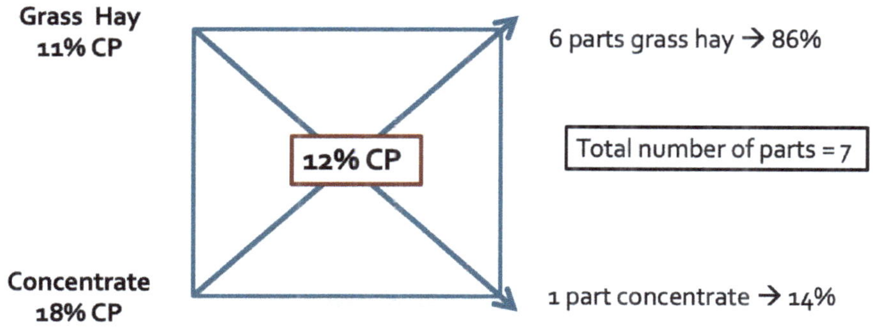

Figure 6. Pearson Square completed using better quality grass hay to reach the same target crude protein of 12%

case that would be 60% grass hay and 40% concentrates (*Figure 5*).

Now, supposing the animals you want to feed need to be fed 2% of their body weight as DM, and they weigh 70 kg each. They will need a total of 1.4 kg of dry matter (0.02 x 70). You would need to feed 40% of their dry matter requirement (0.02 x 70 x 0.4) as a concentrate – that is 560g of concentrate! This is *a lot* of concentrate, and concentrates are generally expensive compared to forages.

Therefore, consider what might happen if we fed better-quality hay with a crude protein of 11%. If you substitute this figure into the square above and redo the math, you would reduce the need for concentrate to 196 g (*Figure 6*).

While you can only input two items at once into the Pearson Square, this really helps you understand the value of knowing your forage quality. If you were to feed only poor-quality hay to lactating females, they wouldn't reach their target protein without adding a lot of concentrates, and you would see them lose weight. Adding concentrates can cause problems for the gastrointestinal system while also being expensive.

How Effective Is Your Feeding Strategy?

By far and away, the best way to monitor the effectiveness of your feeding strategy is to monitor body condition. By performing this monthly (and keeping records!), you can quickly establish whether you're feeding enough or too much. There will often be individuals with their own particular issues, but with feeding, most of the animals in the group will consistently maintain, lose or gain weight over a period of time from a consistent level of feeding. Monitoring body condition will allow you to adjust feed quality or quantity according to need. Body condition scoring is discussed in detail in Chapter 3. You can also weigh animals to see more subtle changes over shorter periods of time.

Tommie keeps alpacas in California. She has a small herd of 10 females and 8 crias. Her problem was that most of them had quite loose poop - not diarrhoea, but the faecal quality was of wet clump consistency, like cow pats rather than the regular distinct faecal beans (*Figure 7*).

The problem would rotate around the herd, with at least half affected on any given day. They were fed hay (orchard grass and alfalfa when needed) but had no grass due to the dry climate in her area. They were also fed about 14 oz (400 g) of a pelleted camelid feed. It had been very hot, and their water was being changed two or three times daily to keep it cool. Faecal testing at Oregon State University had not pointed to parasite issues, and the females were reportedly in good body condition. They were bright with no apparent issues, and the crias seemed to be growing well. Tommie wondered if this could be a nutritional issue or heat-related.

Although the measured amount of pelleted feed was actually within the label directions for this particular feed, I was surprised at the amount being fed. I thought that this could potentially be disrupting the microbial populations, resulting in the looseness. I thought it would be useful to consult with Dr Bob Van Saun because this is a fairly common question from alpaca owners, and perhaps he could shed some light on this issue. He also has more regional-specific knowledge of alpaca feeds in the US.

He agreed that the amount of feed supplementation seemed high, given the quality of forage in California, but he did have much more insight to impart. Clearly, this wasn't an individual animal issue, so he wondered whether there might be an altered microbiome in the hindgut that might be resulting in the more fibrous material there, bringing extra water into the hindgut and thus producing the softer faeces. Because of the high level of grain feeding alongside presumed high-quality forage, this might result in a faster rate of passage of gut content through the forestomachs, leaving extra fermentation to take place in the hindgut.

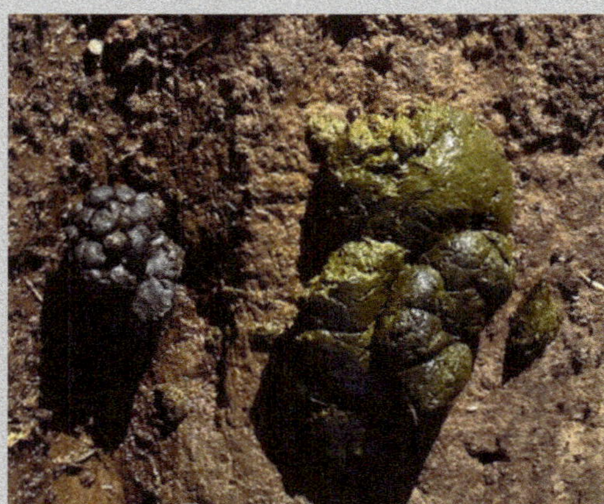

Figure 7. This image shows the soft, cow-pat-like faeces that were a regular feature in Tommie's herd, which caused her concern.

He agreed that reducing the level of concentrate provision while increasing grass hay would be a good first step and that monitoring the effectiveness of this change was necessary. Another recommended option he proposed was to add some yeast product, as in ruminants, yeast supplementation has recently been shown to improve microbial populations, alongside optimising rumen pH and fermentation.[2]

Following the suggestions, Tommie reduced the amount of pelleted supplement feeding, and just over two weeks later, without having yet added any yeast, she reported that just making this small change had fixed the problem of the loose faeces! I recommended that she monitor their body condition and weight to ensure that this hadn't resulted in them being undersupplied with nutrition. After one month, she reported that the females were maintaining their condition and weight well.

Sometimes, feed labels can suggest feeding rather high levels of supplementation to alpacas and llamas. This can result in minor problems such as the above, or sometimes worse problems, including C3 ulcers. If Tommie had an analysis of the hay she was feeding, it might have been possible to plan her feeding more accurately from the start rather than relying on label instructions for the supplementary feed, which in this case was excessive. Unfortunately, this hadn't been an option for her as she had to buy only small quantities of hay at a time from her supplier due to a lack of space and the supplier could not provide the analysis.

If this is also an issue for you, I suggest starting at a lower level than you think on any supplement feeding, building up to this level slowly to avoid upsetting the microbial populations and monitoring body condition scores and weights weekly to help you appreciate the effectiveness of your ration in supplying appropriate energy and protein levels. Increase supplementation if necessary to increase weight/condition, or back off a bit if they start gaining when you don't need them to.

Blood sampling can also measure serum concentrations of various minerals and vitamins, which can help determine the adequacy of the mineral content of your forage and feed.

Hay Analysis

Measuring the quality of your feed, particularly stored forages, will help you determine which foods are best fed to which animals. Very few owners actually do this routinely, either because they think it's too expensive or they constantly have to buy in different batches. However, because concentrates and supplements are the most costly part of a nutrition programme, providing higher-quality forages in a targeted way to the animals that need them most in your herd can save money on supplement costs over time.

You can save the higher-quality first-cut hays for those with higher energy demands and give the poorer-quality second-cut hays to those with maintenance energy requirements. Various companies can analyse forages. Do your homework, though, and make sure that they will give you the information that you need. There are also strict processes to follow when submitting forages for analysis. Most companies will probably be able to provide information on how best to sample, but here are my top five tips:

1. Take a representative sample from each lot of hay. A "lot" is the hay harvested in a day from one field or a specific variety.
2. Due to variation among bales from each lot, it is important to sample 20 small rectangular bales or 8–10 large bales.
3. Using a bale corer provides a better sample than grabbing from the surface of the bale because this causes less separation of stems and leaves. This works with either a hand brace or a variable-speed drill. The core sampler should have an internal diameter of at least 3/8 inch and a length of 12–18 inches. If you don't want to buy your own, consider hiring one from an analysis company or feed merchants, or collaborating as a regional group of owners to purchase one for shared use.
4. The best place to core sample
   - Small bales - through the centre of one end
   - Large rectangular bales - any place on the bale end or side at a 45° angle
   - Round bales - perpendicular to the circumference of the bale
5. To take a sample, test each lot separately and take multiple samples from bales that are separated from each other physically. Mix the cores and place them in a clean plastic bag, seal them tightly and label them before sending them to the lab.

Managing Fat or Skinny Camelids

Overweight Camelids

What to do about overweight animals is an ever-present problem outside South America. In small herds with animals in different physiological states, those with only maintenance requirements may easily gain weight, while those with higher needs risk losing weight. While it is possible to individually manage the feeding of these individuals in small herds this way, it does require attention to detail and partitioning in some way at feeding times. It may be relatively straightforward to manage the feeding of supplements this way, but if the grazing itself is of very high quality, no amount of feed-bowl management will help an overweight female lose weight!

Feed restriction is the obvious solution to helping overweight animals lose weight. However, if these are females who are either lactating or in the last few months of pregnancy, I would caution against dietary restriction. These animals have quite high energy and protein requirements. If they get into a negative energy balance (insufficient energy to meet demand), these girls will start mobilising their body fat as an alternative energy source. The fat is transported to the liver, and if this process overwhelms the liver's ability to cope with it, then metabolic syndrome and fatty liver (hepatic lipidosis) may occur.

Kate Brookes of Mullacott Alpacas (Devon, UK) struggles to manage the condition of some of her animals. She started doing forage analysis back in 2018. At that time, her hay had only 6.8% crude protein, which is very low, so she decided to seek help to improve this and provide her herd with better nutrition.

They reseeded the pasture to improve the grass and then used fertiliser, increasing protein to 12.1% in 2019 and 17.9% in 2020. A grass analysis in January 2023 revealed it to be quite lush, with 25.6% protein, and her 2024 hay had 18.9% protein. About six months before that grass analysis, some soil conditioner had been added to break down organic matter and increase the amount of nitrogen available.

You can see from the data that she achieved a great deal in improving the quality of the forage. However, Kate will need to be careful which forages are provided to the different physiological groups in her herd. Her current concern is having many overweight females. One consideration is that excessive nitrogen from very high protein intake can be detrimental to fertility.[3]

After giving birth, the increased energy demands of lactation will naturally help these females lose some weight. It is safer not to restrict their diet during this period and instead manage any potential dystocia issues related to excess weight if they arise. Pregnant females up to eight months of gestation who are not also nursing have energy requirements close to maintenance levels and can be placed on a restricted diet. However, this should be done cautiously, with their weight and condition closely monitored. Any animals on a restricted diet must be carefully observed, ideally through weekly weighing, which provides a more sensitive measure of weight changes over time than body condition scoring.

Concerning overweight animals, the easiest groups to manage are the males and non-pregnant females. Managing this group should be the first step, as any supplements for these groups can be completely cut back or even stopped altogether. Ultimately, whether or not you can stop feeding will depend on whether they can meet their vitamin and mineral requirements in other ways. For example, in the UK, we have a supplement called Camelibra™ (GWF Nutrition) that is designed to be fed in low quantities to supplement a forage-based diet, providing vitamins and trace elements. It is possible to continue feeding this at a low level to overweight camelids to maintain vitamin and mineral supplementation without overloading them with concentrates. This approach also allows for human interaction during feeding times and enables monitoring of the animals.

If possible, overweight groups should also be receiving poorer quality forages. This could include putting these animals on poorer areas of pasture or, when grazing is poor anyway and hay is provided, then providing them with the worst quality hay. If cutting back on concentrate/supplement feeding does not achieve the desired effect, cutting back on access to forage is the next step. Where animals are grazing, this might be restricting access to that grazing. One way to manage this is to bring them onto hard standing or concrete for a few hours to limit their grazing time. If you don't have these areas, minimise the size of the pasture they can access or fence off a small, heavily grazed section of a paddock to use as a feed-restriction area. Monitor the effect of these measures. If their weight doesn't decrease, extend the restriction period. Because camelids primarily graze during the day, the restriction should occur during daylight hours. If this isn't reducing their weight, restrict them for longer periods. Since camelids graze mainly during the daytime, this restricted period will need to be during the daytime hours.

Underweight Camelids

When dealing with underweight camelids, the first thing to consider is what is causing them to be underweight in the first place. Where most of the animals in a group are underweight, this is likely due to underfeeding or insufficient quantity or quality to provide for their needs. Since forage is such an important component of the camelid diet, forage analysis can be incredibly important in assessing the adequacy of the diet, especially for animals in the higher requirement groups.

Multiple animals in a group may also be affected by parasitism, although it is likely that a small proportion of any group is more susceptible to these than the rest. Nevertheless, faecal testing of individuals and a representative selection of the group is always warranted as a first diagnostic step.

When an individual is in poor condition, it is important to consider individual animal concerns. For example, check for dental issues that might be causing oral discomfort and check for swellings on the jaws that could indicate tooth root abscesses. Bloodwork can be a helpful diagnostic tool to determine whether systemic issues are present. Consider the social position of that individual within the group in case they are struggling to get in to feed - these animals can be fed separately to resolve this.

Regardless of the underlying cause, to encourage weight and condition gain, it is important to ensure that these animals receive the best quality forage, whether in the form of grazing or stored forages. Forages bought bagged often have nutritional information provided and are of consistent quality, so these can be helpful in these circumstances. Chopped dried grass purchased in the UK often has a crude protein of 16% and is highly palatable. Alfalfa hay or chopped alfalfa provides high protein content, too. Sugar beet or beet pulp is an excellent energy source. Whatever you do, it is important to ensure that energy and ammonia (from protein) are present at the same time so that they can be utilised properly and promote microbial growth in C1. In other words, increasing protein provision without ensuring adequate energy in good-quality forage creates a mismatch, wasting both energy and protein because microbes cannot store one without the other.

Key Takeaways

Nutrition is such a fundamental part of maintaining the health and productivity of your animals that it cannot be ignored. It involves far more than simply letting them graze on pasture, tossing them some hay when needed, and adding a concentrate as a supplement. Here are some key takeaways from these two chapters to help you manage the nutritional provision for your herd.

- Take time to plan the nutrition for your herd. Nutrition is the basis for ensuring that your animals are fit and healthy, productive and able to resist disease to the best of their ability.
- Consider the requirements of each physiological state in your herd. Growing animals, those in late pregnancy and lactation, and those no longer growing and not breeding need to be considered separately and managed accordingly.
- The microbial population of the gut is a primary consideration. Keep the microbes happy, and you'll keep your animals happy. Feed them with this in mind.
- Aim to provide at least the maintenance requirements of your animals as forage and make up the rest in supplements where needed.
- Use forage testing to assist in planning your nutritional programme. Since forage is the primary part of their diet, having an analysis, as Dr. Bob Van Saun puts it, "is the single best measure of your nutrition program and its adequacy."
- Blood testing should be used to assess trace elements and vitamin status, thereby assessing the diet's adequacy in providing these.
- Body condition score your animals regularly (at least monthly) to monitor the effectiveness of your feeding programme and make adjustments as required. Weighing should be used as an additional tool to monitor growth in young animals and as a more sensitive indicator when trying to add or reduce weight in individuals.

If you take the time to collect the data you need to manage your herd's nutrition and adjust your plan based on routine data collection, you'll see improvements in your animals' health, productivity, and disease resistance. In the next chapter, we will talk about biosecurity and a key part of reducing the impact of disease is to have healthy animals.

7

Biosecurity (Part 1): Keeping Your Animals Safe

According to the Animal & Plant Health Agency, "biosecurity refers to a set of precautions that aim to prevent the introduction and spread of harmful organisms."1. From your perspective as a farm owner, biosecurity involves protecting your existing herd from diseases that new animals may bring, reducing the risk of disease spread among newly introduced animals, and limiting exposure to potential pathogens already present on your farm.

In 2001, the UK faced an outbreak of Foot and Mouth Disease (FMD). This outbreak was hugely damaging for the farmers in the UK. By the time the disease was discovered at a slaughterhouse, it had already taken hold on 57 farms in 16 counties around the UK. The costs of the outbreak were the compulsory slaughter of 6.5 million animals and £8 billion to the UK economy. The outbreak originated from infected, illegally imported meat used in a restaurant, with leftovers fed to pigs that subsequently developed the disease.

While we're fortunate not to have to deal with this day-to-day, the outbreak prompted the UK as a nation to reevaluate biosecurity in the livestock industry and implement necessary improvements. This example highlights that it is infinitely preferable to think of what you can do to protect your herd *before* it's too late and you have a disease outbreak to deal with. I love this quote from James Thurber, the American author and cartoonist: "Let us not look back in anger, nor forward in fear, but around in awareness." In other words, we must learn from our mistakes to prevent problems in the future. If we prepare in the present for every eventuality and have a plan in place, we can feel better for having done what we can.

It was previously thought that camelids were quite resistant to many diseases. However, the emergence of several infectious diseases has expanded our knowledge in recent years. Globally, we have seen bovine viral diarrhoea virus (BVDV) and Johne's disease. Vector-borne diseases such as Bluetongue Virus, West Nile Virus, and Eastern Equine Encephalitis Virus have also affected camelids in different parts of the world. Climate change has contributed to the spread of these diseases, as the range of their vectors has expanded into previously unaffected areas. In Europe, particularly the UK and Spain, bovine tuberculosis has increased in prevalence, leading to camelids being affected. We now know that camelids are highly susceptible to this disease. Meanwhile, in the US, an outbreak of alpaca coronavirus caused an acute respiratory syndrome.

For most of these diseases, little is known about the epidemiology and pathogenesis of these diseases in camelids, leading us to extrapolate from other species - which isn't always accurate. However, our biosecurity precautions aim to minimise the spread of all diseases within and between herds, reducing losses from disease, lowering overall costs, and lessening the emotional distress experienced by owners.

The biosecurity section of this book covers two chapters. I will divide this first chapter into two parts. In Part 1, we will discuss the infectious agents that can cause disease in camelids and the potential sources of biosecurity threat to your animals. In Part 2, we will discuss measures to help minimise the impact of disease events on your farm by preventing their spread to other animals. This not only improves animal welfare but also reduces the cost of disease. The next chapter will focus on keeping disease off the farm entirely - ensuring you don't unintentionally acquire disease from neighbouring livestock or roaming wildlife, or actively bring problems from newly purchased animals, visiting animals or animals travelling to shows or events.

Part I: Potential Diseases and Their Sources

The Diseases

Table 1 lists the organisms that might cause disease in camelids. They are listed by group, from largest to smallest. Examples and the potential source of infection are given. Those at the top of the table are the easiest to control but tend to cause the most problems in camelids worldwide.

Strep equi subsp *zooepidemicus,* more commonly known as *Strep zoo* or "Alpaca Fever," is an interesting one. This bacterium is a normal commensal organism carried in the upper respiratory tract of equines but is not normally present in the respiratory tract of camelids. When alpacas have been diagnosed with *Strep zoo,* there has often been a history of contact with equines, though not always.[2] [3] [4] [5] The disease is recognised as one of the most significant camelid diseases in South America, where camelids frequently intermingle with other species.

Outbreaks there are often linked to stress. For example, a European owner reported the death of a stud male following transport with horses in a vehicle. The journey from the UK to Spain was lengthy and undoubtedly stressful. However, other alpacas on the same transport did not develop the disease, suggesting that individual susceptibility may also play a role.

We in the UK have been unfortunate to experience how highly susceptible camelids are to bovine tuberculosis, as the disease increased in prevalence during the first twenty years of this century. Badgers and deer act as wildlife reservoirs of the disease, so minimising contact with cattle and wildlife is important for excluding tuberculosis from camelid herds.

The viral diseases listed largely have a geographically limited distribution, often associated with the presence of insect vectors. However, bovine viral diarrhoea

Disease-causing Group	Examples	Source
Ectoparasites	*Sarcoptes, Chorioptes, Psoroptes* mites	Other camelids, foxes *(Sarcoptes)*
Gastrointestinal parasites	Nematodes, trematodes, cestodes	Other camelids, sheep, cattle
Protozoa	Coccidia	Other camelids
	Giardia, Cryptosporidium	Other camelids, livestock
Bacteria	*Strep equi* subsp *zooepidemicus* ("Alpaca Fever"	Equines
	Salmonella	Horses, cattle, other camelids, poultry
Mycobacteria	*Mycobacterium bovis* (TB)	Cattle, badgers (UK), infected camelids
	Mycobacterium avium subsp *paratuberculosis* (Johne's Disease)	Cattle, infected camelids
Viruses	Llama adenovirus, coronavirus, resp viruses, WNV, EHV-1, BVD, BTV, FMD	Other camelids, cattle, horses, sheep, pigs, birds, etc.

Table 1. Infectious diseases of concern in camelids. Examples of pathogens and their potential sources are listed.

virus (BVD) has been diagnosed in camelids globally due to its spread from cattle, and Bluetongue virus (BTV) comes in many serotypes that are prevalent in different parts of the world. The only known FMD virus infections were in a group of 30 experimentally infected llamas. Only 3 of the 30 llamas showed evidence of infection, and only 2 of those had mild clinical signs. There was no transmission between llamas or from llamas to susceptible livestock.[67]

The Sources of Biosecurity Threat

Camelids most often encounter other camelids, making them the most obvious source of threat. There is also potential to control and manage contact with infectious agents through this source. Any animals that die on the farm should be removed efficiently, and a postmortem examination should be carried out to investigate the possibility of any infectious diseases that may spread to other animals in the herd. The postmortem examinations can potentially allow farmers to limit spread at an early stage. Any fear about what is found is irrelevant because the consequences of not detecting it will only increase the losses experienced.

Livestock on neighbouring farms can also be a source of disease. Limiting contact using double fencing or solid hedge lines is a helpful precaution. Other animals can also carry disease: Poultry can spread *Salmonella,* cats can spread toxoplasma when defecating in haystacks, rodents spread *leptospirosis* through their urine, and dogs can leave *neospora,* sarcocysts, and tapeworms in their faeces if they defecate on pastures.

Any object that comes onto your farm from another can be a potential source as it may carry infectious organisms on board. For example, vehicles and trailers from other farms may carry diseases whether animals travel on them or not. Feed delivery vehicles may also be travelling from farm to farm. You would be advised to ensure that vehicles arriving from other farms do not enter the areas of your premises where your animals might be grazing or may transit through. Loading and unloading should take place outside these areas. This may require setting up secure spaces, such as gated areas, to allow unloading without the need for halters if necessary. If it is absolutely necessary for vehicles to enter these areas, then make sure they will not be dropping organic material onto the ground from wheel arches or the underside of the vehicle, and make sure that the wheels are cleaned and sprayed with an appropriate disinfectant before entering areas that are trafficked by animals. Second-hand farm equipment such as trailers and farm machinery should likewise only enter your premises if cleaned and disinfected from other livestock farms.

Visitors from other farms, vets and any farm workers coming onto the farm may be a source of contamination if their clothing and footwear are not clean. Staff working on the farm with their own animals at home, visiting shows or other farms must also be aware of the potential for cross-contamination. Owners or staff moving from group to group can also transmit disease. On one farm with multiple groups of animals, owners treating one group of alpacas for sarcoptic mange inadvertently spread the disease to multiple groups via clothing.

Consider your own farm equipment.

Farm utensils such as buckets and cleaning equipment can act as fomites, meaning they can transfer infection from one part of the farm to another if not cleaned in between transfers.

Finally, live vaccines should never be used in camelids. Live vaccines can potentially revert to virulence, meaning they can *cause* disease. Since no vaccines are licensed for use in camelids, the effects of live vaccines would be entirely unpredictable, potentially increasing the likelihood of reversion to causing disease.

Part II: Prevention and Management of Disease Events on Your Farm

The best strategy for preventing disease events on your farm is to ensure that your animals are maintained in optimum health, as this will make them less susceptible to disease. Body condition scoring is an essential element in this, but you also need to ensure that their immune systems are supported by good nutrition to help their bodies respond to potential threats. Additionally, you will need to implement preventative management strategies. These strategies can be divided into two categories: those focused on preparing your animals and those focused on preparing their environment.

Preparing Your Animals to Be Disease-Resistant

Regular Body Condition Scoring

Body condition is a measure of overall health. It permits the identification of over or underfeeding while also allowing you to detect individuals who may be having trouble due to disease or a low position in the social hierarchy. I recommend that you monitor and record body condition on a monthly basis and recognise that both over *and* under-conditioning can cause problems.

Loss of body condition over a cross-section of animals in a group can indicate a possible parasite issue or under-provision of food. For the latter, this might be in terms of quantity or quality. Hay or grass may sometimes not have the nutritional value that you expect or meet the higher demands of groups needing support for foetal growth, maintaining body weight, growth, or feeding a hungry cria.

Loss of body condition in individual animals may indicate similar issues but on an individual level, such as insufficient food intake or other clinical problems like dental disease, abscesses, pneumonia, tumours or chronic illnesses. Once you've ruled out simple problems, you may need a veterinary evaluation to investigate these individual concerns. Overconditioning can predispose animals to heat stress, lead to birthing difficulties, reduce milk production and increase the likelihood of hepatic lipidosis, a secondary effect of other disease conditions. Any animal that is not eating sufficiently to supply its needs can end up with metabolic syndrome that ultimately can lead to hepatic lipidosis.

Optimal Nutrition

You should ensure that your animals receive optimal nutrition in terms of the feed and minerals provided. For this, think about grass quality. At certain times of the year, the quality may be poor, resulting in the need for supplementary hay and/or feed. Laboratory forage analysis is highly recommended as the most reliable way to assess the adequacy of provided forages, which form the foundation of the feeding program.

Be sure to check feed sources to maintain quality control. Ensure your feed comes from mills that do not process products with ionophore additives, which will help avoid contamination. These are used to control coccidia in pig and poultry feeds. Blood samples can also be submitted to evaluate the adequacy of vitamin and mineral provision. Mineral deficiencies are often a cause of disease in herds.

Vitamin D Supplementation

As mentioned in previous chapters, camelids are prone to vitamin D deficiency when kept outside South America, away from the high ultraviolet radiation found there. Therefore, you may need to establish a vitamin D supplementation programme for young stock during winter to prevent rickets. Adults may also benefit from supplementation, as vitamin D supports the immune system, and adequate levels can help protect against disease. In addition, vitamin D is known to improve foetal growth, mammary development and milk production in other species.

Water

Ensure unlimited access to fresh, clean water and regularly check that it is always available. Water sources may include the main supply, wells or boreholes. While water from fast-flowing streams is fine, you must remember that quality will vary and the water may be contaminated beyond your control.

Never use marsh or stagnant water that could harbour liver fluke. If using well water or water from an open dam, check the quality and ensure appropriate filters are used to control unwanted pathogens such as Giardia and Salmonella. If ponds or rivers overflow following heavy rain, remove animals from flooded areas and ensure their drinking water is not contaminated. In cold weather, maintain water sources, removing ice from buckets and troughs.

Shelter

Protection from the elements is important, and it includes access to shade in summer and shelter from rain, wind, cold and snow in winter. Appropriate bedding, such as straw, may be necessary for insulation against the cold. Additionally, coats can be useful for certain individuals in colder conditions, helping them conserve energy that would otherwise be used to stay warm.

Colostrum Management

Ensure that newborn crias obtain sufficient colostrum. This is vital in preventing neonatal diseases and will give crias the best start in life. Partial failure of passive transfer can result in chronic ill thrift and poor fertility once they reach reproductive age.

Vaccinations

Vaccinate against preventable diseases that are prevalent in your area. This should always include protection against clostridial diseases, at minimum. Other diseases, such as bluetongue (various serotypes), rabies, West Nile Virus and leptospirosis, may be prevalent in certain areas.

Disease-resistant stock

We know that genetics plays a key role in the susceptibility of animals to disease. There are many studies that highlight this. For example, cattle have been shown to have considerable genetic variation to many diseases,[8] and lines of Merino sheep that had been selected for increased resistance to *Haemonchus* showed significantly lower egg counts than those that had not been selected for this characteristic.[9]

It is often stated that 20% of the animals in a herd account for 80% of the herd's parasite problems. If you do enough faecal worm egg counts, you will start to identify the camelids in the herd that are more susceptible to worm burdens. Likewise, this may also be true for susceptibility to chorioptic mange. Such animals may pass this susceptibility on to the next generation, and you may notice these characteristics running in family lines. If you do notice this in your herd, you may wish to honestly consider whether these are genetics that you wish to perpetuate in your herd. While it may be a difficult decision, especially when selecting for excellent fleece characteristics in stud males, consider the broader implications. If offspring frequently succumb to *Haemonchus* or suffer from recurrent mange that requires weeks of effort to manage, this is far from ideal for you or your potential buyers. Stud males, in particular, can spread their genetics widely, as they sire numerous progeny each year. Therefore, stud males with strong disease resistance should be considered superior.

Control Gastrointestinal Parasites

Gastrointestinal parasites are probably the number one health threat within any camelid herd and represent an ever-present biosecurity risk on the farm. They cause more illness and death than any other disease, yet people can be quite laid-back about them and not be aware of what a proper parasite control strategy entails.

Your parasite control strategy is a critical component of your herd health plan, essential not only for within-herd biosecurity but also for preventing problems from entering the herd from outside. I come across supposedly "experienced" breeders who still think a suitable parasite control strategy is a twice-annual injection of ivermectin or doramectin. I will cover parasite control in a lot more detail in the next chapter, but here are the essentials – alongside regular body condition scoring and mucous membrane checking – for what a parasite control strategy should involve:

Periodic Faecal Testing

Perform routine herd-level faecal testing *at least* twice a year. Start with testing in spring and autumn and do additional tests for any animals of concern between these herd tests. The frequency of herd screening can be increased depending on the problems experienced. Wet summers can result in the need for screening tests to be added earlier than autumn due to a build-up of eggs on pasture.

Choose the Right Faecal Testing Method

The Modified Stoll's Test is the optimum test for camelid faecal testing as it incorporates a float solution having high specific gravity with double centrifugation. These test features greatly enhance its sensitivity, resulting in better floatation of larger and heavier eggs and oocysts such as *Nematodirus, trichuris* and *E mac.* These are known to cause significant clinical problems in camelids at relatively low levels of infestation, and therefore, it is important to be able to detect them. Other tests, like the commonly used McMaster's test, are excellent for counting eggs when burdens are very high, but they are less sensitive for detecting the lower burdens of larger, heavier eggs and oocysts that are often a concern in camelids.

Sample as great a proportion of the herd as you can afford to submit for testing. This will result in fewer missed problems as alpacas can be quite individual in their susceptibility to parasites. If the entire herd is tested, this permits targeted treatment and reduces the use of anthelmintics (and therefore the development of resistance). As an absolute minimum, you should test 10% of the herd or 10 animals - whichever is the highest number.

Select older animals or animals aged 16-18 months and in poorer body condition, as they are more susceptible and do not pool samples. Otherwise, the eggs will be diluted among the group sample, resulting in a failure to detect individuals with parasite problems.

Some animals may also be prone to parasite problems. Identify these individuals, always include them in routine screening, and keep them away from susceptible young stock and their pasture areas.

If you find parasite problems in faecal samples and must treat them, always do follow-up faecals (usually 10–14 days later) to ensure that your treatment has been effective. Always try to dose animals individually based on their body weights. In fact, I strongly encourage you to purchase a set of scales for your farm.

Pasture Management

Design your farm with ease of management and parasite control in mind. Divide larger fields into smaller paddocks that can be grazed in turn ("pasture rotation"), allowing some areas to remain ungrazed to allow parasite eggs to die off and the grass to recover. The period in which pastures must rest to become "clean" depends on the contamination level, type and environmental conditions. After four months, you would expect contamination to have declined significantly, though not necessarily eliminated.

When designing your farm layout, include management aisles that permit the movement of animals and vehicles around the farm without having to cross other paddocks. If these aisles are placed around the edge of the property, they can serve as physical barriers against mollusc incursion in areas where Meningeal Worm is a concern (such as in the US). Concrete or gravel surfaces are particularly effective, as they are less attractive for molluscs to cross.

The double barrier also prevents nose-to-nose contact with neighbouring livestock that may transmit disease.

Stocking density, or the number of animals kept on an acre (or hectare), should be kept under control. In areas with good pasture, I recommend a *maximum* stocking density of 5 alpacas or llamas per acre (0.4 hectares) of pasture, but this may vary widely depending on location and climatic conditions. Higher stocking densities may be possible, but these increase grazing pressure and contamination and require animals to be moved more frequently; thus, an increased proportion of resting pasture is required. Otherwise, there will be an increased reliance on supplemental forage provision.

The best parasite control method is removing faecal material since this removes the eggs from the pasture. Under optimum conditions, strongyle-type eggs may hatch on pasture in 3–5 days. Therefore, pasture should be cleaned every other day (or stretched to 3 days if required, such as over a weekend) before eggs hatch onto the grass. Various mechanised options exist to achieve this, depending on your budget and pasture size. Farms I work with that regularly clean the pasture have virtually no problems with parasites and often rarely have to use any wormers.

Lastly, the susceptibility of different groups of animals should be considered. Weaned crias are likely the most susceptible group, so they should be placed on the cleanest pastures. Crias, with their dams, are another susceptible group that will need special attention.

Preparing the Environment to Prevent Disease

The following practices are suggested for biosecurity on alpaca farms.

General Cleaning and Disinfection

Personal hygiene is vital to prevent the transmission of pathogens between animals and from animals to humans. When a disease in an animal can cause disease in humans, it is called zoonosis or zoonotic disease.

Personal hygiene should include frequent and effective hand washing with alcohol-based formulations or soap and hot water. Use hot water and soap when hands are soiled. [World Health Organisation (WHO) guidelines recommend that handwashing between hospital care workers for human patients should take 40–60 seconds and cover all hand surfaces. This guideline is also reasonable for those working with animals. Alcohol-based formulations have a place where hands are not obviously soiled. These are more convenient for hygiene and can be placed at sites where you want to ensure their use. For example, at the entrance to an office area for workers coming in off the farm, by the exit to a barn or treatment area or at an entrance to a food preparation area. WHO guidelines suggest that handwashing using alcohol-based formulations should be 20–30 seconds, again including all surfaces of the hands.

Cleaning and disinfection of boots with appropriate disinfectants. It is advisable to use boots around the farm that are *cleanable*. Rubber boots are ideal, particularly in the winter. If you prefer canvas footwear or lace-

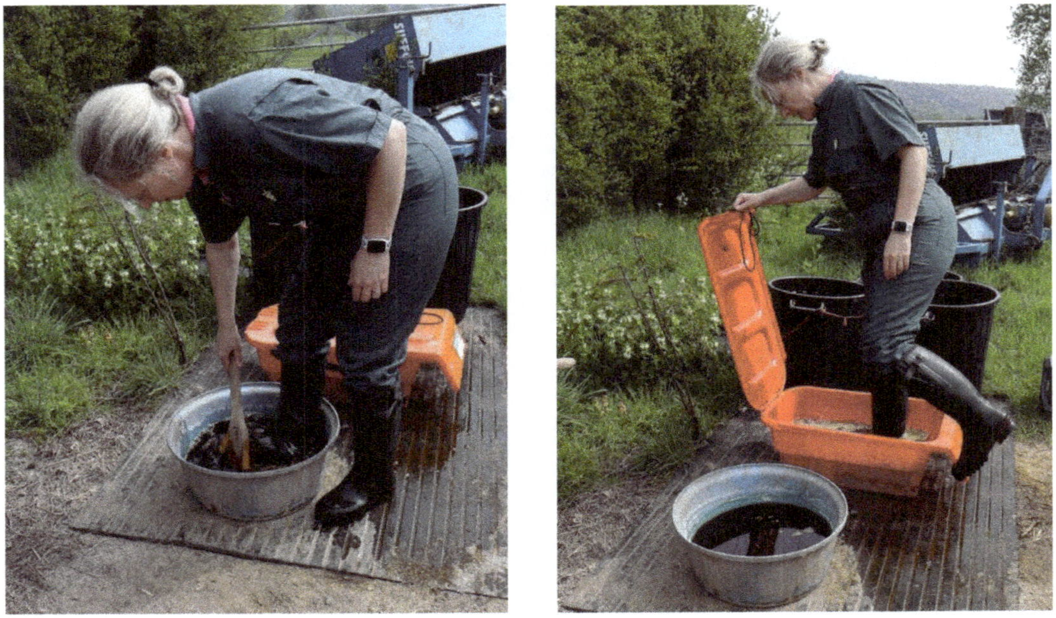

Figures 1 and 2. Using a boot dip properly. First, use a brush and water to remove all organic debris like mud and faeces (1a), then dip clean boots into disinfectant (1b).

up footwear, be aware that these are not readily cleanable. However, unless you are dealing with something infectious (and your boots are not getting covered), ensure that the treads are properly cleaned. Boot covers and disposable overalls are an alternative option used in veterinary isolation facilities.

Boot cleaning encourages good general hygiene around the farm and should be a routine part of the working day rather than only for special occasions. Good brushes and buckets should be available in locations that are easy to access and encourage their use. For example, they can be placed outside the farm office or near the farm exit for workers returning from the fields. Single-use disinfectant sachets are also a convenient option—they require no measuring and are particularly useful when travelling.

If using boot dips, make sure they are replaced daily or when dirty. Organic material soon renders disinfectant inactive. It helps to have a bucket of water or hose next to the boot dip so that the mud and faecal material can be physically removed before dipping in the disinfectant bucket. Ensure that treads are properly cleaned of all dirt, not just the visible parts of the boots. Having a lid on the boot dip prevents dilution by rainwater (*Figure 1*). Boots should always be cleaned if travelling to other farms and on return to the home farm.

Thoroughly wash clothing worn when caring for animals. A top tip is to use overalls over your everyday clothing. Sturdy overalls will protect your clothing and are more readily cleanable. Have at least two pairs so one can be washed while the other is in use.

Wear waterproof clothing when working with alpacas with mange. The clothing can be washed down if you move on to handling unaffected alpacas. This also reduces the likelihood of mites being transferred from one animal to another.

For convenience, consider using disposable overalls for some situations, such as mange cases. After handling affected animals, the overalls can just be thrown away. Ensure coats and other outerwear are also washed regularly.

Colour-coding utensils can reinforce on-farm biosecurity protocols. For example, different areas can have different feed buckets and shovels. This is particularly useful for allocating tools that cannot be used elsewhere to a sick pen area.

Disinfection requires surfaces to first be clean. All organic matter, including soil, mud, faeces, urine, milk and spit, must be removed before disinfecting fences, floors, walls, clothing or hands. Disinfection of certain organisms, such as *Cryptosporidium,* may be difficult (which can also cause disease in humans), so it is best avoided in the first place by following optimal biosecurity on the farm.

Also, note that surface type influences your ability to disinfect a surface properly. Smooth or impervious surfaces such as metal or plastic are easiest to clean. Washing with soap and water will remove 99% of microbes in these areas. On the other hand, unfinished plywood retains 15x more microbes than painted/varnished plywood, and painted/varnished plywood retains 15x more microbes than plastic.[10]

Different disinfectants are available for different applications. Check that the disinfectant you want to use is appropriate for the application and organism(s) you are concerned about. Sodium hypochlorite, or household bleach, is cheap and environmentally safe. When used at the correct concentration and with adequate contact time, it is effective against most bacterial and viral pathogens, though not against *Cryptosporidium.* FAM30 is a versatile disinfectant frequently used on farms for boot dips, wheel dips and surface cleaning, as it is effective against a wide range of pathogens, including tuberculosis.

You can check whether a particular disinfectant is approved for a specific use on this UK website: disinfectants.defra.gov.uk. This website gives the concentrations required for statutory use in the UK, though other countries may have different regulations for the concentrations used. Additionally, always ensure you follow the instructions on contact time and application temperature, as both are crucial for effective disinfection.

Control of Wild & Domestic Species

Wild and domestic species have the potential to introduce disease and may gain access to the farm. Control programmes to limit their access must be written and implemented.

Rodents. Rodents can be responsible for transmitting many pathogens, such as leptospirosis. Thus, vermin control is a vital part of farm management. You can implement this yourself or employ a specialist to do it. However, ensure these practitioners know your specific biosecurity protocols and use clean clothing and footwear. Your farm can also provide them as necessary.

Cats can also be very efficient at rodent control but must be adequately wormed. The key points in rodent control are keeping animal feed in rodent-proof areas and making areas less attractive for rodent infestation. See *Table 2*.

Insects. Flies, midges and mosquitoes can spread vector-borne diseases such as bluetongue virus, West Nile virus and *Mycoplasma haemolamae*. Keep muck heaps away from animal areas to minimise flies. Fly traps and sticky tape can be used to trap flies, and fly-zapping ultraviolet lights can be installed in animal accommodation areas.

Various fly repellents licensed for use in sheep and cattle are safe for camelids but may have variable efficacy depending on the agent and vehicle used. Those that rely on coat oils to spread the agent over the animal may be less efficient in camelids. For these, rather than relying on a single strip down the topline of the animal, it can be more effective to apply thinner strips at 2, 4, 8 and 10 o'clock positions as well. The recommended dose can be applied to the skin after parting any fleece via a syringe and artificial insemination pipette.

Domestic Pets. Cats and dogs may pose a biosecurity threat to camelids. Feral cats may be a particular risk to pregnant alpacas due to toxoplasmosis as it causes abortion. Toxoplasmosis may also result in blindness.[12] Alpacas may also become infected by eating feed or hay contaminated with cat faeces, and young cats and kittens are more likely to shed oocysts. Therefore, feral cat populations can be controlled by neutering. De-worm all domestic cats and dogs regularly. Dogs can spread *neospora*, which can lead to abortion and reduced fertility; sarcocystosis, which can cause abortion, neurological signs, and reduced growth rates; and tapeworms. To prevent these risks, restrict dogs' access to your pastures, keep them wormed, and promptly remove any dog faeces from paddocks.

Wildlife. Badgers and deer are known to carry tuberculosis in endemic areas such as the UK. Camelids are highly susceptible to TB, and if you are in an area where TB is a potential risk, badger-proof fencing should be seriously considered. There are generally two types of badger-proof fencing: electric fencing, which is cheaper but requires significant maintenance and is more practical for shorter stretches, and dug-down fencing, which is buried into the ground to prevent badgers from digging underneath. A combination of dug-down and electric fencing is recommended, and a line of electric fencing can be added to the tops of the fencing to prevent climbing. In the next chapter, we will address specific biosecurity measures for TB in more detail.

Farm Equipment. Do not share equipment between farms. Ideally, purchase new equipment that has not been in contact with other animals if it will be in contact with your own stock. It should have been properly cleaned and disinfected if it is bought second-hand. Be particularly

1	Rodents don't like being exposed, so remove all rubbish and overgrown vegetation around buildings. Keep weeds and grass short or have hard-standing around buildings.
2	Keep feed bags off the floor on pallets and away from walls.
3	Store feed in containers that can be closed and stay closed even if they fall over.
4	Sweep up any spilt food.
5	Fix dripping pipes and troughs – seal water cisterns and tanks to prevent rodent access.
6	Place rubbish in rodent-proof containers.
7	Block holes in walls to exclude rodents. Windows will require 6 mm mesh to keep mice out (e.g. feed storage areas).
8	Map out the farm and examine for evidence of rats. Include areas outside the farm boundary. • Mark out positions for permanent and clearance baits • Permanent baits: Place bait in drain pipes at the base of straw or hay stacks and check every 2 weeks. If signs of feeding are found, replenish bait and re-survey the premises • Clearance baits: check weekly and continue placing bait for a week after they've stopped being taken
9	Pay attention to health and safety. • Burn all dead rodents found and any unused bait boxes • Prevent access to bait by children and other animals • Wear gloves when handling bait or dead rodents and wash hands thoroughly • Do not re-use bait containers for any other purpose • Make sure you know the safety rules for any baits/rodenticides being used

Table 2. Rodent control protocol. Adapted from Carr, "Biosecurity beyond the boot dip", Nov 2014. [13]

cautious with any equipment used to handle faecal material.

Management of Disease

Record Keeping

Record keeping is an essential part of general farm management as well as disease management. You should keep good records of everything that goes on on your farm. Records should be accessible and logged in a way that makes them easy to use and the data easy to extract.

Computer software programmes permit all sorts of records to be kept, which should always be backed up in case of data loss. However, old-fashioned paper and pen methods have their place, as do simple spreadsheets, if you prefer. A medicines or treatment book should be kept accessible in any treatment area, and health records for individual animals should be kept up to date. Any movements on or off the farm should be recorded in a movements book so that these can easily be found if needed. In addition, farm visitors should be logged, and this can be a separate book.

Keep records of the dates on which various husbandry procedures are performed, such as shearing, toe-nail trimming, tooth trimming and faecal checks. These records can be useful for evaluating growth rates, monitoring reproductive performance, tracking body condition or weight, and identifying recurring problems. When you keep records of these characteristics, it may be possible to spot positive or negative trends that you can respond to if needed. For example, if all animals are losing weight in a group, you may want to evaluate your nutritional plan or collect some faecal samples to assess parasite loads. If individual animals are identified as having lost weight, different possibilities may need to be considered.

Protocols for Dealing With Sick Animals

Isolation

When sick animals are present, they should be isolated from the rest of the herd while diagnostics are performed. Until the nature of a condition is confirmed, always assume that it is infectious and potentially transmissible to other animals. This will allow you to adjust biosecurity measures as needed.

Depending on the problem, affected individuals may need to be isolated in a small pen, stall or paddock. Remember that if sick animals have access to pasture areas, these areas are not cleanable. For camelids, complete isolation is highly stressful and can worsen their condition – they may even refuse to eat, preferring to starve rather than be alone! Therefore, when you need to isolate a camelid, this will normally be with a buddy of some sort because we need to minimise stress.

For dams and crias, the company of either the cria or her dam is usually sufficient and is clearly necessary. Where the sick animal isn't part of a mother and cria pair, it may be a related animal or friend. However, if you are concerned about infectiousness, avoid pregnant females or crias who are likely to be more susceptible. Animals can be penned singly if they can still see other animals to socialise. Whether or not you allow them to interact directly over a fenceline depends on the potential transmissibility of the disease in question.

Sick Pens

You should always have pens available and ready for sick animals. These should be in a well-ventilated area, preferably on cleanable flooring such as concrete or rubber matting. They can be stables, fixed wall structures or temporary stalls made from hurdles. The latter is better because the hurdles can be periodically disassembled, any bedding removed and the entire area properly cleaned. They can also be erected anywhere.

- Sick pens should always be thoroughly cleaned and disinfected between individual sick animals. This includes floors and walls (or fencing/hurdles, if applicable).
- Use dedicated pens for newborn crias if they are brought into a stall to facilitate nursing or because they are weak and need additional care. These should be clean and freshly-bedded with straw for warmth.
- Depending on the type of problem being experienced, consider the possibility of transmission to other animals. Isolation of the affected individual is pointless if its caregivers continue to move freely from treating this sick animal to other areas of the farm where there are healthy animals. Dedicated protective clothing may be required for treating the sick animal, along with a boot dip outside the stall (or dedicated boots or boot covers). Keep a selection of materials, such as gloves, needles, syringes and medications, in a separate, cleanable container at the stall side.
    - An example is tracking organisms that cause neonatal diarrhoea (e.g., *Cryptosporidia* and Rotavirus) via footwear from a pen splattered with diarrhoea to an area with healthy crias and their dams.
    - Another example is animals that are diseased but not normally ill, such as those with mange. Mange mites (particularly *Sarcoptes*) are very contagious. Transmission of mites from animal to animal is relatively easy via clothing and entirely avoidable.

Written Protocols for Dealing with Sick Animals

Written protocols are there so that you don't forget anything! They should be clear and ensure that everyone follows the same rules. These protocols should outline the steps to take when an animal is found unwell or affected by a specific disease, where the animal should be moved, how the area should be prepared, and what needs to be ready (e.g. foot dips, equipment) for different issues. They should also include contact details for the veterinarian and specify any signage needed to warn others.

Managing a sick animal often involves numerous daily tasks. A written checklist with boxes to tick for each completed task ensures nothing is overlooked. This is even more important when multiple people are involved in caring for these animals. I have shown an example treatment sheet in Figure

3. The supplementary PDF that accompanies this book can be downloaded.

Deaths

If an animal dies, remove it from the paddock or barn as soon as possible and move it to a site where other animals do not have access. This should be close to the perimeter fence but not visible to passers-by. You should arrange for the animal to undergo a post-mortem examination at a pathology facility, veterinary surgery or on your farm – I listed these in order of preference. A pathology centre is preferred, although it may take more effort on your part because there are better facilities there that will enable a more complete examination. For example, the tools available will permit a complete evaluation of the brain and central nervous system, which is difficult for vets working in practice to achieve. In addition, pathologists are skilled in performing postmortem evaluations and may be able to interpret findings with greater accuracy. It is always important to know why an animal died in case there is a disease risk to other members of the herd. Any deaths should be recorded and the cause of death noted, if known. If a postmortem examination is done on the farm or isn't done at all, arrange for disposal of the carcass as soon as possible.

Different countries and regions may have different regulations for disposing of dead animals, so familiarise yourself with those applicable in your area.

FARM CARE TREATMENTS SHEET

Animal Name/ID: ______________________________ Farm: ___________________________________

Gender: _____ Age: _______ DOB: ____________

[List treatments along with route of administration and volume: then place a circle at each time the medication should be administered. Owners to initial or tick the circle when complete.]

DATE	TREATMENT	Route	VOL (ml)	08	10	12	14	16	18	20	22	00	02	04	06

Figure 3. This is an example of a treatment sheet that can be used when caring for sick animals on a farm. (A downloadable version is available on the PDF accompanying this book.)

Key Takeaways

In this chapter, we have discussed the diseases you need to be concerned about and potential sources of biosecurity threats. Some diseases will not be prevalent in your country, but others may be and are common to all locations where camelids are kept. Disease-specific considerations may also apply to your biosecurity preparations. For these, perform your own risk assessment, consider where the threats may come from, and develop a plan suitable for ameliorating the risk.

Some key takeaways from this chapter:

- A great deal of your disease preparedness involves ensuring the health of your herd and giving your animals the best chance to resist any disease that comes their way.
- There are practical management steps that you can take to reduce transmission of any disease within the animals of your own herd and to manage wild and domestic species that may introduce problems.
- Good record-keeping is essential for tracking any problems.
- Preparations can be made to manage any sick animals on the farm.

In the next chapter, we will discuss in more detail how to manage and prevent incursions from outside your biosecurity barrier.

8

Biosecurity (Part 2): Keeping Disease *Off* the Farm!

"Awareness is the greatest agent for change."
– Eckart Tolle

"External Biosecurity" relates to the protocols in place to prevent disease from acquiring access to a particular farm from outside. Outside of your farm, you can have very little influence over what happens, and it must be assumed that all animals off your farm carry a risk of disease, whether or not they actually have a disease. It must also be assumed that the environments they may encounter potentially carry infection risk. This includes exposure to diseases brought in by new animals or animals returning from shows or breeding activities and minimising the risk of disease spread among newly introduced animals. We will, therefore, focus on this particular aspect of biosecurity.

Figure 1 shows the potential pathways for disease transmission that should be considered when planning your biosecurity for *your* farm. On an "open" farm, animals may move between your herd and others through sales, purchases or breeding activities, either by visiting other herds or hosting animals from elsewhere. Your animals may also come into contact with animals from other herds at shows and events. At any of these contact points, there is the potential for disease transmission from an animal carrying the disease, the vehicle transporting it or fomites (inanimate objects that may carry infection, such as utensils). In addition, the disease may enter your herd via the farm boundaries. For example, by contact with neighbouring livestock or roaming wildlife, windborne viruses or vector-borne pathogens.

Different levels of biosecurity are used on livestock farms to prevent disease transmission from outside (*Figure 2*). The high-health pig and poultry units are at the top of the biosecurity pyramid. These units have high stocking densities and a high stock turnover rate. They also have highly host-adapted pathogens that thrive in these units and cause devastating disease outbreaks, causing massive morbidity and mortality rates.

One example of these diseases is the porcine epidemic diarrhoea virus (PEDV). This virus spreads quickly among pigs,

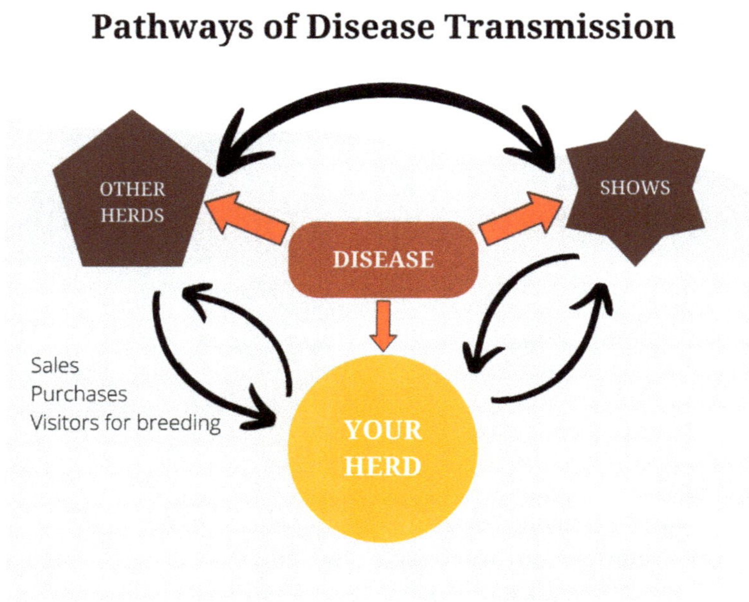

Figure 1. The pathways for disease transmission between herds.

causing watery diarrhoea and dehydration. With severe strains, the virus will kill 30–100% of young piglets. Clearly, the impact of having poor biosecurity on a pig farm could be severe, and biosecurity protocols are needed to reduce the risks of this sort of virus taking hold on the farm. In high-health units, vehicles are not permitted beyond a fenced boundary, strict protocols are enforced for moving pigs off the unit, and staff and visitors are required to shower in and out. Additionally, visitors such as veterinarians moving between units must observe a three-day interval between visits to sites housing other pigs.

The next level of biosecurity on the pyramid is the "closed" herd. In a closed herd, no stock is brought in. The farm uses its own breeding males or artificial breeding techniques such as artificial insemination (AI) and embryo transfer (ET) with frozen embryos. You may find closed dairy, beef, pig and sheep farms. Some camelid herds could be closed if they used their own males exclusively, but this would prevent them from offering stud services. In a small industry, running a closed herd is a difficult prospect. The difficulty for camelid herds is the lack of advanced reproductive techniques allowing AI or ET. Camelid semen is difficult to freeze, and even if freezing was effective, its low volume and concentration mean a single ejaculate provides only one or two AI doses. While ET works well with fresh embryos, there is no commercial trade in frozen embryos due to the difficulty of freezing embryos that can survive the freezing and thawing process.

The "open" herds are most similar to camelid herds, where animals may be

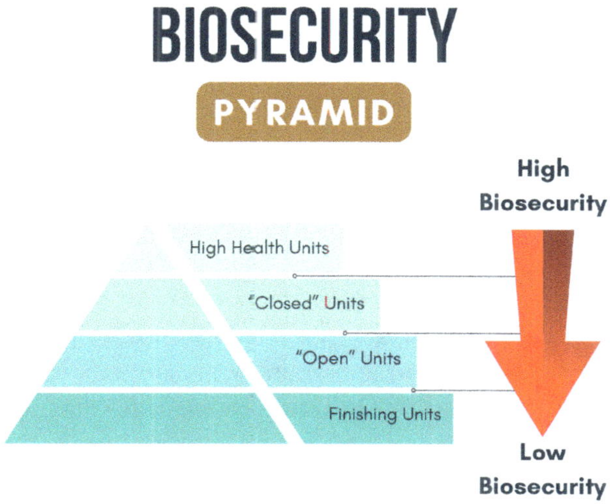

Figure 2. The biosecurity pyramid shows the relative level of biosecurity practised within each level.

brought in, and there is contact with other herds through purchases and other activities, including breeding. In the fourth category of biosecurity, which has the most potential risk, animals are brought in from multiple sources and mixed. There may also be animals added or removed over time. This is a typical set-up for finisher cattle units and beef feedlots. Some camelid holdings may fit this description, particularly where animals are bought and sold regularly and quarantine is not practised. This scenario is most common for dealers who collect animals from multiple farms for export. Such a system creates a melting pot of potential diseases, as animals without obvious signs of illness may carry infections that become apparent due to the stress of transportation and social mixing, leading to the spread of disease.

Biosecurity Recommendations

The following six practices for external biosecurity on alpaca and llama farms regarding planned contacts with other camelids and people are suggested.

1. **Avoid sick animals.** Avoid introducing animals that do not appear healthy to the rest of the herd. This seems obvious, but it is not uncommon for well-meaning owners to take on "rescue" animals and find that they've taken on more than they've bargained for. It's okay to help out, but you must be aware of what you may find. Take appropriate precautions and be prepared to take extra measures to ensure that the animals are healthy and won't cause problems for the rest of your herd. Sometimes, rescue animals require rescuing because they've not

While I was a vet student, I "saw practice" at a local vet practice that did a lot of pig work. This included visiting the high-health pig units for routine work such as blood testing. On arrival at the units, we would have to strip off and pass through a shower to the "clean" side, where there would be clean clothes to use while in the unit. We were required to wash our hair on the way in and out of the unit, but there were no brushes, hair driers or scrunchies on the other side to tie up long hair! I have always had long enough hair that I would look like a scarecrow without those luxuries! Fortunately, I usually found an elastic band somewhere on the other side. The main issue was that the clothing on the other side wasn't really designed for female visitors. There would be long johns, a long-sleeved t-shirt and a pair of overalls to wear. Plus, a selection of rubber boots that were at least two sizes too large to clop around in. Underwear was just not an option! I literally cannot imagine having to do this now. I've never been particularly poorly endowed in the mammary department, and you can imagine the embarrassment of wandering around a pig farm without even a little support as a female vet student in her early twenties!

been cared for properly, either because of a lack of will, time, financial resources or illness. They may also come without medical histories. Poor care is more likely to result in disease issues, such as internal and external parasitism, or animals in poor body condition experiencing mineral deficiencies and being more vulnerable to disease due to stress-induced immunosuppression.

If you are buying animals from an outside source or feel obliged to take on any rescue animals, always have a thorough veterinary health examination performed. You must also follow the isolation and testing protocols outlined below. *Never* introduce these animals directly into your own herd - always follow quarantine measures!

Be particularly careful to look over any new acquisitions for evidence of mange. Where it exists, it would be recommended to have the animal treated to your satisfaction prior to collecting it. Proper treatment for mange requires a lot of work, and you don't want to buy extra work. If you are taking on rescue animals with mange, be aware that this will consume a lot of your time to treat it. These animals must be kept isolated and treated thoroughly before introduction to the home herd to prevent the spread of the disease.

2. **Inquire about the health status of the farm.** Know the disease status of any herd from which animals are being bought or where animals are being temporarily housed. Ask about the current health status of the farm as well as any past issues with diseases, such as gastrointestinal problems (including diarrhoea or parasites), respiratory disease, abortion, ill-thrift or failure of passive transfer. Knowing that a particular farm had a problem with a disease or health is not necessarily something to worry about. Knowing that

the problem was identified, diagnosed and treated correctly, with prevention measures employed afterwards, should be reassuring. It shows honesty and that the farm has good health control practices and potentially good biosecurity. I would be a little more wary of a seller who insists they've never had any problems. Do they even know what to look for? A farm with perfect husbandry and animals in top condition will still have *some* issues to deal with.

For those in countries where bovine tuberculosis can be a concern, ask what sort of contact a herd has with other herds (usually for breedings) and how they manage those contacts to minimise disease transmission. Also, inquire about what biosecurity measures are being used to prevent TB and if these include perimeter fencing. These questions become especially relevant when you know if the area you are buying from has a local problem with TB. You can easily check the local TB situation in the UK by looking at the interactive bovine TB map at ibtb.co.uk. This map shows the location of all active TB breakdowns in cattle herds in the UK, the date the breakdown started and, if relevant, when restrictions were lifted. It does not show affected camelid herds. Camelid herds are not required to be tested for TB, but they may take part in voluntary surveillance testing for TB in their herd. A history of whole-herd testing with negative results provides greater confidence that purchasing an animal from that herd is less likely to result in disease transmission or subsequent TB-related tracings.

3. **Insist on pre-movement testing.** Ideally, the testing and treatment for any illnesses are done before the animal arrives. This is to show that they are at least as healthy as the farm's own animals, provided that optimal health screening and disease prevention measures are in place for the existing herd. Demanding to test for incoming animals is pointless if the home herd is not healthy to begin with!

Veterinary health examinations should be performed within days of animal movement to reassure you that you're not bringing an obviously unhealthy animal to your herd. When engaging a vet for this service, you should be clear about what you wish to check. You are entitled to choose your own vet if you wish. For breeding soundness, you should arrange a separate test, usually done by a vet experienced in camelid reproductive techniques. Preferably, you schedule these tests before purchase or at least before taking the animal onto your property. If you've already had the animal on your property for some time, the cause of any infertility may arguably have resulted from an event on your own farm.

It should be noted that a veterinary health certificate only shows that the animal appeared healthy *at the time of the examination* and does not certify it as free from disease. It is also important to understand that the stress of moving animals between farms, attending shows, or experiencing changes in environmental conditions or social status can suppress the immune system. This suppression can make a previously healthy animal more susceptible to developing disease or cause it to begin excreting a virus, bacterium or parasite. For example, an animal can have a negative faecal evaluation for parasites before transportation and then, several weeks later, find that the same animal has a clinically significant parasite burden. Quarantine deworming can help minimise this problem.

Pre-movement testing might include the following tests, but other tests might be indicated in your country:

- Blood testing for BVD. The best test to request for this is one that tests for the presence of the antigen itself (the virus) rather than antibody testing, which merely tells you that an alpaca has been exposed and doesn't tell you whether it is infected. PCR testing is the best and most economical way to test for BVD as it detects the actual virus in the animal, confirms active infection and can be done as pooled testing. This means

It is standard practice in the equine industry to perform a pre-purchase examination (PPE) when you're interested in buying a horse. The purpose of the examination is to confirm that the horse is suited to the purpose for which you are buying it. The testing can be fairly basic for a child's pony or it can include x-rays of all feet and the hocks for horses required for competition.

The PPE is always done by someone other than the horse's own vet to remove a potential conflict of interest. In the camelid industry, many PPEs are done by the seller's own vet. This may be on the grounds of practicality if there are no other vets nearby, but the seller can influence the vet if it is not in the buyer's best interests. It is perfectly normal to request a vet of your choice to do the examination if you wish. A refusal to allow this should be viewed as questionable.

I was once asked to examine a group of alpacas by a potential buyer. We discussed what they wanted, but the buyer later called back to tell me that the seller would not permit me to do the examinations and insisted they were very confident in their own vet. I suggested that that sounded suspicious, but they were keen to progress the purchase. A few months later, the buyer had an alpaca with respiratory problems that they wanted my help with. Unfortunately, it was one of the purchased alpacas and was diagnosed with bovine TB traced back to the area that these alpacas had come from. During a discussion with them later, the owner commented that they had all been in poor condition when they first arrived. Although I do not know the motivation for refusing my attendance on the farm, it seems that the seller thought I might be more likely to ask questions and spot problems on the farm that might have prevented the sale.

you batch serum from up to 10 blood samples and test them together in one test rather than 10. If the pooled test is positive, all samples will then be tested individually. However, for screening purposes, the high sensitivity of the test helps keep costs down. On the other hand, the cheaper antigen ELISA tests are not accurate. They are prone to false positive test results in camelids due to high background reactions.[1] If you want to test camelids for antibodies, request a serum neutralisation test.

- Faecal testing. If required, *appropriate* treatment for endoparasites should be performed before arrival, and animals should be retested before release onto your pasture. You can retest usually 10-14 days after dosing, and you want animals to have zero egg counts before release onto your pasture. It is better to make sure that any animals about to move onto the farm are treated just before the move while off grazing so that they are not re-infected following treatment. They will then drop any worms onto the ground at the source rather than at your premises. You can carry this out on your own farm if you prefer to be responsible. It is more important to check that the new arrivals have a zero egg count before moving on to your grazing than to test them before dosing. However, if you do both, you can also see if there is any resistance to anthelmintics in the incoming animals by looking at pre- and post-treatment egg counts. However, the tests should be completed at the same lab for consistency. See below for a "quarantine deworming strategy."
- Skin scrapes on animals exhibiting any skin lesions to check for mites. No farm without an obvious mange problem should accept a new animal with active lesions.
- TB testing. This test is always a requirement for pre-export testing. In the UK, where there is a serious bovine TB problem in cattle spilling over into camelids, pre-movement TB testing is a potentially useful tool, and serological testing gives greater sensitivity over traditional skin tests. Ideally, the TB test should be carried out within 30 days of the animal movement. A test is only valid at the time of testing, so the closer it is done to movement, the better. However, this must be balanced with the time it takes to receive test results. Export testing requirements change over time and vary depending on where the export originates and ends up, so it is best to check the current regulations for the areas you wish to export to and from.
- Skin testing is fairly well recognised as having poor sensitivity when used alone.[2] [3] Serological testing has much better sensitivity but will still fail to detect around a third of potentially infected individual animals.[4] Boosting the antibody response by skin testing prior to blood testing is recommended to improve the sensitivity of detection, but it adds to the cost.[5] This effect was demonstrated in a large outbreak of bovine TB in alpacas in Spain. Serology

alone is the minimum suggested for pre-movement testing for domestic alpaca movements. But knowing that a herd has an annual herd-level negative TB test will provide greater certainty that a negative test is still likely to be negative at pre-movement testing. In my opinion, trusting a stand-alone test that can incorrectly diagnose an animal as healthy when actually infected a third of the time is a little risky. Post-movement testing can be done in addition to pre-movement testing 42–90 days after arrival. Animals that tested negative at a pre-movement test could become positive over time, especially due to movement stress. A repeated test can provide further confidence. If the animal has remained in quarantine from the main herd when it is post-movement tested, you will not have put your herd at risk if it tests positive.

4. **Isolate and quarantine new animals.** Ideally, all new animals brought to a farm should be isolated and quarantined before introducing them into the herd. This includes animals that have been to shows or have been off-farm for breeding purposes since they have been commingling with other animals. If solitary animals are being introduced, placing one or two of your own animals in the quarantine area may be advisable to reduce separation stress. These animals are treated as isolated like the animals just arriving on the farm. Consider what type of animal would be appropriate to use for this purpose, as they should be animals that are less likely to succumb to any diseases they might carry. Or if they do, it wouldn't be as disastrous if you were to lose that animal. Less valuable animals, such as geldings, could be chosen for this purpose, but avoid using pregnant or lactating females. Pregnant animals are more at risk for problems associated with viral transmission that may result in birth defects or abortion. Young animals are also unsuitable as their immunity is lower.

   The recommended minimum quarantine period is 6 weeks, but 8 weeks would be preferred. Six weeks will allow any previously prepatent *Eimeria macusaniensis* to be detected in faecal tests at the end of the quarantine period. The prepatent period for *E macusaniensis* is approximately 34 days.[6] Other parasites and viruses are likely to be apparent on faecal tests or due to clinical disease within this period; however, this might not be the case for Johnes, BVD, or TB.

   Consider post-movement testing for TB, as this will further reduce the risk that you may introduce TB into the rest of the herd from a purchased animal. This should be done between 42 and 90 days after arrival. Animals should remain in quarantine until the test results are known.

   Operate an all-in, all-out policy such that all animals housed in the quarantine area enter and leave quarantine at the same time. The quarantine period commences on the date the last animal entered. Do not have animals moving in and out of the quarantine area on an individual basis.

The location of your quarantine site should be physically separate from the main herd as well as its handling facilities and housing. This should be several hundred yards away, if possible, and positioned to be downwind from the main herd. At the very least, there should be a double fence line between the groups to prevent direct contact. This may be unrealistic for most situations, but would be desired for a quarantine area for imported animals. For regular animal movements such as a show group, these animals should be kept together and separated from the main herd for the duration of the show season. Ideally, a separate paddock area should be allocated to them and separated from the home herd by a double fence providing at least a 3-metre separation. On larger facilities with more animals and staff, allocate different staff to work with the quarantine group and do not have the same staff return to the main herd. If this is not possible, tend to the main herd *before* tending to the quarantine group.

Wear clothing and footwear dedicated to the quarantine group when tending to this group. These must be washable. Rubber boots are perfect because they can be properly cleaned and disinfected, while suede or fabric work boots are not. Colour coding of overalls is an obvious and visible reminder. Have separate utensils for the quarantine area – shovels, forks, brushes, buckets, etc. These can be colour-coded for the quarantine area.

Animals in quarantine should be monitored at least once daily. Monitor attitude, appetite, water consumption, urination and defecation, as well as coughing, discharge from the eyes or nose, diarrhoea, etc. Animals showing any signs of disease should be further separated from the rest of the quarantined animals and evaluated by a vet.

With regard to parasite control in newly purchased animals, it would be best to eliminate all parasites in newcomers for the following reasons. Firstly, it will prevent any subclinical worm burdens from becoming clinical due to the immunosuppressive effects of stress; secondly, it will prevent the introduction of drug-resistant parasites. A suggested protocol is the following:

- Have the alpacas wormed with at least two different wormers (and Baycox) a few days before leaving the herd of origin. My current suggestion is to use Cydectin oral drench at 2x label sheep dose and a choice of fenbendazole (e.g. Panacur) at 4x label dose or levamisole (8 mg/kg oral drench). Monepantel may also be selected for this purpose but needs to be used at 3x the label sheep dose. Speak to your veterinarian for their recommendations, availability and suitability in your area. You could also do this worming on arrival at your herd if you prefer to be in command of this yourself, but you must also be able to do the following steps.
- Keep the new arrivals on hard standing (preferably concrete) until

a faecal can be checked 10–14 days post-treatment. Remove faeces daily to prevent eggs from hatching out of deposited faeces.

- Confirm zero egg count in new arrivals (10–14 days post-dosing) before releasing onto previously grazed pasture. Use a sensitive test to be more certain of your zero-egg count. Ideally, keep new arrivals quarantined from the existing herd for 60 days, as above. Recheck a faecal at the end of quarantine and before introducing the animal to the main herd.

5. **Employ protocols for natural breeding.** At the current time, most alpaca and llama breedings are carried out as natural matings. There is a small amount of embryo transfer being done on freshly collected embryos, but artificial insemination has yet to be well-established for routine use. This means that if owners of females want access to stud males on other farms, contact is required between animals from different breeding herds. Contact between animals does constitute a biosecurity risk and should be managed to minimise that risk. One of the greatest risks of natural breeding behaviour in camelids is spitting. This is because food particles from the first stomach are aerosolised with expelled air from the lungs. In TB endemic zones, since camelids are prone to having "open" TB lesions in the lungs with open abscesses communicating with the airways, spitting constitutes a potential risk for transmission. Therefore, wherever possible, it would be ideal to spit off females at the farm of origin prior to transport to ensure that females are not going to spit at the male.

   The Table 1 on page 135 contains some guidelines for managing disease transmission risk during breeding.

6. **Minimise exposure of the herd to human visitors**. As Part 1 of Chapter 6 describes, human visitors can unintentionally transmit disease to the animals on your farm. It might be that the only visitors to your farm are family and friends or other camelid owners, or you may operate a tourism business from your farm and offer alpaca walking or experiences, or have accommodation on site for visits. Regardless of why they are visiting, it is crucial to make sure that they are aware of your biosecurity arrangements. It may be appropriate to brief them on these prior to their visit so that they can ensure that they bring the correct kit with them. People might not want to dip their suede brogues into a bucket of disinfectant on arrival!

   When visitors come to your farm, it may be appropriate to question them before allowing them access to animal areas about where they have come from, about exposure to any other livestock and to make sure that they come to the farm wearing clean clothes and boots. Don't forget to make provision for vehicles to try to avoid vehicles crossing areas where animals graze. Depending on what your visitors are

Type of Farm	Interaction	Recommended Biosecurity Precautions
Stud Farms	Females travel to the male for breeding; high numbers of animal movements.	Isolated breeding pens away from the resident herd
		Concrete floor surface to enable cleaning/ disinfection
		Spit masks for females, which is the responsibility of the female's owner and must be clean. Males can use spit masks, too, if desired. Note that a spit mask with large holes in it will not prevent disease transmission. All it will do will prevent the spattering of C1 material around the breeding area.
		Minimise time spent hanging around in the breeding pen with males. Transfer the male to the farm, or transfer the female when finished to the trailer and go.
Smaller Farms	Males are travelling to outside farms; low numbers of animal movements	Isolated breeding pen to be provided for stud services, preferably outside the main field. If it is not possible to do this, then a pen should be created just inside the entrance so males don't have to cross the field. Other animals must be in another field, or a double 3-metre boundary must be present to prevent fence line contact and spitting.
		Foot dip or cleaning of male's feet on and off the farm
		Spit mask for females (and males) – the responsibility of the female's owner
		Ensure the pen floor surface is clean from faecal contamination.
Agistment	Females (usually) stay on the breeding farm until pregnant. Best avoided if possible.	Try to keep non-resident animals isolated from residents and use separate breeding areas.
		Perform risk assessment based on knowledge of herd locations and practices.
		Use of foot dips for general biosecurity, and spit masks as above.

Table 1. This table contains some guidelines for managing disease transmission during breeding.

doing, you may wish to provide visitors with overalls and either rubber boots or over-boots or shoes kept on the farm for this purpose. Also, make sure that hand-washing facilities are available and that they are used.

Consider providing dedicated protective clothing and boots for the vet on the farm, particularly if they visit frequently. Vets visit many different farms in a single day, and this simple measure could be very useful in limiting potential transmission.

One potential measure to consider is having a visitors' book. This can serve multiple purposes. If you ever need to track who is visiting the farm, you have an easy record to view any time you wish. You might also ask them to include a contact phone number. Visitors should be briefed regarding farm biosecurity arrangements upon arrival. When they sign the visitor's book, this can also be used to confirm that they have been briefed and know what is required of them.

Additional Biosecurity Recommendations for TB

In the UK, we are unfortunate to have had a severe problem with bovine tuberculosis that has worsened over the first 20 years of the 21st century. Bovine TB can be spread via the movement of infected cattle and also infected wildlife, notably badgers and deer in the UK. Camelids are extremely susceptible to bovine TB when exposed, and some will develop clinical signs of weight loss and respiratory problems, which ultimately result in death (*Figures 3 and 4*).

Other outcomes of infection are that they effectively clear the disease from their bodies, or they might be able to contain the infection but not eliminate it completely. This may be in visible lesions in their organs or at a cellular level. TB is a complex disease that has some challenges in terms of diagnostics. It is best to avoid it entirely, and the optimum way to do that is to have excellent biosecurity. This should be individualised to your own farm, so if you are not in an area where TB is endemic, you might not need badger or deer-proof fencing.

Badger-proof and Deer-proof Fencing

If you live in an area with a moderate to high risk of TB, I strongly recommend installing badger-proof fencing and, if necessary, deer-proof fencing. This will help you control the introduction of TB through wildlife. Badger-proof fencing needs high-tensile wires specifically for badgers, with the mesh having a vertical spacing of no larger than 8 cm. The fencing either needs to be continued into the ground or electric fencing added outside of the fence.

- For dug-down fencing, at least 45 cm of the fence must be dug into the ground, with the buried section extending in the direction from which a badger would approach. The height must be at least 1 metre. To be extra safe, add a single electric wire at the top of the fence outside to stop badgers from climbing over it.
- For electric fencing, this uses four strands of electric wire at heights of 10, 15, 20 and 30 cm from the ground.

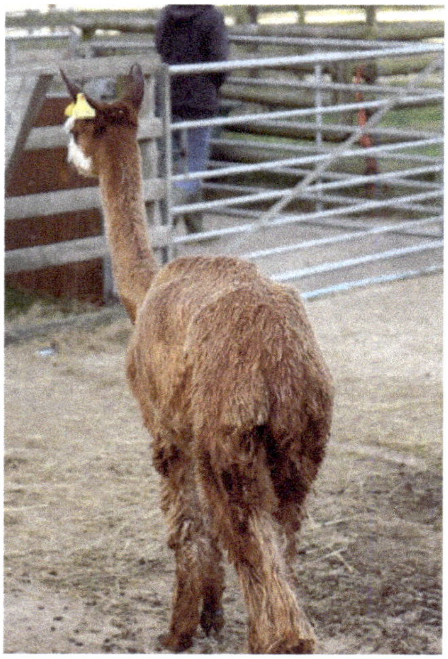

Figure 3. Alpaca with clinical tuberculosis exhibiting severe weight loss.

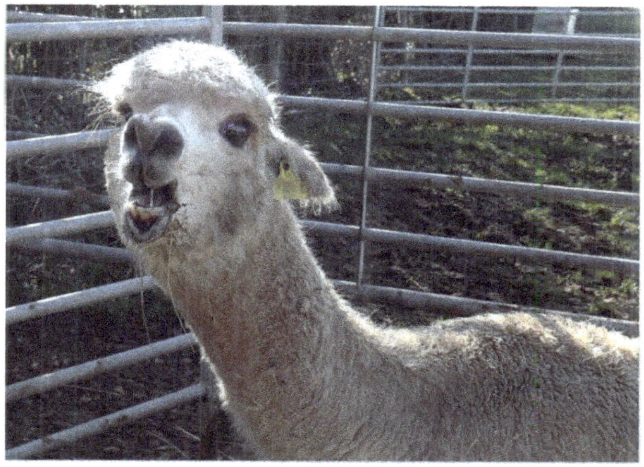

Figure 4. Alpaca with clinical tuberculosis in respiratory distress shortly before euthanasia.

This can be used alone to deter badgers from entering certain farm areas, such as around hay and feed storage areas. Or it can be used outside of paddock fencing. However, it is important to remember that grass or weeds below the electric fencing are kept down by strimming or using a weedkiller because any vegetation will cause the electricity to short out or reduce the voltage transmitted. Therefore, this type of fencing requires quite a lot of maintenance. It is easier to use for shorter distances.

- It's important to consider farm gates as a point of access. Gaps greater than 7.5 cm below gates should be avoided, as this will allow badgers to gain access. Concrete should also be placed under the gates to prevent them from digging under. Metal sheeting can be added to existing gates to badger-proof them.
- Deer are thought to have less of a transmission risk than badgers. However, if you wish to exclude deer, fencing must be at least 8 ft.

Boundary Buffer Zones

You should install double fencing or use an equivalent boundary, such as a large hedgerow, that provides a gap of at least 3 m between animals in your fields and any neighbouring livestock. This prevents nose-to-nose contact and the direct transmission of TB and other infectious diseases over the boundary.

Manage Feed and Water Access

If you don't have badger-proof fencing, you need to restrict badger access to your feed store areas and troughs. Avoid putting feed onto the ground on pasture, and clean up any spilt feed. Make sure that any leftover feed is removed. It's a good idea to turn troughs over after use to prevent rodents from accessing them and prevent the troughs from filling with rainwater.

It has been shown that badgers can access troughs that are 115 cm high, but 95 cm height restricts most climbing badgers. Feed and water troughs on cattle farms should be raised as high as possible to minimise this. They should also not be placed next to a structure that allows them to climb up and gain access to the trough. For most camelids, this may be too high, so badger-proof fencing may be a better idea to prevent access in the first place.

Avoid Introducing Infected Animals

Don't buy animals that appear unhealthy. Be particularly cautious of underweight animals and/or have increased respiratory rates.

The ibtb.com website allows you to check for local TB breakdowns in cattle herds in the UK. This allows you to determine the amount of TB circulating in an area where you wish to buy alpacas.

Find out what biosecurity protocols are in place on the farm that you wish to buy animals from, and also precisely what they do to monitor for TB in the herd, bearing in mind the relative risk from TB in their area. If a herd is doing routine whole-herd annual testing for TB with negative results and has appropriate biosecurity precautions in place to minimise TB incursion, you can feel quite confident that you will not be buying TB into your herd.

However, you should also consider requesting pre-movement TB testing for the animals you wish to purchase and post-movement testing within quarantine. Do *not* introduce new purchases directly into the main herd. Receive negative test results from post-movement testing before mixing.

Specific Guidelines for Breeding Activities

It is difficult to avoid contact with other herds for breeding activities, either because of selling stud services or needing to use them. Natural breeding requires contact between animals and is, therefore, a risk for disease transmission, particularly if females are spitting. Several precautions can be taken to minimise the risk:

- Perform spit-offs or behaviour tests at home. This reduces the possibility of the stud male being spat at. Consider having your own males on the farm to enable this, because some stud farms will not do spit-offs for you due to the risk to their own males.
- Use spit masks that will stop the aerosolised spread of infectious agents. Commercially available spit masks will only block green gunge, not infectious particles. You can use medical face masks inside spit masks to reduce this transmission.
- Breed in areas away from the main herd, whether the female visits the stud farm or the male travels to the female. The floor surface should ideally be concrete to facilitate cleaning and disinfection.
- No fenceline contact with other animals from the herd.
- Minimise contact time between the

male and female. Remove the visiting male or female from the pen as soon as breeding has finished and remove them to the transportation ready for travel.

Colostrum and Plasma

Using fresh/frozen colostrum and plasma carries a risk of disease transmission, such as TB, Johnes and BVD. So, if you are sourcing fresh colostrum from local cattle or goat farms, ensure that the source is free of these diseases, or consider using a freeze-dried colostrum substitute (such as Immucol Platinum, which you can find in the product section of ukalpacavet.com)

Plasma should be prepared from your own animals in your own herd. Plasma from another herd carries the risk of transmission of TB.

Key Takeaways

Biosecurity can be a scary topic when you consider the potential diseases, their sources, and the steps needed to prevent problems. Remember that not all the risks and diseases will be relevant to you, and you don't have to do everything! However, it's important to at least think about all the potential risks for your own herd and decide what level of risk you are willing to accept. A consideration of the costs will also be required.

Some key takeaways from this chapter:

- Develop a farm-specific strategy and ensure that everyone working on the farm follows it and visitors respect it.
- Research the disease risks in your area to help you understand the potential problems that you may face.
- Be aware of the risks of disease incursion and understand what risks you are prepared to accept and those you are not. Some decisions will involve weighing cost versus benefit, which is okay as long as you understand the implications of not following a particular recommendation.
- Never introduce obviously unhealthy animals into your herd or manage these animals separately in quarantine while their health problems are addressed.
- If you are prepared, in the event of a disease outbreak, you can feel reassured that you did everything possible to prevent it. You will also know how to minimise the outbreak's effects on the herd.

In the following chapters, we move on to the health problems that your animals might experience. We discuss how you can identify them, potentially prevent them from occurring in the first place and what you should do when they occur.

9

Gastrointestinal Parasites

South American camelids are generally affected by the same types of gastrointestinal parasites as sheep, cattle, and goats, including worms, protozoa, and flukes. They share the same worm populations, which has implications when co-grazing with these species. They have their own species-specific coccidia and are susceptible to both the small and large types of liver fluke that affect ruminants.

Compared to other species, there has been relatively little research done regarding the gastrointestinal parasites affecting camelids, particularly those affecting camelids outside of South America. However, the life cycles of South American nematodes that have been studied are like those found in ruminants elsewhere. It has not been shown definitively that camelids experience a periparturient reduction in immunity that results in a "rise" in faecal egg counts around the time of parturition, although this is certainly likely. We've observed increases in worm egg counts and coccidia burdens due to stress as a consistent feature. This can be due to stress that occurs for camelids subjected to weather changes, animal movements and hierarchical disruption both within and between herds, as well as from stress on the immune system that results from concurrent disease.

The Pareto Principle, also known as the 80/20 rule, states that 80% of outcomes come from 20% of causes. This Principle can be seen in action in gastrointestinal parasitism in all livestock as well as camelids where it is often stated that 20% of the animals in the herd carry 80% of the problems. This is an important phenomenon to consider in the control of parasites. At the turn of the century, it was commonplace to worm all animals in a herd or flock at certain intervals – so-called "blanket worming". Unfortunately, this has led to the emergence of resistant worms in our populations. We have since developed a far greater understanding of this concern and how to better manage parasites. Identifying 20% of animals that require treatment is a critical feature of how we deploy parasite control strategies, covered in the next chapter.

In this chapter, we will examine each parasite group individually, discussing the clinical syndromes that may occur when your camelids are affected and providing a breakdown by parasite species.

Worms

The worm populations affecting camelids include the following groups:

1. Nematodes, which is divided into three types:
   a. Roundworms
      i. Strongyles, also known as trichostrongyles
      ii. *Nematodirus*
   b. Whipworms (these are also roundworms, but I like to think of them as a separate group)
      i. *Trichuris*
      ii. *Capillaria*
   c. Threadworm - *Strongyloides*
2. Tapeworms
   a. Moniezia

The strongyles are a large group of worms, including *Haemonchus, Ostertagia, Teladorsagia, Cooperia, Bunostomum* and *Trichostrongylus.* Their eggs are indistinguishable from one another, so on faecal egg counts from the lab, they are normally grouped as "strongyles" or "strongyle-type eggs." Larval cultures can be used to differentiate the hatched larvae: however, this takes 10–14 days to perform so it is largely irrelevant by the time the results are obtained. Instead, a rapid staining technique with fluorescein-labelled peanut agglutinin can be used to differentiate one particular type of strongyle egg, *Haemonchus contortus,* that causes anaemia.[1] This can be useful information to assist in managing herd outbreaks. *Strongyloides* eggs are slightly smaller than strongyle-type eggs and are always passed larvated within the egg, unlike strongyles that still must undergo some development to larvae within the egg after being passed out in the faeces.

As far as camelid-specific nematode infections, there are a few host-specific nematodes affecting camelids in South America, such as *Lamanema chavezi, Graphinema auchenia, Nematodirus lamae* and *Camelostrongylus mentulatus.* The first two of these have rarely been reported outside South America until recently when *Graphinema auchenia* was reported in a small proportion of alpacas in Australia.[2] There have been several reports of *Lamanema chavezi* in New Zealand, the United States, Germany and Switzerland.[3-6] In a recent publication out of Germany, it was shown that this parasite was capable of maintaining itself locally in Europe, so there is potential for this to become an issue following the importation of camelids. *Lamanema chavezi* larvae migrate to the liver where they develop into L4 larvae and cause liver damage there before migrating to the bile ducts and back to the intestine. It is considered to be the most pathogenic roundworm that affects South American Camelids.[7] It causes haemorrhages and focal necrosis within the liver that results in the formation of small abscesses: affected animals may also become anaemic, anorexic and suffer from marked weight loss. This parasite may account for some of the evidence of parasite migration found within the liver of some necropsied llamas and alpacas that have been exported from South America. *Nematodirus lamae* has been identified in alpacas in the UK and New Zealand.[8,9] The roundworm *Camelostrongylus mentulatus* has been the subject of investigation in the UK. Its presence in the UK was reported in 2008 as a finding at necropsy in two young animals that had high worm burdens.[10] It has been thought to be fairly host-specific although its eggs have also appeared in the faecals of other domestic and wild ungulates, especially those in wildlife parks where camelids are kept (E Flach, Personal communication). The significance of this gastrointestinal parasite is unknown at present. It has also been documented in Australia more recently.[2] In a series of studies based in Australia, *C mentulatus* was the second-most common worm found in the alpacas studied.[2,11]

Parasitic gastroenteritis may result in a variable number of clinical signs including ill-thrift, weight loss, diarrhoea, colic, anaemia, lethargy and anorexia. Anaemia is more specifically associated with *Haemonchus*, and sometimes *Trichuris* infestations. Death is also a potential consequence of gastrointestinal parasitism in animals in which parasites are not detected and treated early enough. In sheep, worm burdens may not be suspected in animals with normal stool. Since camelids have an extra-long spiral colon that enhances water retention – an adaptation to arid climates – diarrhoea is uncommon. Therefore, it should not be considered a prerequisite clinical sign when suspecting gastrointestinal parasitism. In other words, it can still be worms, regardless of what their faeces look like!

Heavy parasite burdens with *Haemonchus* may result in severe anaemia. An important feature to understand regarding *Haemonchus* is that both larvae and adult worms suck blood from the third stomach compartment. Together, they can suck 1.4% of blood volume daily per 1000 worms which can soon accumulate to cause anaemia in affected individuals. Since the larvae are not yet able to lay eggs, it is possible to detect clinical anaemia before increases in egg counts where large numbers of larvae are present. Once you understand this, it is clear that you cannot rely on faecal egg counts alone to screen for *Haemonchus*.

As responsible owners, you must always evaluate body condition scores and the colour of the mucous membranes around the eyes, along with faecal egg counts, to ensure a more accurate interpretation of the herd's parasite status. These should be checked monthly whether or not faecal egg counts are planned. Any abnormalities should initiate faecal testing to rule out parasite burdens. Mucous membrane colour should normally be a healthy pink colour. Paleness suggests anaemia and can be an indicator of *Haemonchus* infestation, regardless of egg counts. Likewise, if you find anaemic animals, while I would suggest performing an egg count in any case, you should also conduct faecal testing on a representative sample from at least that group to assess egg counts within the group or across the herd to establish the severity of the problem. This will allow you to initiate control measures where necessary to prevent the problem from spreading.

To learn how to tell if your alpaca or llama is anaemic, there is a video available in the Resources section of my website at www.ukalpacavet.com/resources.

I do advocate immediate worming of severely anaemic animals regardless of egg counts, but I would not support doing this in the absence of sampling the individual and others in the herd. And never blanket worm the rest of the group - faecal test first and find out which animals actually require treating.

Since camelids are well-adapted to high altitude and low oxygen conditions, this makes them excellent at dealing with anaemia. This means that it is possible to find a camelid patient that has coped very well with the loss of its red cells from parasite infestation until it presents with acute collapse with a packed cell volume (PCV) as low as 3-4%. Often a stressful event such as a sudden change in the weather, herd changes or routine husbandry procedures may precipitate this acute decompensation. Although these animals may seem near death upon examination, a blood transfusion, combined with parasite treatment and other appropriate symptomatic therapies, can have a dramatic clinical effect. This procedure is essential for survival and relatively straightforward with the proper equipment. However, it must be emphasized that further stress to such animals, such as transportation or even just the placement of an intravenous catheter may result in distress and potential death - but without this treatment, affected individuals will probably die in any case, so these interventions must still be attempted.

Nematodirus and *Trichuris* (a whipworm) are associated with significant pathology, even at low egg counts. Nematodirus can lead to severe weight loss, while Trichuris primarily affects the large intestine and is more commonly linked to diarrhoea, colic, straining, and occasionally anaemia, as it is a blood-feeding parasite. The anaemia resulting from *trichuris* is not likely to be as severe as that caused by *Haemonchus.* Eggs from these worms are often found at low levels in the faecal samples of animals up to 18 months old. If the animals are clinically normal, with good body condition and normal faeces, this is generally considered a normal finding. Older animals tend to have stronger immunity to these parasites, making these eggs less commonly observed in their faecal samples. Where they are found they can indicate immunosuppression due to underlying disease or stress.

Tapeworms in camelids (e.g. *Moniezia*) are relatively common but are not thought to be primary pathogens. However, heavy infestations can result in weight loss, ill-thrift and diarrhoea, especially in younger animals. Therefore, finding tapeworm segments in the faeces of affected animals could direct the need for treatment.

Protozoa

The protozoal organisms affecting camelids include the following:

1. Coccidia
2. Giardia
3. Cryptosporidium

Coccidia

Coccidiosis is most diagnosed in neonatal and juvenile camelids. Adults are more resistant to clinical disease due to prior exposure and their mature immune systems being able to mount an appropriate immune response to control it. Adult camelids that have not been exposed to coccidia as young animals may be more susceptible to disease, and those that are immunosuppressed by concurrent disease or stress may also succumb to clinical coccidiosis.

Outbreaks of coccidiosis tend to occur where there are large groups of crias and are exacerbated by warm and wet weather that allows for the persistence and sporulation of coccidial oocysts on pasture. The pathogenesis and severity of the clinical signs observed are associated with the number of coccidia ingested. The higher the number of oocysts ingested, the more severe the resulting clinical syndrome. Re-infections from a contaminated environment can cause an excessive coccidia burden that may be fatal.[12] Following ingestion of sporulated oocysts, motile stages called sporozoites are released which penetrate epithelial cells in the small intestine. The sporozoites then undergo both sexual and asexual reproductive stages within the gut wall producing merozoites and eventually oocysts, which are then shed in the feces. The release of each of these stages causes direct damage to the epithelial mucosa of the small intestine, resulting in enteritis and diarrhoea. Straining may also be observed. Heavy infestations can cause extensive damage such that the gut may struggle to absorb sufficient nutrients and affected crias may experience poor growth. Diarrhoea may rarely be haemorrhagic and contain shreds of sloughed mucosa. However, Cheney and Allen (1989) report that since the lesions are primarily in the small intestine, fresh blood is rarely seen in affected llamas.[13]

Coccidiosis in camelids is caused by several different species belonging to the genus *Eimeria*. Coccidia are highly species-specific, meaning camelid *Eimeria* does not infect other species, nor do coccidia from other species, such as poultry or sheep, infect camelids. Six species of coccidia have been identified that affect South American Camelids and these include *Eimeria lamae, E. alpacae, E. macusaniensis, E. ivitaensis, E. punoensis* and *E. peruviana*.[12,14-17] A distinguishing feature of the *E. macusaniensis* oocyst is that it is much larger than the other four species, measuring 81-107μm in length, and has a very thick wall.[15] Likewise, *E ivitaensis* is also larger and thick-walled but more oval in shape. In contrast, the other four main species measure 17-40 μm in length and have a thin-walled oocyst.[14]

The life cycle is not particularly well-established for coccidia specific to South American Camelids. However, Foreyt (2001) lists prepatent periods for four out of the five species that affect South American Camelids (not including *E ivitaensis)*.[18] The prepatent period is the time following ingestion of the oocysts and before oocysts are detected in a faecal sample. During this period, the sporozoites released from oocysts invade the gut wall where they undergo both asexual and sexual reproduction stages of their life cycle which then produce the male and female gametes. These are fertilised and oocysts are then excreted in the faeces. The prepatent periods vary from as short as 10 days for *E. punoensis* to 33-34 days for *E. macusaniensis*. The prepatent periods for *E. alpacae* and *E. punoensis* were established from experimental data using faecal samples from four llamas.[19] I've diagnosed clinical coccidiosis in alpacas as early as 21 days of age based on finding oocysts on faecal tests, but crias can exhibit clinical signs of coccidiosis before this age, as oocysts may not yet be being shed. The early appearance of clinical disease suggests that neonates exposed to contaminated environments can become infected in the first few days of life. *E. macusaniensis,* often just called *"E mac"* for short, has been associated with significant pathogenicity. During its long prepatent stage, it can cause significant damage to the bowel wall when burdens are high. This may result in rapid weight loss and low blood protein concentrations, normally without anaemia, and before the appearance of oocysts in faecal samples. Therefore, *E mac* should be a top differential diagnosis in camelids with weight loss and hypoproteinaemia (low protein) on bloodwork, particularly when anaemia is not present, even if a faecal test does not show *E mac.*

For diagnosis of *E mac*, the method used for faecal examination technique can affect the yield of oocysts detected.[20] Flotation solutions with a specific gravity of ≤1.20 (such as saturated sodium chloride which has SG of 1.20) may fail to allow detection of *E. macusaniensis* oocysts which are large and have a relatively high specific gravity. In comparison, a sugar solution with specific gravity of 1.28–1.30 (used at a 1:10 dilution for oocyst detection by centrifugal flotation) gave more reliable results in that study, especially when low concentrations of oocysts were present. Therefore, it is important to check which method is being performed if you are sending off samples to an outside lab. If performing your own analyses, make sure that you are performing a test that is sensitive enough for *E mac.* Otherwise, you may get a false negative test result and incorrectly believe that *E mac* isn't a problem when in fact it is. The Modified Stolls test is also reliable – it uses a concentrated sugar solution combined with double centrifugation and can float the dense or larger eggs and oocysts including *E mac, Nematodirus* and *Trichuris.* This is the test we use in our laboratory.

Effective treatment of clinical coccidiosis is achieved using anticoccidials. It is important to realise that most anticoccidials will *control* coccidiosis but do not fully eliminate the organism. There are different anticoccidial medications available in different parts of the world. In Europe, Australia and New Zealand, treatment of camelids is usually achieved using diclazuril (such as Vecoxan, Janssen Animal Health) or toltrazuril (Baycox, Bayer or Tolracol, Krka UK Ltd). These are both triazine drugs: ponazuril is the major metabolite of toltrazuril and is available in the United States, licensed for use in horses and poultry. Single doses are usually sufficient for treatment. However, for heavy infestations of *E mac,* you can sometimes see an increase in oocysts at a retest faecal, because of its longer life cycle. This means that there were stages of the coccidia that were not treated effectively at the time of initial treatment. Treatment may need to be repeated two or more times at 10–14 day intervals to target stages of development that were not susceptible during the initial dosing. Interestingly, toltrazuril can act on intracellular stages of the life cycle: in other words, it affects the stages within the gut wall that are undergoing development into schizonts and gametes. Other practitioners have used shorter intervals between treatments, and I would suggest giving at least 5 days between doses to aid in treating sequential waves of coccidia.

In the United States, treatment is achieved using oral sulfadimethoxine (Albon, Pfizer USA) at a dose of 15 mg/kg twice daily for 5 days. Amprolium (Corid, Merial) may also be used orally at the treatment dose of 10 mg/kg once daily for 5 days. Ponazuril can be used at a dose of 10-20 mg/kg orally.[21]

Clinically affected animals such as those with diarrhoea should be isolated and treated. Unaffected young animals from the same pen or pasture should also be treated since they will have been exposed and may be harbouring coccidian stages at various stages of development in the gut. It is not normally necessary to treat adults pastured with these crias due to their better immunity to coccidiosis. However, you may find that some adults have "spillover infections" from crias in groups with heavy infestations. These animals may be suffering some sort of stress and may be worth treating. At the same time, also consider what might be causing that "stress." Any animals that are affected more severely may require other supportive therapy depending on the case, such as IV fluid therapy and nutritional support.

Good management practices and maintenance of hygienic facilities for young animals should be considered the most important factors in the prevention of coccidiosis. Where you have larger numbers of crias pastured together, you will have a good breeding ground for coccidia. These groups are immunologically naïve to coccidia and will permit reproduction of coccidia in the gut. If conditions are also warm and wet, then coccidia burdens are more likely to proliferate. Quarantine of visiting and newly purchased animals with faecal examinations performed at the beginning and end of the quarantine period should help reduce the spread of coccidia within susceptible populations.

Strategic use of anticoccidial drugs may also be considered as a supplemental means of controlling coccidiosis. It should be used on a herd basis but is rarely necessary in smallholdings where proper monitoring is taking place. Since outbreaks of coccidiosis are common in the wetter months, prophylactic drug regimens should be used during these times of year on farms experiencing problems with coccidia. Consideration should be given to the application of preventative measures before and during stressful events such as weaning, shearing or herd movements. The oral products mentioned (diclazuril, toltrazuril) can be used for this purpose. Amprolium (US) may be used prophylactically and is added to water at the label dose over 21 days. Correct dosage of amprolium is important since overdosing causes thiamine deficiency and can produce neurological signs of polioencephalomalacia.

Alternatively, decoquinate (Deccox®, Alpharma) may be used more safely and added into feed at 0.5 mg/kg/day for 28 days. Ionophore antibiotics such as monensin or salinomycin should not be used to prevent coccidiosis in camelids since they are susceptible to the toxicity of these drugs.

Cryptosporidiosis and Giardiasis

Cryptosporidium species are protozoan pathogens and can cause severe and sometimes fatal outbreaks of diarrhoea in neonatal animals as well as in immuno-compromised individuals. *Cryptosporidiosis* may affect humans; therefore appropriate hygienic precautions should be used when handling affected animals.

Infection occurs by ingestion of contaminated food or water. *Cryptosporidium* oocysts are extremely resistant to decay in the environment and to most disinfectants. As few as 10 oocysts are capable of inducing disease in susceptible individuals. A malabsorptive diarrhoea occurs in cryptosporidiosis leading to dehydration and electrolyte imbalances. Maldigestion also occurs such that weight loss and emaciation in neonates are typical. Renal failure is a potential sequel in crias with cryptosporidiosis. The cause of this renal failure is presumed to be a prolonged state of subclinical dehydration, and this suggests that rehydration therapy is important in treating this disease.

The simplest method of diagnosing cryptosporidiosis is by examination of faecal smears using modified acid-fast stains (Chen et al 2002, Tzipori and Ward 2002).[22,23] Recently, ELISA tests for both *Cryptosporidium* and *Giardia* oocyst antigens have improved sensitivity and can be easily applied in practice situations as there are simple kits available for test. PCR testing may be a useful diagnostic tool that is more readily available these days.

Effective treatment for cryptosporidiosis is difficult. There is no specific treatment for crypto. The mainstay of therapy involves supportive care with intravenous fluids and/or intravenous feeding due to the malabsorption and maldigestion which occur in this disease.

Diarrhoea in crias affected with *Cryptosporidium* may be profuse and watery. If *Cryptosporidium* is not diagnosed and appropriate supportive therapy is not initiated early on, chronic disease resulting in kidney failure and emaciation may result. In addition, a failure to diagnose means that appropriate control measures may not be put in place to prevent transmission to further animals in the herd and highlights the importance of getting the diagnostic testing performed.

Giardia infection primarily occurs from contaminated water sources and is a zoonotic disease. The oocysts can survive about 3 months in water at 4° C. This organism affects the small intestine and results in malabsorptive diarrhoea leading to dehydration and weight loss. Larger farms with higher numbers of young stock seem to be at higher risk. Also, those using on-farm water sources such as ponds to supply water tanks also have an increased risk, but water filters can be used with success.

Oral fenbendazole (e.g. Panacur) at 50 mg/kg once daily for 5 consecutive days appears clinically to be effective at treating giardiasis in llamas and alpacas. This corresponds to 5 ml per 10 kg bodyweight of the 10% oral solution and 10x bodyweight using equine paste syringes.

Liver Fluke

Two types of liver fluke affect livestock and camelids: the large liver fluke known as *Fasciola hepatica* and the small liver fluke known as *Dicrocoelium dentriticum*. Both are trematode worms or "flatworms." All grazing animals are susceptible to liver fluke including cattle, sheep and camelids although the species exhibit slightly different clinical syndromes. In both, the life cycle involves an intermediate host and free-living stages. *Fasciola hepatica* is the predominant liver fluke affecting livestock in the UK and the Pacific Northwest of the US. Both areas have a temperate and wet climate. There are reports of acute, chronic and fatal forms of fascioliasis in camelids.[24-27] *Dicrocoelium* has been reported as more of a problem in drier, more mountainous locations such as Switzerland, Austria and Sweden.

Fasciola Hepatica

The disease caused by this type of liver fluke is known as "fascioliasis." To understand how to manage liver fluke, it is important to understand the life cycle of the parasite (*Figure 1*). Adult fluke living in the bile ducts of susceptible livestock lay eggs that are passed out onto pasture in the faeces. Under suitable conditions (>10 degrees and wet), the miracidium develops inside the egg and then hatches. It migrates through moisture to find the intermediate snail host. This is a mud snail rather than a normal garden snail. The most common one is the dwarf pond snail, Galba truncatula, which is tiny and measures only 3-5 mm. If the miracidia find a snail host, they undergo further stages until the infective cercariae stages emerge from the snail onto the pasture. If livestock, including camelids, ingest the infective metacercariae from the pasture, the larval fluke stages migrate to and through the liver causing extensive damage within the liver. Fibrosis is the result of this, and this can occur in camelids within 3 weeks or so. The fibrotic change is then irreversible. The migrating larvae eventually turn into adults that live within the bile ducts of the liver, potentially blocking the flow of bile, and the adults lay eggs.

The period from the ingestion of metacercariae by grazing livestock to the production of eggs by adult flukes typically takes 10–12 weeks. The whole life cycle from egg to adult producing eggs is around 18–20 weeks.

The hatching of eggs and development stages depend on day and night temperatures being greater than 10°C (50°F), as well as sufficient moisture being available. These conditions will occur at varying times at different locations. For example, in the UK climate, they may occur potentially as early as March or April in the south of the country, or as late as the end of May or early June in Scotland. Liver fluke is not present all over the UK, although the incidence and distribution are reported to have increased over the last 10 years and is now found in previously "dry" areas. In wet summers, conditions are ideal and massive numbers of cercariae are shed by snails onto pasture, resulting in massive infections in grazing livestock. If it's dry from May to July, there are fewer snails and fewer eggs, and contamination is reduced. The ingestion of large numbers of infective metacercariae normally occurs from July to October, after wet May-July conditions, and then results in clinical fascioliasis. Alternatively, snails may become infected later in the summer or early autumn, leading to shedding the following spring and resulting in earlier cases of fascioliasis during that season.

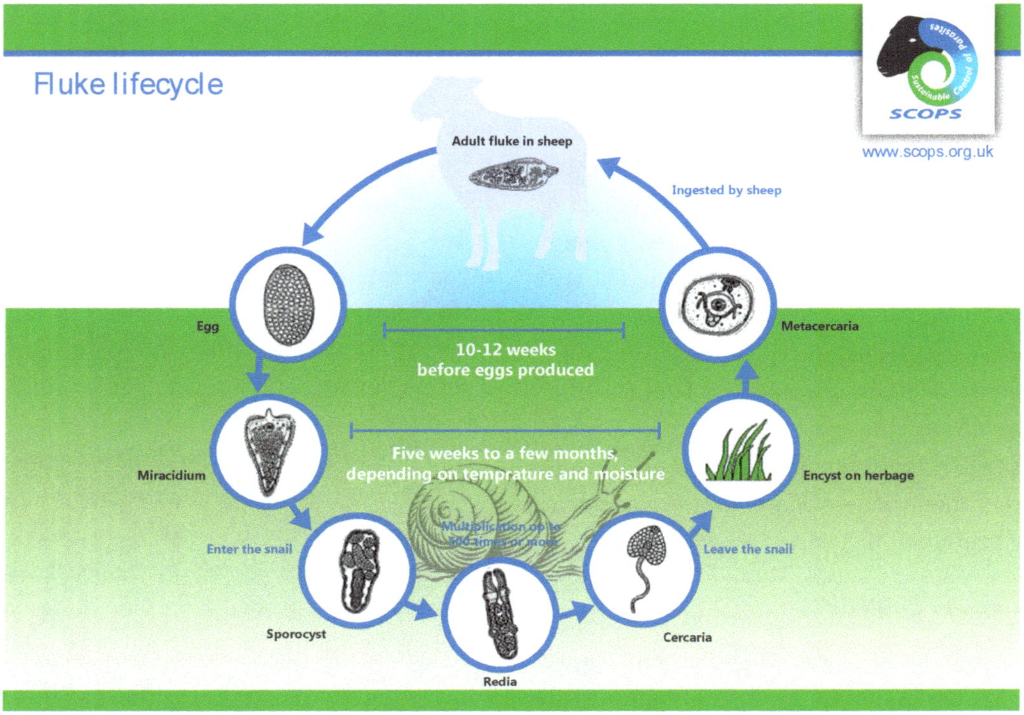

Figure 1. The life cycle of the liver fluke Fasciola hepatica. Reprinted with permission from SCOPS, Sustainable Control of Parasites at www.scops.org.uk.

Diagnosis of Fluke

Clinical signs of fluke can be extremely vague including lethargy, weight loss, inappetence and weakness. If fluke is a possibility in your area, specific faecal tests can identify fluke eggs. This needs to be a sedimentation test which maximises the chance of detection rather than a standard faecal egg count. If fluke is a possibility, request a specific fluke test when submitting a faecal sample for analysis. However, it should be noted that eggs are only shed by adult fluke and shedding of eggs is variable. Therefore, a negative faecal test does not rule out fluke as a diagnosis. Based on the life cycle, adult fluke are most likely to be present over the winter if not killed by previous flukicides. Winter is therefore a good time to include this in testing. Pooling samples for fluke testing (only) is permissible - this can increase the chances of detection in a herd because it is more cost-effective. It is not necessary to test all animals individually because if fluke eggs are found, you are likely to treat all animals for fluke. After all, a negative test doesn't rule out infection.

Bloodwork may be helpful in the assessment of clinical cases of liver fluke. During the migration of fluke larval stages, liver enzymes may increase due to the damage being caused to liver parenchyma. Once adults are present in the bile ducts, obstruction of bile ducts can cause increases of the specific enzyme GGT on bloodwork which can be suggestive of fluke, although is not definitive.

Serological tests for fluke that are used in cattle have not worked well in camelids while the coproantigen test (faecal testing for antigens excreted by fluke) is not validated for use in camelids. However, the coproantigen test should still work as it's specific to the organism rather than the host.

Fluke may be found at post-mortem examination – depending on the stage of fascioliasis, the finding of either migrating larvae or adult fluke in the bile ducts is definitive. Furthermore, evidence of damage consistent with fluke migration may be found in histopathology. Occasionally extensive liver damage may be found at postmortem that is consistent with fluke but adult fluke are not seen due to recent flukicide treatment.

Dealing with Fluke

Since fluke problems can be severe in camelids, reliance only on pharmacological agents is unrealistic and ultimately may result in the development of resistance to the very few drugs that we have at our disposal. Therefore, environmental control is also warranted.

Because the life cycle of liver fluke requires an intermediate snail host, if animals don't graze areas with snails, they will not become infected. Therefore, environmental control is a key part of fluke control. Draining wet pasture areas may be one option where this is allowed, or simply moving livestock off wetter pastures in late summer, autumn and winter can reduce the risk of ingesting infective metacercariae. Otherwise, fencing off high-risk wet areas such as marshes and bogs can help. Using natural water sources, particularly those that provide habitat for the intermediate snail stages, would be discouraged.

On farms where there is a recognised problem with fluke based on postmortem examination and fluke faecal tests, control may be warranted. It is not advisable to use flukicides "just in case" but rather based on an epidemiological assessment by your local vet. Most flukicides will only kill adult fluke while triclabendazole (e.g. Fasinex, Elanco Animal Health) is the only agent that can kill the migrating larval stages of fluke. Since resistance to these drugs can develop if they are used often and repeatedly, it is important to use these drugs only where necessary and based on knowledge of the life cycle. Monitoring via faecal tests and post-mortem examinations of any animals that die unexpectedly will help guide fluke control programmes.

In summer and autumn, triclabendazole would be the drug of choice if available because it can kill migrating fluke larvae. In contaminated environments, dosing can be repeated at 10-week intervals, starting in the summer depending on environmental conditions, through until December time. For animals that remain on fluke pasture over the winter, treatment using a drug that kills adults only in Spring as day/night temperatures approach 10°C would be advisable, to kill any adults that remain after the winter and prevent eggs from being excreted onto pasture which start the cycle over again. For camelids, adulticide drugs would include albendazole (e.g. Albex, Chanelle UK or Endospec, Bimeda) and closantel (e.g. Flukiver, Elanco Animal Health).

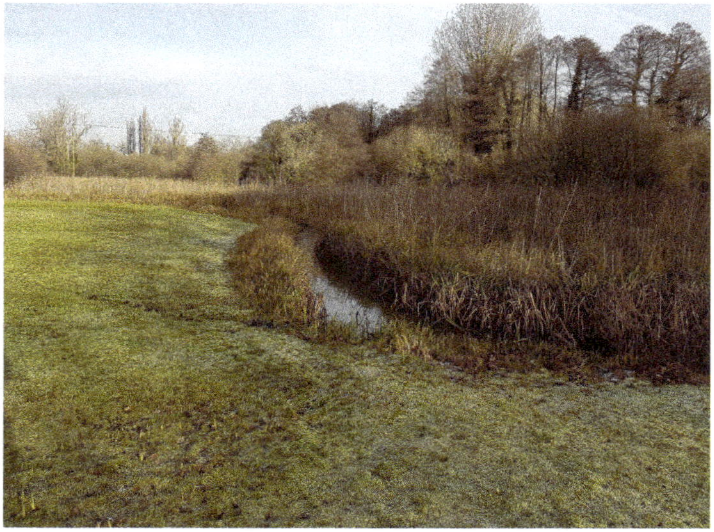

Figure 2. Marshes are ideal fluke territory. Water from marshes should not be used as drinking water. This farm was experiencing heavy losses from liver fluke.

Quarantine Measures for New Stock

If buying new animals, quarantine measures aimed at fluke control depend on the risk posed by the incoming animals and the presence of suitable snail habitats on the destination farm. In circumstances where the farm has a potential snail habitat but no history of fluke infection, you absolutely do not want to introduce it! Therefore, animals should be treated to remove all fluke stages before introduction. If there is no suitable snail habitat and no history of fluke problems, the risk of fluke establishing on the farm is low. In such cases, treatment of incoming animals would focus on those coming from fluke-endemic areas to address any infections they might carry and minimise health problems. Triclabendazole is recommended where available, as it is effective against all fluke stages.

Although triclabendazole resistance is still not that common in the UK, there are some areas where resistance exists, notably in the Scottish Borders. Clearly, treatment with triclabendazole will not kill any resistant flukes, so treatment with two agents may be considered. However, these treatments should not be administered simultaneously; a gap of 6–8 weeks between treatments is recommended. In addition, since animals can continue to shed eggs for up to 3 weeks after killing adult flukes, incoming animals should be kept quarantined (off infected pastures and in quarantine) for at least 4 weeks after treatment.

Dicrocoelium Dentriticum

Dicrocoelium dentriticum is a smaller fluke than *Fasciola hepatica*. It has been known to cause severe disease in camelids in

Europe, particularly Switzerland, Germany and Austria, but is rarely mentioned elsewhere. The life cycle for the small fluke is a rather interesting one and includes two intermediate hosts: the terrestrial snail and a species of ant. The snail ingests fluke eggs within the faeces and the larvae develop into a juvenile stage within the snail. Cercariae are released from the snail in a slime ball that is consumed by ants that are attracted to the slime trails and they then develop into metacercariae. These forms then take over the ants' nervous systems and manipulate the ants into climbing up blades of grass at nighttime to hopefully be grazed by unsuspecting herbivores. If they don't get eaten, the ants return to the safety of the ant colony but repeat their ascent to the top of the grass each night. This is so they don't get killed by the heat of the sun. In the herbivore, whether it's a ruminant or camelid, the fluke migrates up the bile duct. Chronic or heavy infestations cause hypertrophy of the walls of the bile duct that may be evident on ultrasound examination, and this may cause bile duct obstruction. Secondary bacterial infections may occur.

Clinical signs of small liver fluke infections are non-specific and include weight loss, lethargy, weakness, poor growth in youngstock, recumbency and death. Faecal diagnostics for small fluke are challenging – neither routine flotation nor sedimentation methods are reliable. A combination flotation-sedimentation method using a zinc sulphate solution with a specific gravity of 1.2 to 1.3 has been suggested.[28] However, eggs are only excreted intermittently. On bloodwork, affected animals may have anaemia, low protein concentrations and increased liver enzymes (particularly GGT and GLDH or SDH). On ultrasound examination, there may be thickening and calcification of the bile duct walls and an enlarged or fibrotic liver while liver fibrosis may result in the accumulation of fluid in the chest and abdomen.

The treatment of choice for small fluke is praziquantel at a dose of 50 mg/kg. There is a concentrated formulation of praziquantel available in Austria that was developed by clinicians at the Veterinary School in Vienna (www.richter-pharma.com).[29] Early initiation of treatment before the development of fibrosis will have a greater chance of success.

Key Takeaways

There are a number of parasites that affect camelids causing a variety of clinical signs. It's important to have an understanding of what the different parasites are, what problems they can cause in your animals, how to diagnose and treat them, and also what their life cycles are so that you can develop parasite control strategies to minimise the effects of these in your animals.

Key takeaways from this chapter:

- The main gastrointestinal parasites affecting camelids are worms, protozoa (including coccidia) and fluke.
- Camelid worm populations are similar to those affecting ruminants and can be shared between species while coccidia is species-specific.
- *Haemonchus* can cause severe anaemia in camelids even before eggs show up on faecal tests. It is therefore a primary differential diagnosis for anaemic camelids.
- Coccidia mostly affects young animals and those that are immunocompromised. Adults develop acquired immunity to them. *E mac* is a particularly pathogenic coccidia with a long life-cycle and can cause weight loss before the identification of oocysts on faecal tests.
- There are two types of liver fluke affecting camelids, depending on your geographical location. Both cause severe disease in camelids.
- You cannot eliminate parasites. Aim to control them and minimise their impact.

We will discuss how to develop a parasite control strategy for your farm in the next chapter.

10

Parasite Control Strategies

The parasite control strategy is one of the most important aspects of your whole herd health plan. As such, it deserves an entire chapter dedicated to it! A crucial point to grasp is that parasite control is not about obliterating parasites into oblivion. This would be a virtually impossible task – parasites have evolved to adapt and survive. Instead, parasite control is about using a collection of tools to minimise the burdens on your animals such that they are affected as little as possible. Monitoring the situation is also essential so that steps can be taken when the little buggers dare to take advantage and multiply without permission!

Every parasite control strategy should be tailored specifically to the individual farm. No one strategy is going to be appropriate for every situation. These are best worked out in conjunction with veterinary expertise – this can be with your local vet or, if preferred, with a specialist consultant like myself.

There are a number of components to any parasite control strategy. In general, these can be grouped into three main categories as shown in the diagram in *Figure 1*. We'll call these the 3Ms of Parasite Control. All three are integral to the parasite control strategy. Actions or findings in each category influence activities that may be needed in the other two categories and vice versa. The sweet spot is where all overlap, there is balance, and the parasites that may affect your herd are under control.

1. **Management of the pasture**. There are several considerations in this category. I also include quarantine of new/travelling stock here because how we deal with this will be crucial in controlling pasture contamination.

2. **Monitoring**. This includes body condition scoring, checking the mucous membranes for evidence of anaemia as well as faecal testing.

3. **Medications**. This involves the use of anthelmintics (wormers) and anti-coccidials where appropriate.

You will notice that in the order I have listed these, the use of medications is last. This is intentional. Pasture management and monitoring must be in place before deciding what medications are needed and when.

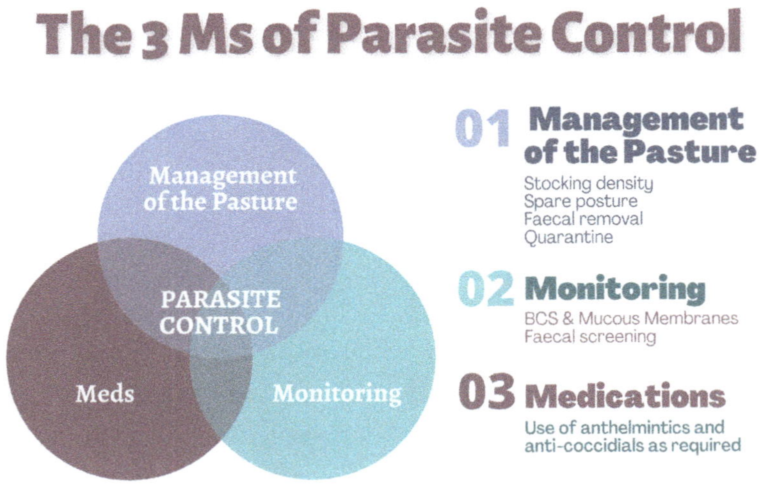

Figure 1. Diagram showing the key features, The 3 Ms, of a parasite control strategy.

You do not have a parasite control strategy if the only thing you do is use medications. We will go into each of these categories in more detail in this chapter. But first, it is important to understand the principles of anthelmintic resistance and refugia.

Principles of Anthelmintic Resistance and Refugia

A fundamental concept to recognise is that worms develop resistance to anthelmintics (wormers) over time. We only have a finite number of wormers available for use and there is not a constant pipeline of new wormers in development that might be available if we use wormers irresponsibly and then find that we have induced resistance in our worm populations. Therefore, responsible use of wormers is not just encouraged but rather, essential.

How Does Anthelmintic Resistance Develop?

Every time a wormer is used in a given population of animals, the worms are exposed to it and have the potential to develop resistance. Worms reproduce quickly, and any mutation that arises during reproduction that gives certain worms a selective advantage over others will persist in the population. If certain worms survive because their genes allow them to survive a worming dose when all the rest die, these are the only worms that will survive to reproduce and that successful gene will be passed on to the next generation of worms. Over time,

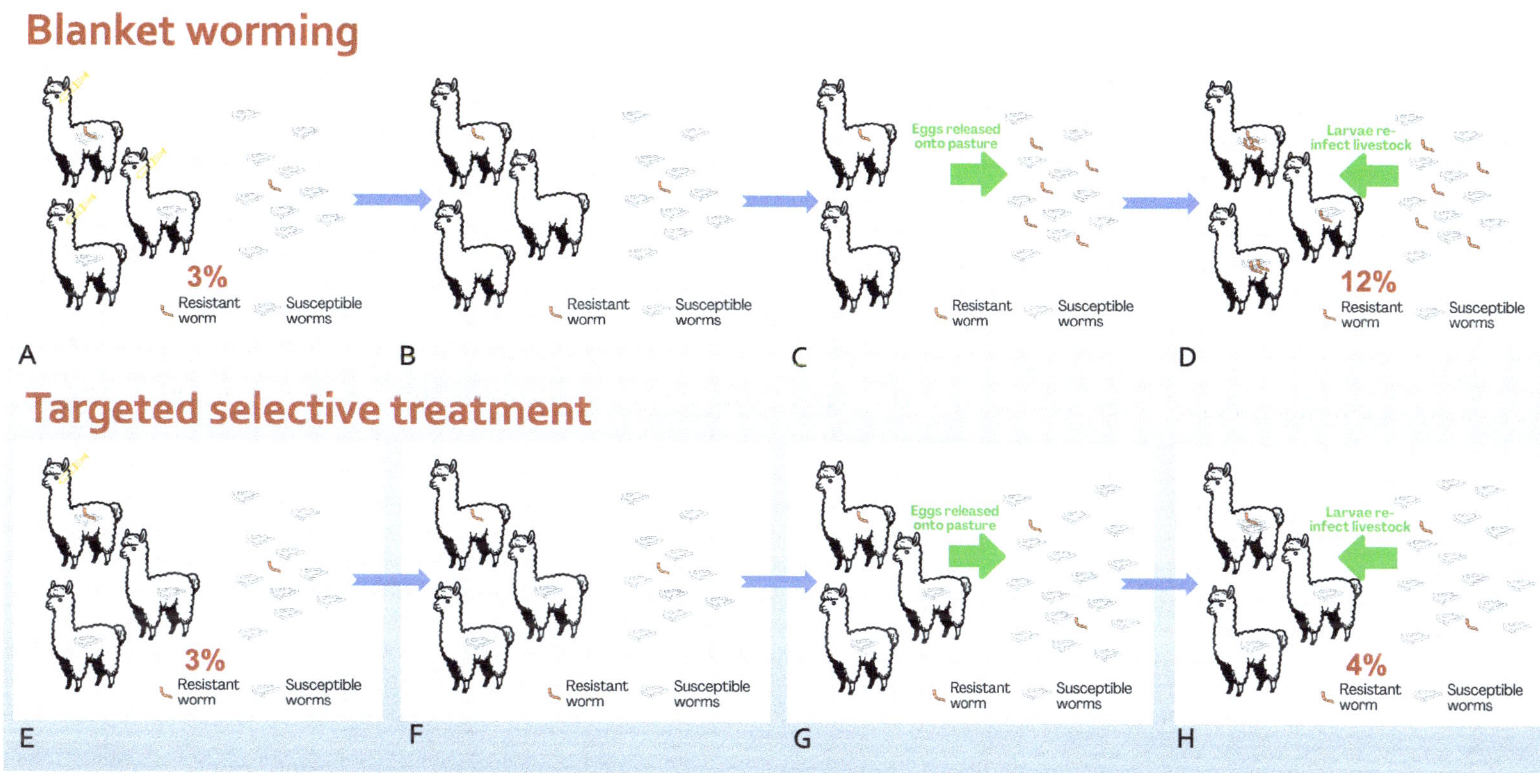

Figure 2. Graphic showing the comparison between blanket worming (A-D) and targeted selective treatments (E-H) on the development of anthelmintic resistance over time. With blanket worming, a low level of 3% resistance quickly becomes a significant 12% while with TST, the resistance only increases to 4%.

this gene will predominate in the population until all worms become resistant.

How Can We Reduce the Development of Anthelmintic Resistance?

If you worm every animal in a population (called "blanket worming"), you kill all the susceptible worms, but the resistant ones survive to reproduce. Since only the resistant worms survive and reproduce, the resistance genes will spread rapidly. If you leave some animals untreated, susceptible worms will also be present in the population, and these will dilute out the resistance genes such that the development of resistance across all worms is slowed down. The susceptible worms in the population are known as the *refugia* population. The lower the proportion of animals that are wormed, the lower the exposure to the wormer and therefore the slower the development of resistance. Therefore, this targeted and selective worming is now recommended. This is achieved based on a combination of faecal testing, body condition scoring (BCS) and mucous membrane colour checking.

Another old-fashioned strategy that people used to employ and that you may have heard of was to "dose and move," in which case animals would be dosed and then moved straight onto clean pasture. Based on the above information, you can see that this would result in only the resistant worms being present in that population, again hastening the development of resistant worms in the whole population. Instead, if you need to move a group of animals to fresh pasture to enjoy fresh grazing, or to allow one pasture's grass to recover, I recommend that you first do faecal testing to see what the level of infestation is before deciding whether or not dosing is necessary. If you have to dose any animals, then dose based on that testing alongside evaluation of BCS and mucous membrane colour. If you find worm burdens, it is suggested that you move the animals first and then dose them so that some susceptible worms contaminate the pasture before you treat them. How long you leave these animals on the fresh pasture before dosing depends on the worm burdens. If burdens are very high, the interval would be shorter because you don't want to increase infection pressure by allowing too much contamination of the pasture. An alternative is to treat first, then wait before moving so that the animals are exposed to the susceptible worm population again before moving. These delay strategies don't work when you're using a long-acting wormer like moxidectin because it protects reinfestation for around 5–6 weeks. When using moxidectin, you can practice selective worming by treating only the individuals identified as needing it based on faecal test results, body condition score (BCS), and mucous membrane colour. This approach maintains some untreated animals in the herd, which helps preserve a refugia of susceptible worms, rather than relying solely on timing to control exposure.

In small herds, you can easily faecal-est every animal and selectively dose only those individuals that are identified as needing to be wormed. In larger herds, where a significant proportion of individuals remain untested, greater reliance on body condition scoring and mucous membrane colour assessment is necessary to determine which animals need worming. This approach is more practical than performing egg counts for every animal. You want to leave at least 15% of the herd or group untreated, but the greater the proportion that you do not worm, the better. You will monitor the effects of that worming (and not worming) by monitoring the individuals' BCS and colour monthly. If concerned, you can faecal test again. Remember that it is not just worms that may cause weight loss so do consider other differentials for this.

The Features of a Parasite Control Strategy: The 3 Ms

In this section, each of the components of your parasite control strategy will now be discussed in detail.

1. Management of the Pasture

A good parasite control strategy should always include pasture management. This is probably the most neglected area of parasite control and one of the reasons I have placed it first. In addition, the measures used in this category reduce your reliance on medications as they will naturally reduce exposure to parasites. This category includes:

Pasture Rotation

As the grass gets eaten down, you should move animals off that area of pasture to allow the grass to recover and to allow any parasites on that pasture to die off. However, you do need to ensure that you are not just moving to another clean area to contaminate with worm eggs. It is therefore best to check faecal egg counts and treat them where necessary before moving them. Again, remember that you should not treat all animals in a group as this will hasten the development of anthelmintic resistance. You want to leave some animals untreated to maintain the refugia of anthelmintic-susceptible parasites.

If you have one large field, it is better to have these large pastures split into smaller ones as that permits some pasture management. If you have only a single large field, but no other paddocks and your animals develop hefty parasite burdens, it will be difficult to manage them as there won't be any cleaner pastures to move them to that will allow them to recover. If you don't want to invest in permanent fencing, temporary fencing can be used to move alpacas around a larger paddock, but this should only be a short-term option. If you do divide larger paddocks, consider how you should do this. Square paddocks allow more efficient use of grazing than long thin ones where the animals tend to graze more heavily at the end, closest to where their supplements are provided. A single shelter can still serve multiple paddocks if you place it at the centre and use fencing and gates to manage access.

Resting of Pastures

One question I am often asked is for how long should you rest a pasture? This is extremely variable and depends upon the parasite that you're trying to get rid of and also the environmental conditions. In general, worms and coccidia thrive in moisture and temperate conditions. The UK climate is perfect for parasite persistence because it is mild and wet. Once eggs have hatched into larvae, these stages are actually quite resilient, and they can survive for months. You should be aiming to get to a point at which at least 90% of the larvae have died off. In general, rest periods can be shorter in hot/dry or very cold weather. Larvae will quickly die when it's over 40°C (104°F) but it's only ever got that hot for one day in England in 2022![1] They are not very tolerant of freezing conditions either. In practical terms, you should aim to rest pastures for long enough to allow the grass to recover, and as long as you can for parasite die-off. After 4–6 months in the usual British climate, you should see substantial reductions in burdens, although they will not be eliminated completely. In places with hotter climates such as Australia, you should aim for a minimum of 2–3 months during hot conditions but 5–6 months when it's cooler.[2]

Although not strictly related to resting pastures, some nematodes including *Haemonchus* larvae have an additional adaptation that you need to be aware of because it can have a significant impact on your animals and isn't controlled by resting your pastures. *Haemonchus* larvae been shown to become dormant (a phenomenon known as "hypobiosis") in the gastric glands of the abomasum of sheep when conditions outside the host are not favourable for the development of eggs into infective larval stages. Once conditions change to being more favourable, then you see a sudden increase in clinical disease and egg counts.[3] To my knowledge, this phenomenon hasn't been demonstrated in camelids, but I believe it does occur. This is often evident when camelids experience a sudden rise in egg counts and clinical anaemia following a period of hot, dry weather that is then interrupted by wet conditions. These conditions often occur in August in the UK. Colleagues in Australia have observed the same and tend to drench sheep once the dry season begins to reduce the problem. If you notice these conditions, it is important to check your animals regularly for evidence of anaemia and consider checking egg counts within a few weeks of the change in weather.

One nematode that behaves differently than strongyles is *Nematodirus,* where larval development occurs within the egg. The eggs of *Nematodirus battus* (which is a species prevalent in the UK, but also in some northern European countries, the USA and Canada), require a period of cold weather before they can hatch in temperatures above 10°C (50°F) or more. If there are large numbers of *Nematodirus* eggs present on the pasture, and the cold-to-warm events occur within a short timeframe, it is possible to see a mass hatching of these larvae that may result in problems in grazing youngstock who are especially susceptible to *Nematodirus*. Other species of *Nematodirus* do not appear to require this cold spell and can cause disease year-round. However, it is predominantly young animals affected – adults develop immunity to this parasite after exposure. For sheep, where *Nematodirus battus* is a particular issue, it is recommended not to put lambs out to graze on the same pasture in consecutive years where they may be exposed to the mass hatching phenomenon. If you are in an area where *N battus* is a concern, you may wish to consider avoiding these pastures, too. Of course, if you practice faecal removal as in the next point, this will be less of a problem.

Removal of Faecal Material

Removal of faecal material from the pasture before the eggs hatch is by far the best method of parasite control. If the eggs are removed before they hatch, there is nothing left to be ingested by grazing animals.

Under optimum conditions, strongyle-type eggs may hatch into first-stage larvae (L1) within 1–2 days on pasture.[4] Therefore, ideally pasture should be cleaned every day or two before eggs even hatch onto the grass. If you do not manage to keep to this frequency, the faecal removal will provide a cosmetic result but not a result that also aids in parasite control.

There are various mechanised options to achieve this depending on your budget and pasture size. See *Figures 3* and *4*. Paddock vacuum cleaners are far more effective than paddock sweepers. The latter uses brushes to sweep up the faecal material, but this isn't very effective for individual camelid faecal beans. Essentially, they provide a cosmetic clean but do not provide an effective reduction in parasite burdens. On the other hand, vacuum cleaners have a hose, the nozzle of which is placed directly over the faeces, and it is sucked up into the hose and a storage vessel. They are more time-consuming but more effective unless the faecal material has been trodden into the ground. The longer you leave the faeces on the ground, the more likely it is to get trodden in, so this favours more regular cleaning.

Stocking Density Control

As a general rule where you have good quality pasture, a stocking density of 5 alpacas or llamas is acceptable. Higher stocking densities can be tolerated as long as the animals are moved on more frequently to fresh grazing or fed supplementary hay. Higher stocking densities increase the likelihood of parasites becoming a problem because the animals are more likely to be exposed. Under those circumstances, faecal samples should be checked more frequently for evidence of eggs.

If you find that you have higher stocking densities than this, you should consider reducing your numbers or finding additional pasture space. Increased stocking densities will otherwise result in increased costs of providing stored forages and feed and increased parasite burdens, especially if faecal removal is not practised.

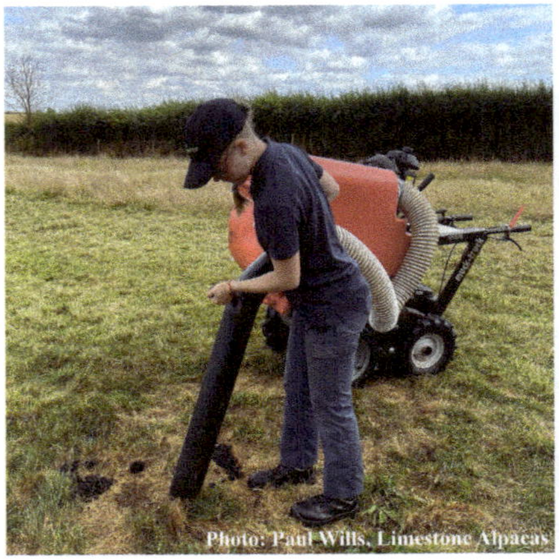

Figure 3. Self-propelled paddock cleaner. Photo courtesy of Paul Wills, Limestone Alpacas.

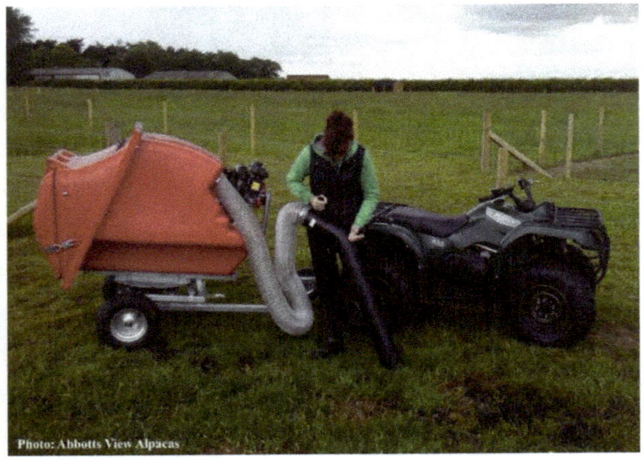

Figure 4. A larger model of towable paddock cleaner. Photo courtesy of Abbotts View Alpacas.

Remember to always have spare pasture available so that you can move animals around, allowing the grass to recover and the parasite larvae to die off. Consider whether you perform effective and frequent faecal removal and assess the number of pasture spaces you can rest at any given time. This will help determine the amount of pasture space required for a herd of a specific size. Because of the duration of time needed in the UK to permit larval die-off, you probably want to allow 2 acres for every 5 alpacas. Let's say you have 10 alpacas divided between 2 paddocks, and you then need to rest each paddock for 6 months, you will need twice the available space than you had the alpacas in at the start of the period (*Figure 5*).

Allocation of Grazing Space

Weaned crias are likely to be the most susceptible group in the herd to parasites: make sure that you put them onto the cleanest available pastures. Crias with their dams are another susceptible group.

Co-grazing With Other Livestock

Sheep are much better adapted to dealing with worm burdens than camelids, having evolved to climates that favour parasites over a longer period. Ideally, sheep should not be on the same pastures or should follow camelids if using rotation of grazing. However, if camelids share the same pasture with sheep, perhaps as guard animals, it is especially important to be vigilant regarding parasite control, particularly the removal of faecal material and faecal screening.

Avoid Grazing Grass That Is Too Short

Most parasite larvae will only climb about an inch from the ground.[5] It is therefore

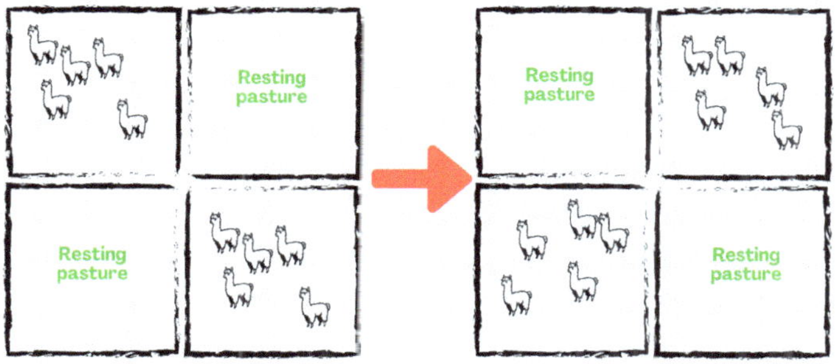

Figure 5. A graphic showing that you might need to allow twice the pasture space than your stocking density of 5 alpacas per acre of land to allow 6 months' resting. In this figure, each square of pasture represents one acre of land.

advisable not to let your animals graze pasture shorter than about 4 cm as this will reduce the ingestion of infective larvae from the base of the grass.[6]

Quarantine of New/Travelling Stock

This is a key feature of parasite control in its own right, but I have included it under pasture management because it involves controlling pasture contamination. By managing incoming animals, you help prevent them from introducing problems or being affected by the stress of moving onto your pastures from elsewhere. It is unfortunately commonly neglected by owners who are excited to receive their new purchases and rush to make them a part of the herd. However, this is not best for your herd or the animals themselves.

In the camelid industry, another important aspect to consider in terms of parasite control is newly acquired animals, visitors and animals returning from shows and breeding farms. These animals may well be harbouring parasites from their previous location. The stress of moving these animals may also precipitate a clinically apparent infection in an animal that was previously doing well. For this reason, a quarantine period is recommended for all animals coming onto the farm. During this period, they should be kept isolated from your existing stock. This should ideally be at least 6 weeks in duration (to cover the possibility of *E mac* that has a long pre-patent period) and the animals should ideally not be in contact (over the fence) with your existing stock. This will help reduce the spread of any viral infections picked up elsewhere, most of which will have been dealt with by the animal's immune system during this length of time.

To both protect incoming animals from the multiplication of parasite burdens due to stress *and* minimise the transfer of anthelmintic-resistant parasites from farm to farm, current thinking is to ensure that new arrivals on the farm carry no worms with them. To reduce the risk, it is suggested that animals should receive at least two different types of wormers on arrival at the new farm. The idea in using different classes of wormer is that parasites may be resistant to one wormer but not multiple wormers. One of the wormers should at least be a broad-spectrum wormer with very little resistance known. In the UK, monepantel (Zolvix, Elanco) and moxidectin (Cydectin, Zoetis) are excellent for this purpose. I rarely use Zolvix for any other purpose than to maximise its use at preventing the transfer of anthelmintic resistance.

On arrival at the new farm, animals should be kept on concrete for at least 48 hours so that faeces can be easily cleaned away daily and any eggs will not get to hatch onto pasture. They should ideally be kept on concrete for 10 days. If this is not available, then limit them to a small area of hard standing or pasture and be especially careful to clean the pasture daily.

10–14 days after quarantine deworming, a faecal should be tested to confirm a zero egg count before animals are released onto previously grazed (not clean) pasture. They will then acquire a population of worms from your own farm. Be careful that you do not put new animals on any pasture that is known to be heavily contaminated, as the new arrivals will be experiencing stress which reduces immunity and results in an increased susceptibility to parasitism. If any parasite burdens are identified at that initial check, animals should then be re-treated. Re-check the animal 10–14 days later to make sure that the treatment was effective before introducing the animals onto the new pasture.

Keep the incoming animals separated from your home herd for a minimum of 6 weeks for parasite control purposes. They can then be introduced to the main herd. At this point, social stresses may ensue as the new animals have to establish their hierarchy within the group. In addition, the effects of the quarantine deworming will have worn off. Therefore, you may wish to recheck faecal samples for egg counts 3–4 weeks after mixing. Consider testing any home herd animals who may have been observed trying to assert their dominance or other individuals who may have been knocked down a peg or two by the incoming animals.

2. Monitoring

After pasture management, the next critical component of your parasite control strategy is monitoring. This includes monitoring your animals by way of body condition scoring and checking the mucous membrane colour for evidence of anaemia. You also need to monitor the faeces for evidence and quantification of parasite burdens. Information from all three monitoring steps is used to assist in determining whether parasite burdens might be an issue. Bear in mind that clinical signs of problems, such as weight loss or anaemia, can occur before eggs and oocysts appear in faecal samples.

Body Condition Scoring

Alpacas should be body condition scored at least monthly, and records should be kept diligently. Any loss of condition may be due to parasites, and faecal screening should be initiated for individuals or groups to see whether parasite burdens are to blame. If not, it may be that the nutrition plan needs adjusting or there may be a medical reason for any weight loss in individuals, but checking for parasites should be the first diagnostic step. Body condition scoring is discussed in detail in Chapter 3.

Mucous Membrane Colour Checking (FAMACHA)

While body condition scoring, I also recommend that you check the mucous membrane colour around the eyes. This can give an indication of anaemia and can be more sensitive at detecting *Haemonchus* problems since this particular worm has larval stages that suck blood from the host: larvae do not produce eggs until they become adults so affected individuals can become clinically anaemic before eggs appear in faecal samples. Mucous membrane colour checking is also discussed in more detail in Chapter 3.

Faecal Screening

Detection of gastrointestinal parasites is achieved by examination of faecal samples for the presence of parasite eggs. It is important to find out exactly which parasites are present so that you can treat them appropriately because there are differences in susceptibilities of the different parasites to different medications (*Figure 6*). Routine faecal screening should always be included as a routine part of any alpaca parasite control strategy. Samples must be taken from individual animals and not from a communal pooping area. This is important for several reasons:

The samples will be as fresh as possible. Once faeces have been passed, eggs start to undergo development into larvae that then hatch. Once the eggs have hatched within a day or two under optimal conditions, testing methods will fail to identify eggs anymore.

Individual sampling allows you to decide which animals to test rather than the poop-pile self-selecting.

You can identify which animals have problems and you can also see the distribution of animals affected. If you collect faeces from a communal pooping area, you do not know which animal it's from.

Avoid pooling your samples. Since only 20% of animals in the herd carry 80% of parasite problems, when you pool samples together, you can fail to detect animals

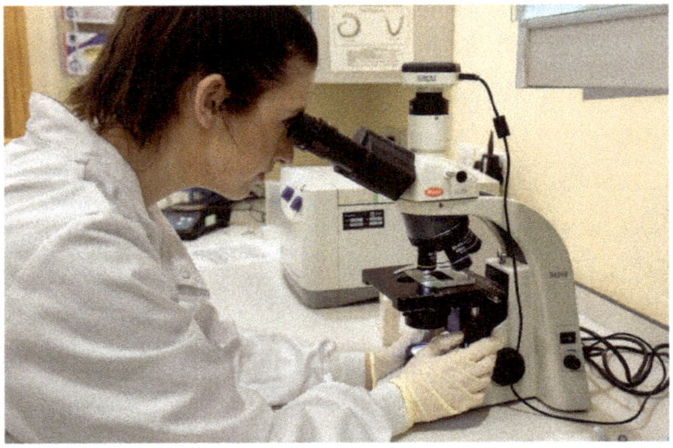

Figure 6. Faecal testing requires the use of some basic laboratory equipment. A good microscope is essential, and a centrifuge is preferable for camelid samples to improve the sensitivity of detection.

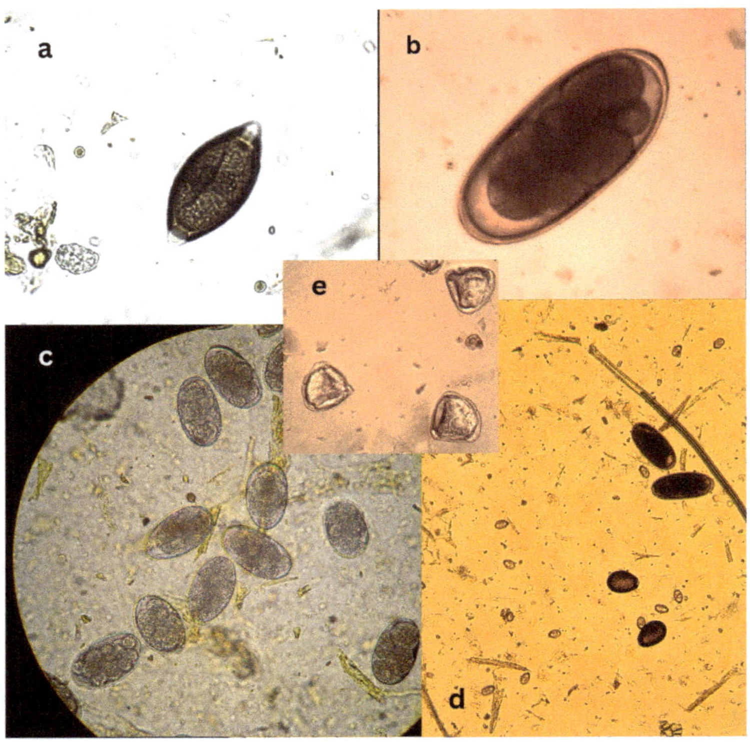

Figure 7. Figure 1 shows a composite picture, not to scale, of the main worm eggs and coccidial oocysts found in camelid faecal samples. A Trichuris, b. Nematodirus, c. strongyles, d. Nematodirus, E macusaniensis and other coccidia, e. Moniezia.

that are heavily parasitized as they may be diluted out by other animals having very low parasite burdens. You also will then have no idea who any "problem" animals are on the farm. Target-selective treatment relies on individual knowledge.

Pooling has mainly been done in sheep farming where animals have low financial value and profit margins are incredibly small. In those conditions, farmers are more likely to accept low-level losses of animals. Camelid owners, in my experience, are not – regardless of the monetary value of the animal. In any case, you should still be collecting individual samples, and the lab then pools the samples by taking a measured quantity from each sample. Otherwise, the lab will merely sample the top faecal beans which are likely from a single unidentified individual.

How Many Samples Should You Check?

When you are screening your herd for parasites, ideally you should check 10% of the herd or 10 animals, whichever is the highest number. If you have fewer than 10 animals, then test all of them and you will have the ideal situation because you will be able to treat each animal individually. In general, the greater the proportion of the herd that is tested, the less likely it is that any problems will be missed: in addition, targeted treatment can be employed if most or all of the herd are tested, and this helps reduce the use of anthelmintics and therefore the development of resistance.

When you have an individual that you want to check, it is always useful to send a representative number of samples from that group. This is because the individual with clinical issues may not always have elevated egg counts, and analyzing multiple samples can provide valuable insights into the level and type of parasite burdens affecting the group.

Which Animals Should You Test?

Consider which animals you are most concerned about because they may have lost condition, are slightly pale, are under stress or are old. Also, consider which animals are likely to have the most problems. Young animals up to 18–24 months of age are more likely to have higher burdens of both worm eggs and coccidia and so are good animals to select. Crias less than 2 months old are unlikely to have worm eggs but may have coccidia identified from about 3 weeks of age. Select a representative number from each group to enable you to make treatment decisions about that group as a whole.

Faecal Testing Methods

There are many different methods available for faecal analysis, with widely varying sensitivities. In general, camelids are sensitive to much lower gastrointestinal parasite burdens than cattle and sheep, presumably since evolutionary development in a cold, arid climate is not conducive to parasite survival on pasture. Hence, exposure levels for the development of immunity may be low. We are therefore concerned with detecting lower levels of parasitism, at egg counts that may be below the level of significance for other domestic ruminants. We want to be able to detect low egg counts, so modified techniques that enable this are superior. Centrifugation of samples alongside the use of a concentrated sugar solution appears to improve detection across all types of worm eggs and the large coccidia *E macusaniensis,* but not the small coccidia. A saline solution McMaster technique was best for maximising small coccidia counts.[7]

The Modified Stoll's test uses a concentrated sugar solution and double centrifugation, which greatly enhances the sensitivity of detection, especially for the larger eggs such as *Nematodirus* and more dense eggs such as *Trichuris.* These are not only significant at low egg counts but also are harder to float. The same is true for *E macusaniensis* as this is a large, dense oocyst. If you want to quantify strongyle-type eggs specifically, the use of the McMaster method will make it easier to be more accurate at higher strongyle egg counts of greater than 300epg – but you will lose the sensitivity of detection of those other potentially harmful eggs and oocysts.

One study evaluated a field-based method, FECPAK[G2], against a modified McMasters solution (using saline with SG 1.20 or sugar solution with SG 1.27).[8] They showed better agreement between tests when sugar solution was used as the floatation fluid, but the type of egg was not reported. However, it should be noted that based on the study mentioned above, the lack of centrifugation appears to reduce the usefulness of detecting heavier or more dense eggs and oocysts that can be clinically significant. Another field-based test, the Mini-FLOTAC, was compared against a high-sensitivity McMaster (using sodium nitrate solution of SG 1.25-1.3), and a modified Wisconsin test using Sheather's sugar solution (SG 1.30), none of which used centrifugation.[9] The McMaster was found to be more sensitive than the Mini-FLOTAC, though the latter has not yet been directly compared to the Modified Stoll's. Based on these studies, the Modified Stoll's is likely to be superior to the field-based testing methods but does require additional equipment to run.

If you find parasite problems in faecal samples that you have to treat, always do follow-up tests on faecal samples from at least some of the treated individuals, to ensure that your treatment has been effective.

3. Medications

We need to be concerned about the potential for parasite drug resistance. For this reason, periodic faecal screening and judicious use of anthelmintic and anticoccidial drugs are recommended. In other words, use the right drug and at the correct dose, based on what is being seen in faecal examinations. Better than choosing a random wormer and hoping it will do the trick!

In Table 1 over the next two pages are the main classes of anthelmintic, anticoccidial and flukicidal medications that are used in camelids.

Name	Active Ingredient	Dose/Route	Spectrum
ANTHELMINTICS			
Benzimidazole ('white')	Albendazole*	10 mg/kg PO (once only)	*Fasciola hepatica, Moniezia,* nematodes, lungworms
Benzimidazole ('white')	Fenbendazole (Panacur)	10-20 mg/kg PO, 5 days 20mg/kg PO, single dose (UK) 50 mg/kg PO, 5 days	Nematodes, lungworms, whipworms: *Nematodirus* (in the US) *Nematodirus* (in the UK) *Moniezia, giardia*
Tetrahydropyrimidine	Pyrantel pamoate	8.5 mg/kg PO 18 mg/kg PO, 3 days	Nematodes Cestodes, nematodes (More used in dogs, cats and horses)
Macrocyclic Lactone (ML, 'clear')	Ivermectin	0.2 mg/kg, PO or SC 0.4-0.6 mg/kg	Nematodes (NB High level of resistance!), lungworms, sucking lice Whipworms, sarcoptic mange
Milbemycin, also a type of macrocyclic lactone	Moxidectin (Cydectin)	0.4 mg/kg PO NOTE this is 2x label dose for sheep	DO NOT USE WITHOUT VET AUTHORISATION
Imidazothiazole ('yellow')	Levamisole	6 mg/kg SC 8 mg/kg PO	Nematodes, lungworms WEIGH ANIMALS TO DOSE CORRECTLY: side effects likely with overdosing
Amino-acetonitrile derivative ('orange')	Monepantel (Zolvix)	7.5mg/kg PO NOTE this is 3x label dose	Roundworms, not whipworms DO NOT USE WITHOUT VET AUTHORISATION

Name	Active Ingredient	Dose/Route	Spectrum
ANTICOCCIDIALS			
Triazine	Diclazuril	1 mg/kg PO	UK, Europe
Triazine	Toltrazuril	15-25 mg/kg PO	UK, Europe, Australia, NZ
Triazine	Ponazuril	10-20 mg/kg PO	US
Sulphonamide antibiotic	Sulfadimethoxine	15 mg/kg twice daily for 5 days, PO	US
Methylpyridine	Amprolium	10 mg/kg, once daily for 5 days, PO	US
FLUKICIDES			
	Praziquantel	50 mg/kg PO	*Dicrocoelium dentriticum*
Sulfonamide	Chlorsulon	7 mg/kg PO	*Fasciola hepatica* (adults)
Salicylanilide	Closantel	10 mg/kg PO	*Fasciola hepatica* (kills adult fluke, + 91% from 5 weeks old), and *Haemonchus*
Benzimidazole	Triclabendazole	12 mg/kg PO	*Fasciola hepatica* (all stages)
Benzimidazole	Albendazole	10 mg/kg, PO	*Fasciola hepatica*

*Table 1. Anthelmintics, anticoccidials and flukicides used in camelids, adapted from Ballweber.[16] PO indicates the drug to be given orally, SC by subcutaneous administration. * indicates not to be used in pregnant animals.*

Where dosing is required for specific worm burdens, animals should also be individually dosed based on weights, preferably actual weights rather than estimates. Under-dosing is an easy way to induce drug-resistant parasites while overdosing (either for single doses or by using multiday courses) can be a problem with certain drugs and cause unwanted side effects. For example, levamisole has quite a low safety index compared to other wormers. It can be dosed at the label dose of 7.5-8 mg/kg (depending on the label) when given orally but is used at 6 mg/kg when given as an injectable product that is available in some countries such as the US. If the oral dose is used for the injectable product, signs of toxicity will be observed that include tremors, head shaking and salivation. Albendazole has been associated with causing severe watery diarrhoea and death in animals that were given multiday courses at multiples of the recommended dose of 10–15 mg/kg given once.[10] Reasonably-priced weigh scales are readily available and weigh bars can be purchased and incorporated into any management system for weighing animals without the need for a handler. These can be walked over a board set securely on top of the bars in a walkway. Having a record of weights is also very useful as a general husbandry tool, to accurately assess weight gain in growing animals or weight loss in adults.

Make sure that you administer the right drug for the job and give it by the correct route of administration *and* at the correct dose. It is most important that anthelmintics are used at the correct dose to achieve successful treatment, but also to avoid the development of drug-resistant parasites. Recommendations on drug use are constantly being updated as new research becomes available, so make sure that you have the most up-to-date information. For example, in recent years worms have become resistant to injectable avermectin drugs such as ivermectin and doramectin (common trade names of these medicines are "Ivomec," "Panomec," "Noromectin," and "Dectomax," respectively). This is most likely because of an over-reliance on these medications for blanket worming during the period when this was a common practice, plus ongoing and frequent use for treatment and prevention of mange and meningeal worms. Pour-on formulations of the avermectins licensed for use in sheep and cattle are not absorbed in sufficient concentrations to be effective. Moxidectin (active ingredient of "Cydectin") is more effective when given orally at twice the sheep dose than when it is used as an injectable, and has less risk of toxicity. Moxidectin should never be used for treating mange or preventing meningeal because if it were, this blanket use is likely to result in rapid development of resistance. Monepantel ("Zolvix") is the most recent class of anthelmintic and should be dosed at 3x the sheep dose, as resistance develops rapidly when underdosed.[11] The latter two drugs are ideal for use in quarantine deworming. Fenbendazole has a high index of safety and is used at 2–4 times the label dose typically. It can be used at up to 50 mg/kg doses for 5 consecutive days for *Giardia* and *P tenuis* – the latter is a "meningeal worm" that causes neurological disease in camelids in North America due to aberrant migration in an atypical host.

Once you have treated a specific parasite burden, you should perform a faecal egg count reduction test (FECRT) to check that your choice of wormer (or anticoccidial) has been effective. Normally you would collect a second faecal sample 10–14 days following treatment, but if using levamisole, the correct interval is slightly shorter at 7 days. You want to see at least a 90% reduction in egg counts, but preferably 95%. If the reduction in egg counts is any less than 90%, then you have significant levels of resistance developing for that particular wormer.

Treatment of coccidia burdens is achieved using one of the triazine drugs (diclazuril, toltrazuril or ponazuril), sulfadimethoxine or amprolium, depending on availability and as detailed in Chapter 9. It is typically young animals that experience the highest burdens and need treatment. You would normally treat all susceptible young stock at the same time.

Some breeders have traditionally used a dosing strategy around weaning time. This may have been using an anticoccidial and potentially a wormer as well. A study by Sue Thomas (a UK-based alpaca breeder) and colleagues actually showed that crias that were treated with fenbendazole (Panacur) at weaning suffered a loss of weight compared to the control group that received nothing at all, a group that received toltrazuril for coccidia only and a group that received both fenbendazole and toltrazuril (wormer and anti-coccidial).[12] Treated groups did show reductions in egg and oocyst counts, but these were only transient, returning to pretreatment levels 4–5 weeks later. Although some individuals will experience stress-related increases in egg and oocyst counts, it is possible that these will remain at acceptable levels and permit immune system development. On farms with low infection pressure, no treatments will likely be required. However, ongoing monitoring of weaning groups is essential. Pre-weaning faecals could be used to benchmark faecal egg and oocyst counts among potential future breeders, not only to guide treatment decisions but also to figure out which animals are more susceptible in the cria group. Susceptibility to gastrointestinal parasites is known to be genetically determined in cattle and other species, and this is likely the same in camelids. More susceptible animals may make less suitable breeding animals.

Liver fluke warrants special mention. In fluke areas, prophylactic anti-fluke medications are recommended because even specialised methods of detection are not necessarily going to detect if infection is present. At certain times of the year, such as winter in the UK, when adult fluke are likely to be present, faecal screening for fluke eggs can be a useful tool. This is when pooled testing is valid because a single positive test indicates the possibility of infection in the herd. On the other hand, a negative test does not rule out fluke – only a positive test is useful and even a single egg is a concern. Always perform postmortem examinations on any animals that die so that fluke can be ruled out as a concern. Once you know you have a problem with fluke on your land, prophylactic medication is warranted along with the other control measures outlined in Chapter 9. Therefore, talk to your local vet about the risk of fluke in your area and adopt a prophylactic drug regime to cover this possibility based on their advice.

Barbervax[R] is a commercially available vaccine against *Haemonchus contortus*. It is available in Australia and South Africa and can be imported under license in the UK. Lambs given 5 doses of vaccine 4 weeks apart, and yearling sheep given 4 doses the following year had reduced egg counts of 84% and 65–84% respectively, compared to control (unvaccinated) sheep.[13] The vaccine has received limited trials in alpacas. Three doses were given at intervals of 3 weeks to young alpacas. The vaccine was shown to be safe, and vaccinated alpacas mounted antibody titres to the vaccine.[14] Another study was able to demonstrate a reduction in faecal egg counts using the same protocol in 7-12-month-old alpacas.[15] Vaccinated animals showed increased body weight gain compared to unvaccinated alpacas, and egg counts were reduced but additional studies are required to evaluate longer-term use of the vaccine under field conditions.

Key Takeaways

In conclusion, establishing your own herd-specific parasite control strategy takes time and effort, but it is worth it for the health of your entire herd now and in the future. Examine each of the 3 Ms and their subpoints, reflecting on your current practices and identifying any areas where improvements or changes could be made. Consider engaging the help of your veterinarian or a specialist consultant like myself to help you develop your own herd-specific parasite control strategy and get you on the right track.

Here are some key takeaways:

- It's crucial to use anthelminthics, anticoccidials and flukicides responsibly, and to ensure that others do the same. Once parasites are resistant to all our available medications, there may not be any other tools in the box and animals that need them may die.
- Keep up to date! Advice is changing all the time as we learn how better to manage parasites.
- Never blanket treat your animals. This is the shortcut to drug-resistant parasites and parasite hell in your herd.
- Don't fill all your available pasture with animals. You will always need more space than you think, especially in a climate that loves parasites! If you don't have room, don't get any more, or sell some that you do have.
- Manage your pasture in a way that controls parasites and manages grass growth.
- Give serious consideration to removing faeces from the pasture before eggs can hatch – this is the single most effective measure to control contamination in your pasture.
- Practise proper quarantine!
- Monitor your animals regularly with body condition scoring, pallor checking and faecal testing. All three are essential and are interpreted together, not in isolation.
- Remember that not all parasite burdens require treatment. You're aiming for balance, with your animals firmly in control.
- Breed away from parasite-susceptible family lines.

11

Skin Problems

Skin problems are among the most prevalent issues faced by camelid owners, and they are certainly the most noticeable. One of the key features of a camelid, especially alpacas, is their wonderful fleece. In fact, their fleece is one of the features that draw new owners to them in the first place. When the skin is affected, the fleece is affected, and this affects a camelid's beautiful appearance. Understandably, therefore, owners want to minimise the effects of skin problems to keep their animals looking great at home, in the show ring and to members of the public.

Most skin problems in alpacas are due to external parasites, mange in particular. However, there are a few non-parasitic causes of skin problems to be aware of that we will also cover in this chapter.

Zinc deficiency may be implicated in skin problems. Zinc is found in numerous body tissues, with skeletal muscles and bones being most abundant in zinc, while the skin comes in third place.[1] Zinc is required for skin formation, maintenance of the skin's integrity via barrier function and involvement in the function of immune cells. In humans, zinc deficiency has been associated with a variety of skin conditions, including atopic dermatitis.

Since my residency, we have often observed zinc deficiency in association with skin problems and supplemented as an adjunctive therapy. When I returned home to the UK, an opportunity arose to investigate this as the herd at home was experiencing skin issues that they had already treated as mange but the problems were continuing. I found that there was a lot of scale and scurf at the base of the hairs and the alpacas were also experiencing hair loss and scaling in the less-haired sites of the armpits, belly, inside hind legs and so on. I had the opportunity to involve a student in a project to investigate this. We enrolled 33 alpacas in the study, 19 of whom had skin lesions and 14 of whom appeared to have normal healthy skin. They all had zinc concentrations that were in the range I would regard as suboptimal, but the average concentrations were not different between the group that had skin problems and those that didn't. We used a scoring system to score the skin lesions at 7 sites on the body for hair loss, crusting and scaling. The alpacas were provided with zinc supplementation for the next seven months and then had their zinc concentrations retested and their skin lesions rescored. Zinc concentrations were significantly increased from pre-supplementation levels, and those with skin problems showed significant improvement in their skin scores (Arnold & Whitehead, unpublished). While it is difficult to properly understand whether zinc deficiency *causes* the skin problems that we see, or is just a contributor to the disease, it is worth supplementing those that are deficient to help the skin heal and perform its protective functions. Further research is required in this area.

Part 1: Skin Problems Due to External Parasites

Mite Infestations and Mange

This group of parasites probably causes the most distress for owners of llamas and alpacas since mange, the major concern, is very obvious. It also causes a lot of distress to animals that are affected and can be quite a challenge to treat. The response of individuals to mite infestations may be exaggerated by a hypersensitivity response in the skin to the invading mites. Often it is in addressing the changes caused by hypersensitivity where we need to spend the most time, to return the skin to its normal appearance.

Camelids can be affected by mange due to *Sarcoptes, Psoroptes* and *Chorioptes* mites, and concurrent infestations are possible.[2-4] The distribution of the lesions is typically similar for all types, that is in the inguinal (inside hind legs), perineum (under the tail), axilla (armpit) and belly regions as well as inside the forelimbs and sometimes around the face and ears. The degree of itchiness experienced by affected animals is variable, although it appears to be worse with sarcoptic mange.

Diagnostically, it is worth performing skin scrapes on all cases because the findings may direct therapeutic choices. Your veterinarian will need to do this. The best areas to do skin scrapes from are those that appear to be the most inflamed. It is crucial to perform multiple skin scrapes from several affected areas to maximise the chances of finding mites. Mites can be hard to find, but take enough skin scrapes and you improve the yield. I would estimate that I find mites on skin scrapes about 80% of the time. Things I do to maximise my chances of finding mites are to do both superficial and deep scrapes, collect from multiple sites and also include a scraping from between the toes, as it has been shown that even animals without mange can carry mites between their toes.[5] If there are mites between the toes, although it doesn't prove that those mites are the type causing the mange, given compatible clinical signs, it is likely that they are the culprits. Mites will drop onto the ground and hop onto the next alpaca that comes their way via the toes, so it is a theory that makes sense. I also take my microscope to the farm if I'm visiting the animal on the farm rather than bringing the slides back to the clinic to evaluate. This means that the slides are fresh and there will be little chance for any mites to have walked off the slide in the interim. The skin scrapes are done in oil to help minimise this risk, but they can still wander about! If no mites are found on skin scrapings, and if the lesions are compatible with mange, a therapeutic trial with mange treatment is in order. In many cases, symptomatic therapy (bathing) will help alleviate some of the itching anyway and help the skin, regardless of whether mites are involved.

Biopsy is a tool that I don't tend to use as a first-line diagnostic, but if a case remains refractory to treatment, it may be worth doing in case there is a different issue. At the very least, it might provide some indication that mites are involved due to finding mites, their eggs or evidence of their presence. Biopsy results may suggest a zinc deficiency type problem which can leave the skin more susceptible to damage by mites and other opportunistic pathogens. In mange cases, the results may be as vague as a non-specific "hyperkeratotic, ortho-keratotic dermatitis," which is why I tend to reserve biopsies for those cases who have failed to respond to mange treatment. Secondary bacterial infections are rare in mange and may suggest a different underlying aetiology. This information also suggests that treatment with antibiotics is unnecessary.

Demodicosis due to the *Demodex* mite has also been reported in a yearling alpaca in New Zealand, but to my knowledge has never been reported since.[6]

In any skin problem, I like to check serum zinc concentrations because zinc deficiency has been associated with an increased incidence of skin problems. Whether the deficiency is a contributor to the disease or an incidental finding is uncertain. However, it is worth checking zinc concentrations in affected animals to see whether supplementation is warranted. Zinc is important in keratinisation, therefore supplementation can aid skin repair and potentially help resist invasion by pathogens such as mites.

Sarcoptic Mange

Camelids affected by sarcoptic mange tend to be intensely "pruritic" (itchy) and infection can potentially be fatal in poorly or untreated cases due to the intense discomfort and reduction in eating behaviour. In a national park in Argentina, wild vicuna and guanaco populations were decimated due to the introduction of sarcoptic mange that was thought to have spilt over from mange-infected llamas that were introduced to land adjacent to the park.[7] In Peru, reports of the prevalence of sarcoptic mange in vicunas varied from 12% and 37% and were thought to be responsible for 64% of vicuna deaths in a recent die-off in Peruvian populations.[8] I have also seen domestic camelids succumb to fatal infestations with sarcoptic mange in my practice.

The source of sarcoptic mange mites can be other camelids, but other species may also be responsible for transmission. While *Sarcoptes* mites may be named with a species-specific sub-lineage based on the species from which it was collected, cross-species transmission occurs and is more likely in some host orders than others.[9] Molecular analysis in the Peruvian vicuna populations found that the *Sarcoptes* mites involved closely matched those found in canid mites, suggesting that there may be cross-species transmission. I would suggest that mange-affected foxes, common in the UK, are responsible for at least some of the sarcoptic mange cases I see here in camelids.

Because of the intensely pruritic nature of sarcoptic mange, affected animals are usually identified relatively early by their owners, although lesions may appear quite

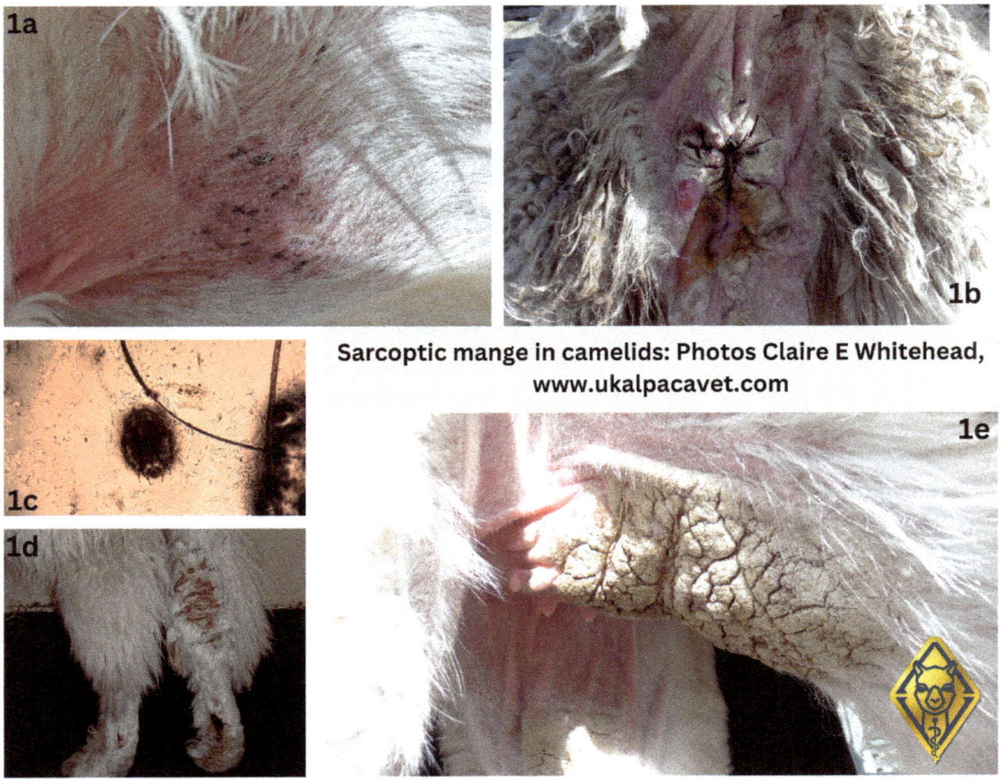

Figure 1. Sarcoptic mange in camelids. Figure 1a shows relatively early lesions with intense inflammation but few scabs. Figures 1b and 1e show more chronic lesions on the perineum and belly with extensive scab formation. Fig 1c shows a sarcoptic mange mite at 40x magnification. Fig 1d shows severe exudative lesions on the forelimbs of a llama.

severe already with extensive crusting and inflammation of the skin, as well as hair loss. Groups of animals may be affected simultaneously. The lesions caused can be extremely inflamed, with oozing of serum and scales/crusts of skin can often be peeled away (*Figure 1*). Sarcoptic mange mites are burrowers and consume intercellular fluid and serum. Even low numbers of mites can cause significant inflammation. This also means that it may be difficult to find the mites on skin scrapes, though this does not mean it's not worth looking for, and in most camelid cases I have found *Sarcoptes* mites to be particularly numerous!

A key difference between *Sarcoptes* and *Chorioptes* mites affects how they are treated. *Sarcoptes* mites consume serum that will contain injected ivermectin while *Chorioptes* mites eat only exfoliated skin cells and will therefore not be exposed to the ivermectin. So ivermectin therapy is far more likely to be effective in treating sarcoptic mange than chorioptic mange. In fact, when you know that chorioptic mange is the culprit, it is virtually pointless to use ivermectin in your treatment regime. It is worth mentioning that the vast majority of mange cases in camelids are NOT *Sarcoptes* related, but a huge amount of ivermectin has been pointlessly administered to camelids with mange.

Sarcoptic mange can affect humans, therefore it is recommended to take appropriate precautions using dedicated or disposable overalls for handling these animals, as well as wearing gloves. I have personally been unfortunate enough to have caught sarcoptic mange from an alpaca that I was treating, and based on my personal experience of 6 weeks of intense itchiness and sleepless nights I would like to encourage you not to repeat my experience! In addition, human dermatology specialists seem remarkably ill-equipped to diagnose zoonotic disease in people, so if you've had contact with mangey camelids, make sure you provide this information to your care provider so that they can treat you more efficiently.

Chorioptic / Psoroptic Mange

Camelids with chorioptic or psoroptic mange tend not to be as itchy as those with sarcoptic mange. Again, multiple animals within a herd may be affected and it seems as though certain individuals appear to be more affected and succumb more frequently. Animals translocated to a new herd may bring mites asymptomatically and then develop mange lesions on arrival, or they may pick up the mites on arrival at the new herd. It can be difficult to know where the mites originated from, but these animals are more susceptible to developing lesions of mange because the stress of moving herd can cause immunosuppression. You should certainly avoid bringing any animals with active skin lesions into the herd without getting them checked by a vet. Be sure to keep them in quarantine for a couple of months before introducing them to the rest of your herd.

Early lesions can be difficult to differentiate from sarcoptic mange lesions without skin scrapes as they begin with inflammation evident as reddened areas of skin and hair loss. Scaling emerges and later lesions become thicker and crustier but tend to remain dry. Longstanding lesions may appear and may have extensive hyper lichenification (thickening of the skin) and pigmentation. It is not uncommon for animals to only be discovered at this stage if owners are not checking their animals thoroughly regularly. Full fleece can mask some lesions until shearing. Most cases have varying degrees of scaliness, crusting and inflammation. The mites can be difficult to find in the more long-standing cases and it's important to find the freshest lesions to scrape for diagnostics. Careful observation under the microscope is required to differentiate chorioptic mites from psoroptic mites. D'Alterio et al demonstrated the presence of *Chorioptes* mites between the digits of alpacas that were not exhibiting clinical signs of mange so between the toes is always a good place to scrape, even when there are no lesions at this site.[5] This may explain the phenomenon

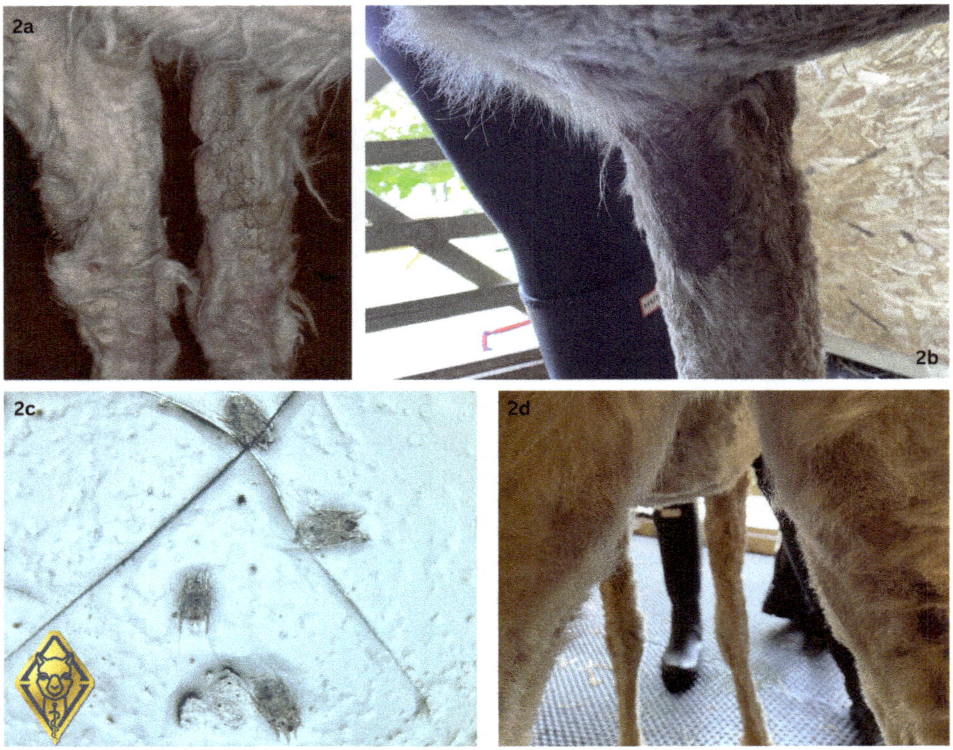

Figure 2. Chorioptic mange in camelids. The images in Figure 2b and 2d show relatively early lesions of chorioptic mange on the upper forelimbs (2b) and back of the hind limbs (2d). In Figure 2d, there is patchy hair loss with a moth-eaten appearance. Figure 2a shows long-standing chorioptic mange lesions with extensive crusting and skin thickening with the formation of thick plaques. The mites in Figure 2c were from skin scrapes from the alpaca in 2d.

of newly purchased animals developing mange after arrival on a new farm in that immunosuppression as a result of stress could result in a previously inapparent mite infestation becoming clinical. Psoroptic mange has been specifically associated with lesions around the ears and face.

Treatment of Mange

In the absence of a specific mite diagnosis on skin scrapes, a therapeutic trial is always a reasonable option if the distribution of lesions is consistent with mange and the animals are, or have been, itchy. I normally treat mange cases with combination therapy that must always include topical therapy. Please remember that when treating any camelids with mange, be aware that mange mites may transfer onto your skin and cause a skin condition on yourself. Therefore, please use gloves when handling mange-affected animals. Also, wear overalls that can be washed after use to prevent any potential transmission onto personal clothing. Disposable overalls are ideal for this purpose. If you experience any skin lesions or itchiness following handling alpacas with mange, you should consult your doctor and tell your doctor about contact with mange.

Topical Therapy

Topical therapy is the most important part of the treatment and one that will result in the most improvement in the animals' condition if it is carried out properly. When the skin is thickened and scaly, you need to use a shampoo that reduces skin thickening. This will need to be a medicated prescription shampoo from your vet. Use a keratolytic or keratoplastic shampoo such as benzoyl peroxide shampoo (e.g. Paxcutol, Virbac) or Sebolytic (Virbac) – these shampoos are particularly good where there is a lot of crusting. You can also use Sebomild (Virbac), or Etiderm if there is any superficial bacterial infection. Etiderm is mildly keratolytic as well as antibacterial but is not going to be the best solution for sorting out crusty scaly skin.

Whatever shampoo is used, it needs to be thoroughly worked into the affected areas of the skin. I use a soft-bristled brush and/or sponge and work it into all the cracks and crevices. Disposable scrub brushes are ideal for this purpose as they have both a sponge and bristles. The shampoo needs to be left on for 20 minutes before rinsing off. During this time, continue to work the shampoo into the skin and pick off any crusts. The shampooing helps to loosen up the crusts and lift them off, in the process making the skin a lot more supple. Clearly, at certain times of the year, warm water and a sheltered/warm area to work are important. After rinsing off the shampoo, the animal needs to be dried off, either by a towel or allowed to drip dry if it's warm weather. Then a topical acaricidal preparation (anti-mite) should be applied to the affected areas. If there isn't much scaling, you can skip directly to the acaricide but the bathing step will be quite soothing for the animal so if you have time, and don't have to treat a whole group, it is well worth doing.

In the UK, I have typically used Frontline spray (fipronil). Fipronil is banned in food-producing animals in North America and Europe. Concerns have been raised regarding environmental toxicity to insects and aquatic life, therefore, alternatives to consider are deltamethrin, or permethrin products (available as pour-ons for farm animals) such as Flypor (Elanco). Both these products would need to use a measured dose smeared directly onto lesions using gloved hands. Deosan Deosect (a horse fly repellent containing cypermethrin) may also be tried, diluted according to directions. Lime sulphur dips and shampoos are also effective against *Chorioptes* mites. However, with the latter, be aware that since this product contains sulphur, it may leave a yellowish residue on the fleece that may be noticeable on white animals. In the US, you can use permethrin (Permectrin III).

This whole procedure of shampooing plus mite-killing treatment needs to be repeated 2–3 times weekly for 2–3 weeks or more depending on how effective the treatment is at addressing skin problems. If the treatment is done correctly, you will normally see quite a big change in 2–3 weeks. But the response

Tips for Bathing

Ideally, when affected animals have really scaly or crusty skin, immersion in water for an extended period (an hour or two) will soften the skin, allowing you to pick off the crusts much more easily. Veterinary hospitals sometimes have large water tanks for floating downer cows, called an Aqua-Cow, which is ideal for this purpose but you have to have a fair amount of warm water to fill it! An alternative for home use would be an old bathtub. You can usually pick up an old bathtub from a local contractor doing renovations, or the local tip. Many alpacas love water and will often try to get into water troughs. If they tolerate it, you could try chukkering the alpaca and lifting it into the tub. You may need the assistance of your vet and some sedation to achieve this. The water in the tub or tank needs to be warm to avoid hypothermia.

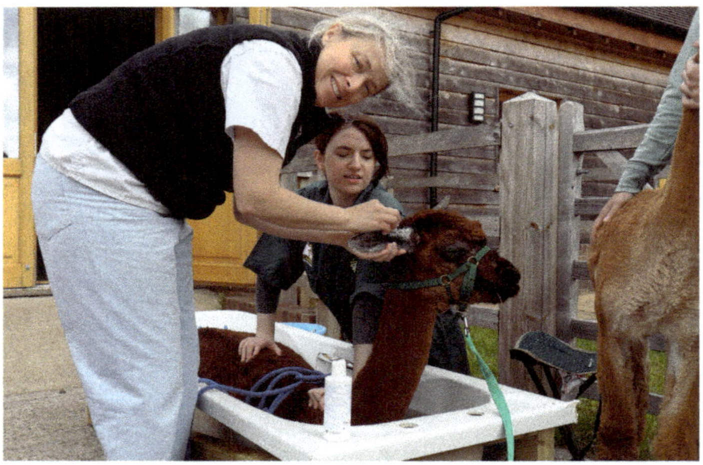

Figure 5. An alpaca being bathed before treatment with medicated shampoo. Bathing for an hour or so softens the skin as well as crusts so that they come off much more easily. It is also super soothing for the animal, and camelids love being in water!

If actual bathing isn't going to be possible, using hosed warm water is the next best thing. If a warm water tap isn't available, you can fill buckets with warm water and use a stomach pump and tubing (I use a stomach tube!) to create a warm water hose. You may be able to get one of these pumps from your vet or source something similar from the hardware store. The hose allows you to get water right up underneath the animal on the belly and in between the hind legs where mange can be quite bad. It's really important to treat all areas effectively. You can do the bathing and shampooing without the hose using just sponges, too.

Finally, if it's cold outside, bring the animals inside to a warm area for bathing as they will get very cold when wet. Use heaters where necessary to improve room temperature.

is highly dependent on the technique, and how enthusiastic you are in performing the bathing!

For sarcoptic mange cases, I have used amitraz (Aludex, Intervet/Schering-Plough Animal Health). However, this product has now been discontinued globally. Instead, a single oral dose of fluralaner has been used effectively to treat sarcoptic mange in alpacas at a dose of 5 mg/kg – this is available as a small animal chewable product (Bravecto, MSD Animal Health UK Ltd or Merck in North America) or as a liquid for treatment of poultry red mites (Exzolt, MSD Animal Health UK Ltd). Efficacy for the treatment of *Chorioptes* mites has not yet been reported. In Canada, off-label use of pesticides such as fipronil is not permitted, but oral fluralaner comes under a different classification as a drug and is permitted – therefore fluralaner may be the only option to try legally.

Ivermectin Injections

Ivermectin injections are useful for sarcoptic mange only, at 500-600 ug/kg body weight every 7–10 days for 3–4 treatments, depending on the severity of the clinical signs. Note that if the mange mite involved is chorioptic, then this is unlikely to be effective. However, if the specific mite has not been identified on skin scrapes and isn't certain based on clinical appearance, then I suggest using ivermectin as a complementary treatment. I do not recommend using longer-acting preparations such as doramectin for these multidose treatment courses as it has a longer duration of effect and repeated dosing may lead to accumulation of the drug in the tissues. You want to aim for repeated peaks of drug concentration in the tissues at intervals that correspond to successive waves of mites as they emerge from their eggs. I would never recommend using moxidectin (Cydectin, Zoetis) because currently, this drug is still highly useful against most gastrointestinal parasites. The more it is used, especially for both mange and worms, the quicker it will become ineffective against gastrointestinal parasites. Cydectin has an initial peak effect that tails off over a long time.

As an alternative, a single oral dose of fluralaner has been used effectively to treat sarcoptic mange in alpacas at a dose of 5 mg/kg – this is available as a small animal chewable product (Bravecto, MSD Animal Health UK Ltd) or as a liquid for treatment of poultry red mites (Exzolt, MSD Animal Health UK Ltd). MSD is known as Merck in North America. As stated above, its efficacy versus chorioptic mange is unknown, but topical therapy is more likely to be effective because of how the mite lives and feeds.

Zinc Supplementation

Zinc supplementation can be helpful when zinc concentrations are found to be low. This needs to be as a chelated zinc rather than zinc sulphate or zinc oxide as this is a much more absorbable form. An example is methionine zinc or zinc methionine (Availazinc, Zinpro) at 1–2 g per head per day for 2–3 months minimum. This is not particularly palatable, so having it mixed in at the feed mill may be possible if you can order enough feed to make it worthwhile. Some feeds already contain quite high levels of bioavailable zinc which may be sufficient. In the UK, one such feed is Camelibra, GWF. The company that makes Camelibra provided us with the zinc-supplemented ration in the study that I described earlier. For any supplementation, whether you mix it into the feed, in a ready-made ration or as an orally administered supplement, you should always check zinc levels again to see how effective the product has been at increasing concentrations.

Vitamin E

Usually packaged with selenium, Vitamin E can be provided as a supplement mainly because of vitamin E's anti-oxidant effect. However, care must be taken with the selenium component as this can be toxic.

Antibiotics

Please note that antibiotics are *rarely* required in the treatment of mange – the only indication would be to treat superficial skin infections (pyoderma) but, in my experience, the presence of a pyoderma should alert suspicion that mange may not be the underlying issue and further diagnostics may be needed. Antibiotics must only be used under the instruction of a prescribing vet and never self-prescribed.

Environmental Management

A crucial part of controlling mange outbreaks is ensuring that the environment does not remain a continual source for re-infestation. *Chorioptes* mites from sheep and goats are known to only survive off the host for a few days, like *Sarcoptes* mites, while those affecting horses have been known to survive up to 70 days in the environment.[10,11] While we do not know the exact life cycle of the *Chorioptes* mites that affect camelids, given the recurrence rate when environmental controls are not instigated, it is my recommendation to err on the side of caution when trying to control the problem and assume that they may stick around for as long as those mites that affect horses. For this reason, following effective treatment (and not before), affected animals should be moved into a "clean" environment, including pasture and shelter space, to avoid re-infestation. During the treatment period, affected animals should ideally be isolated from unaffected herd-mates and confined to an area that can be cleaned, or at least a smaller pasture area that you do not mind being "contaminated" by mites and can be rested for at least 90 days afterwards.

In addition, you need to be aware that in-contact animals may be carrying mites even if they are not clinically affected and have skin lesions. Therefore, check through all in-contact animals carefully for any evidence of mange. If they have lesions, they should be treated. If there are no lesions, these unaffected animals should have your choice of acaricide sprayed below the carpi (front "knees") and hocks to kill any mites that have been picked up from the pasture. Make sure you work it down to the skin and between the toes.

An alternative or additional management tool to consider in terms of dealing with the carriage of mites by unaffected animals is foot-bathing with lime sulphur solution. This has been used with some success in horses, in which *Chorioptes* cause skin disease and particularly pastern dermatitis affecting draught breeds.[12] Lime suphur is keratolytic, bactericidal, fungicidal, antipruritic (stops itching) and antiparasitic. Disadvantages are the sulphurous smell and that it will stain white fleece yellow. Lime sulphur can be bought as a 97.5% sulphurated lime dip (Lime Plus dip, Dechra) and diluted to 5% by using 50 ml in 1 L of water. It has been suggested to use this in a foot dip for alpacas to control *Chorioptes* carriage. Anecdotal evidence is encouraging for this to be included in mange management, although no studies have evaluated its efficacy. The alpacas would need to stand in the solution for 30 seconds or so to allow it to soak in properly: they should stand on hard standing for 20-30 mins post-dip. Dipping would need to be repeated at intervals depending on the clinical scenario and circumstances of the individual farm.

Weekly treatment of mange with topical eprinomectin (Eprinex) has been reported, but after four treatments it was not possible to eradicate chorioptic mange mites.[3] In another study, it was shown that eprinomectin was ineffective at treating mange.[4] In general, the key to treating the chronic crusting and scaling that occurs with mange is to treat the skin. While topical acaricidal treatments will kill mites that come into contact with the treatment, with extensive crust and scale, it may be difficult to kill the mites if the treatment doesn't reach them. Therefore, using a keratolytic or keratoplastic shampoo is very useful for removing the crusts. It also helps to reduce skin thickening and improve the overall appearance of the skin. This is what gives a much more dramatic impression on you as owners who, after all, keep these animals for their fleece and appearance!

One of the most frustrating aspects of mange is the crusty skin on affected alpacas. Owners have tried many different off-the-shelf treatments to try to soften the skin and reduce the thickening. Most of the creams are barrier creams like Sudocreme, which I find a little annoying when you come to treat them, as they are sticky and quite difficult to shampoo off. I found that in animals with very crusty skin, using a cream containing palmitoylethanolamide (PEA-derm cream, Kela Animal Health) was extremely beneficial in removing those crusts and improving the appearance of the skin. It also soaks in really nicely. It can be used in animals that are undergoing mange treatment, and used on the skin on days in between mange treatment days. The cream can also be used in animals that have crusty skin but no evidence of active mange. It won't treat mange by itself, but it can be useful as an adjunctive therapy. Unfortunately, in the UK our Veterinary Medicines Directorate determined that this product needs to be a prescription product, so it is unavailable in the UK. It is still available in Europe, however.

Lice

Lice infestations occur in camelids and can cause "pruritus" (itching) and anaemia. Affected animals may also experience weight loss and some hair loss. Lice may be found over the trunk and down the neck in the hair coat. They like winter fleeces that provide a nice warm environment and naturally decline in the summer months when it is hot and animals are shorn. There are two main groups of lice – sucking lice and chewing lice. The sucking lice have a narrow head and suck blood out of the animal they're infesting: if the infestation is severe, this can result in anaemia. Chewing lice have a larger, flatter head and these lice feed off dead skin as it is shed from the surface. Lice can be seen by the naked eye but you have to look closely as a cursory glance may cause you to miss the diagnosis. Lice can look very like scurf or debris in the hair coat. Sucking lice are almost see-through until they've sucked blood, after which they turn black as their bellies fill with digested blood, making them quite easy to see on a white animal. If you have an anaemic camelid patient, always check for lice as well as *Haemonchus!*

Sucking lice can be treated with injectable avermectins. For chewing lice, use a topical product licensed for killing lice in other species. This can be administered from a 50 ml syringe and applicator tube in several lines, along the topline and also down the sides of the animals, by attaching the syringe to an insemination pipette and applying after parting the hair.

Blowfly Strike

This condition affects camelids in much the same way as other small ruminants. Blowflies are attracted to wounds and moist skin - this can include wet or damp fleece from rain, faeces, urine or other body fluids. Screwworm larvae that are found in South America and Africa may cause primary damage to the skin that will then also be invaded by other blowfly. I once saw a group of animals with sarcoptic mange that were secondarily affected by fly strike due to the serum oozing from the skin lesions. Always keep an eye out for wet patches of fleece on your animals from spring to autumn, when flies are around. If you see wet patches, you must investigate the cause without delay. The animals may already be affected by fly strike or you can take steps to deal with the

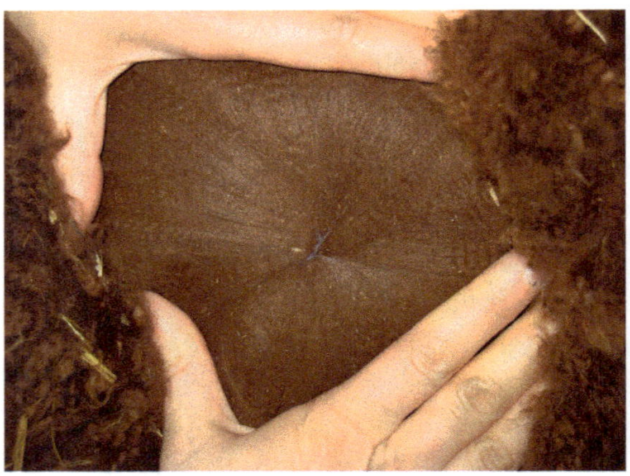

Figure 3. This young alpaca has chewing lice in the fleece. Some of the flecks apparent in this photo are scurf but most are chewing lice.

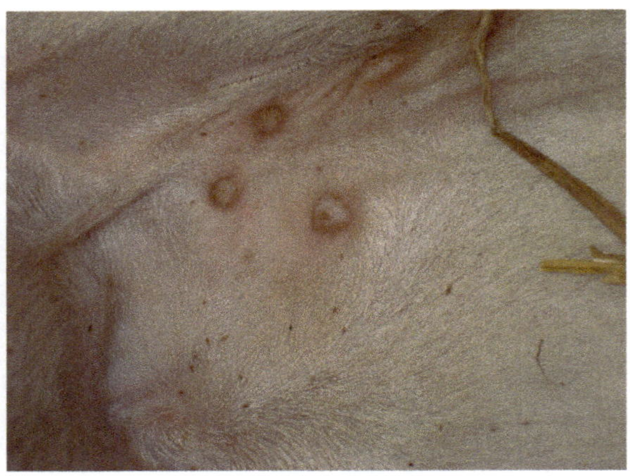

Figure 4. This alpaca has a severe infestation of sucking lice. The alpaca died from anaemia shortly before this photo was taken.

cause of the wetness.

In fly strike, the flies lay their eggs in large batches of up to 300 eggs, hatching within just a few hours. The larvae cause direct and indirect damage to the skin. They feed on the tissue causing damage with their mouthparts and also secrete enzymes to break down the tissues. Toxins are released that may be absorbed into the bloodstream resulting in toxaemia in the affected animals. This can cause affected animals to become dull and listless and they may die if the problem is not recognised and treated quickly.

Treatment does require a strong stomach and involves physical removal of all visible maggots, making sure you check in the fleece surrounding the affected area. There may be larvae of different sizes present. It will help to clip the fleece away from the wound area as this facilitates removal and cleaning of the affected area with iodine or chlorhexidine solution. You may prefer to call your vet and ask for their assistance in treating this, particularly if you have not done it before or do not have the required equipment and treatments. However, once you have learned how to deal with these, you will be able to deal with most cases yourself, except those who are systemically unwell. Following wound cleaning, apply an insecticidal treatment that is licensed for use in sheep specifically for treating fly strike. In addition, in any animal that appears to be systemically compromised with signs of weakness or depression, intravenous fluid therapy for toxic shock is indicated. Systemic antibiotics and anti-inflammatories will be recommended in such cases.

When sourcing a treatment for blowfly strike, you need to make sure that you find one that treats an existing strike rather than one that just prevents the development of larvae. These products contain cypermethrins which may also protect from further strike, or deltamethrin which will only treat an existing strike. Make sure you read the label, follow the directions and use appropriate PPE.

Dermatophilosis

Dermatophilosis is caused by the bacterium *Dermatophilus congolensis.* It is also called "lumpy wool disease" in sheep, or "rain scald" in horses or also "rain rot." It is most frequently found in camelids following periods of wet weather that don't allow the skin to dry out properly, but the lesions may not be noticed for some time, and may only be found at shearing. The constantly wet skin becomes more susceptible to invasion by *Dermatophilus.*

Lesions are found on the topline, particularly at the base of the neck where there are folds of skin that reduce the ability of the skin to dry. Dermatophilus causes crusting of various thicknesses. When crusts are removed, the lesions can be quite sensitive, and crusts often come away with hair attached (paintbrush lesions). Crusts can be macerated on a slide with saline or potassium hydroxide, air-dried and then stained with typical veterinary stains such as Diff-Quik. Characteristic rows of gram-positive cocci bacteria may be identified.

Affected animals should be brought out of the wet environment if applicable at the time of discovery. Lesions should be cleaned with chlorhexidine. Most lesions are already old by the time of discovery, but if you find active infections that are still moist, they can be treated with antibiotics as well – the preferred treatment is penicillin once daily for 5 days.

Ringworm

Ringworms appear to be quite rare to camelids. Rosychuk describes focal areas of hair loss with scaling and crusting that occur primarily in the short-haired areas of skin.[13] I have seen it in young camelids around the face where it caused thick plaque-like lesions and caused difficulty breathing due to lesions around the nostrils. These crias also had scurf in the fleece at the bottom of the chest. Diagnosis is based on fungal culture or PCR. Treatment with fungicidal washes licensed in other species (e.g. enilconazole) is effective.

Midge Hypersensitivity

Midge hypersensitivity has been documented and there are numerous anecdotal reports.[14] Lesions tend to be bilaterally symmetrical and affect the skin of the ears, around the eyes, nose, armpits, belly, groin and lower limbs. Lesions include hair loss as well as crusting and thickening of the skin with occasional papules. If midges are an apparent concern in your area, consider protective housing from dusk til dawn and the use of fly zapping devices, fly collection devices and sprays that contain permethrin.

Part 2: Skin Problems Not Caused by Parasites

Some skin problems are not caused by parasites, although these are less well-defined. I believe that there is a lot of research that needs to be done in this area to find better diagnostics and therapeutics for camelids with skin disease.

Cutaneous papillomas or warts are sometimes found on camelids, normally around the nose. These are caused by papillomavirus and are usually evident in young animals, typically less than two years of age. They usually don't cause any problems and resolve spontaneously.

Skin tumours may occasionally occur, including fibromas, fibropapillomas, fibrosarcomas, trichoepitheliomas and squamous cell carcinoma.[14] Any lumps in the skin can be biopsied or aspirated to obtain a diagnosis and excision may be warranted.

Some alpacas appear to be prone to sebaceous cysts, particularly suris. Owners may notice little scabs on the skin. They appear painful when squeezed, but a thick plug of waxy sebaceous material can be squeezed out of these, leaving a pit usually about 1 cm in diameter that requires cleaning.

I have seen some alpacas with allergic skin disease. These animals may have lesions that appear very similar to those caused by mange, in that the distribution affects all the less hairy areas of the body. For this, you will observe hair loss, itching, reddening of the skin and scaling/crusting. These cases will not have mites found on skin scrapes, but since mites are not always found in mange cases, this failure to find mites cannot be used as a rule out of mange. Since they look so like mange, they should be treated as above for mange. If they fail to respond to appropriately aggressive therapy, then further diagnostics can be attempted.

In these cases, I will consider performing biopsies of the skin and also allergy testing. There are two ways to do allergy testing. One method includes clipping a panel of fleece from the trunk and injecting a load of allergens intradermally and then observing the skin reactions. The other method involves blood testing and submitting samples to a specialised lab for allergy testing. I only have personal experience with the blood testing method. It is important that mange has been ruled out before testing, otherwise it can adversely affect the quality of the results. Also, having worked with one laboratory that used two separate methods at the time, in a single case only, we found that the Greer *equine* assay wasn't suitable as there were too many very high measurements found for them to be meaningful. On the other hand, the Heska assay was more believable. Based on the results, you then look to see what is present in the individual's environment and build an immunotherapy treatment based on a combination of the test results and the allergens present in the environment. If successful, you will start to see improvement within 3–6 months. Lifelong treatment is required.

When owners hear about allergic skin disease, it is common for them all to think that their animals must have allergies when 90% of the time, they have mange that hasn't been treated effectively. It is essential to follow an appropriate mange treatment before allergy testing to avoid interference with test results, and also because the testing and treatment are expensive and lifelong.

Autoimmune skin diseases are also a possibility, although rare, and require skin biopsy for diagnosis. Steroid therapy is required to treat these so is incompatible with breeding females.

Atopic dermatitis is a well-characterised inflammatory skin problem in people and dogs. In other species, genetics, environmental factors, hormonal changes, stress and vitamin D deficiency have been implicated and it likely results from an interaction between genetics and those other factors, particularly the environmental triggers such as exposure to mites and pollens. This remains an unexplored area in camelid medicine.

Key Takeaways

Skin problems in camelids are among the most common experienced by owners. Here are some key takeaway points from this chapter:

- Mange is the most important cause of itching, hair loss and scaling of the skin but is often poorly treated by owners and vets alike. Most cases of mange in camelids are caused by *Chorioptes* mites rather than *Sarcoptes* mites and this means that it will typically not respond to injectable ivermectin, which, although incorrect, is the most commonly employed treatment.
- Topical treatment with medicated shampoos is likely the most effective approach for relieving itching and addressing skin changes caused by hypersensitivity.
- Make sure that your vet performs skin scrapes to identify the mite involved in mange so that treatment can be directed appropriately.
- Management of a mange problem should include screening the rest of the group or herd and taking steps to reduce environmental contamination and re-infestations.
- Consider lice infestation as an important differential diagnosis for anaemia in camelids.
- Be on the lookout for moist patches of fleece on camelids and inspect for blowfly strike as this can have a serious impact on the animal within hours.
- Dermatophilosis is an adverse consequence of camelids being in a wet environment, but this can be easily diagnosed and treated.

In the next chapter, we will talk about neurological problems affecting camelids. These are another important group of problems, particularly in North America, due to the presence of meningeal worm.

12

Neurological Problems

Neurological problems are relatively common in camelids and are interesting to me as a vet, which is why I have dedicated a whole chapter to them. They can cause worrying problems for the affected animals, and this causes a lot of stress for owners. The diagnosis can be narrowed down by careful examination, application of knowledge and diagnostic testing.

However, this can become expensive if advanced imaging modalities such as CT or MRI are required. As an owner, you must first understand whether the problem is potentially treatable and the prognosis. To arrive at this point, the diagnostics may well be required and a worthwhile expense as it is worse to have persisted down a path of exhausting care for a recumbent animal only to find that it didn't make any difference. Be prepared to consider a referral to get the answers you seek.

Two-Minute Overview of Neurology

Before we delve into the different neurological problems affecting camelids, it might be helpful to consider why we see neurological deficits and provide some simple explanations for how they occur. Don't worry, I'll keep it as simple as I can! It is useful to think of the nervous system as a communications highway in the body. Signals travel up and down the "highways" (spinal cord) and "side roads" (peripheral nerves) to control movement, sensation and reflexes. Reflexes do not require conscious control and include things like a withdrawal reflex from a stimulus and the patellar reflex that causes your lower leg to jump forward when a reflex hammer stimulates the patella tendon. The cranial nerves are a specialised group of nerves that control movement, sensation and reflexes around the head. When there is a problem, some of these roads may get obstructed or narrowed, affecting how the signals reach different parts of the body. This may affect the ability of the body to move, feel or how it reacts to stimuli. We can narrow down where the source of the problem is by evaluating the body's ability to perform these normal functions.

Spinal Cord Deficits

As vets, we have to do various tests to localise a spinal cord lesion to a particular area of the spine. One of the things we look for is awareness of body position (proprioception). Typically, an animal will stand with its feet square underneath itself. If you pull a foot out of the normal position by placing it to the side or turning it over so that the animal bears weight on the top of its foot, the animal will put it back to where it should be. If an animal has reduced proprioception, there will be a delay in returning the foot to its normal position. They also have to be able to move the leg, which requires the motor nerves supplying the muscles to be functional. The pathways responsible for proprioception are superficial in the spinal cord, so in the event of a lesion that impinges on the spinal canal, reduced proprioception is the first problem you will see. Reduced proprioception, as well as intracranial (in the brain) problems, also result in uncoordinated walking (called "ataxia"). So, it is useful to observe the animal walking if possible. A few tests can be done to exaggerate subtle proprioceptive problems.

We can also check various involuntary reflexes, such as the patellar and perineal reflexes and withdrawal reflexes of the fore and hind limbs when the toes are pinched. Movement indicates an intact reflex arc, but there are nuances that we won't go into here. Finally, we can check for the perception of pain in animals that are recumbent and unable to stand. Initially, we can check for perception of superficial pain by pinching the skin with forceps. If there is no response, such as pulling the limb away, making head movements, or crying out, we can check for deep pain by squeezing the nailbed. The nerves that carry signals to the brain regarding deep pain are deepest in the spinal cord and are the last tract to be damaged, reflecting more severe injury. So, an absence of deep pain perception would carry an extremely poor prognosis.

Level of Damage

In the simplest terms, we can localise a lesion to a particular spinal cord region based on the above tests, although there are some other tools that we can use to define the lesion further. For our purposes here, though, this simplistic approach is adequate:

- Forelimbs and hindlimbs affected with weakness/paralysis indicate a lesion between the 1st and 5th cervical vertebrae (C1-C5)
- Reduced/absent reflexes in forelimbs and normal/increased reflexes in hindlimbs indicate a lesion affecting the 6th cervical vertebra to the 2nd thoracic vertebra (C6-T2)
- Hindlimbs only affected indicate a lesion after T2.

The cranial nerves are a little more complicated, but each nerve can be evaluated to determine the likely location of the problem. Brain lesions can also cause weakness or paralysis of the limbs, but there will usually be some indication that the brain is also involved, such as central depression, circling and cranial nerve deficits.

Having looked at the basics of neurology, we can now move on to the specific problems that affect the nervous system. There are a number of problems that can cause neurologic complaints in camelids, and I will cover them under the following general headings.

1. Developmental Problems
2. Trauma
3. Infections Of The Spine, Middle/Inner Ear Or Brain
4. Space-Occupying Lesions In The Brain
5. Polioencephalomalacia
6. Degenerative Conditions
7. Parasitic Infections
8. Thermoregulatory Problems

Developmental Problems

Congenital abnormalities that affect the nervous system may or may not be apparent at birth. One of the more common issues affecting the brain is cerebellar hypoplasia. This may be inherited or occur due to infections with viruses that occur during pregnancy, including BVD, bluetongue virus and Akabane virus. Signs of cerebellar hypoplasia include tremors, high-stepping gait, wide-based stance, swaying and seizures. Usually, the problem isn't progressive and affected animals learn to adapt, but consideration should be given to the potential aetiology in a herd setting.

Congenital vertebral malformations may include shortened, misshapen or fused vertebrae. Affected animals may not show clinical neurological signs right away, but as they grow, the abnormality may put increasing pressure on the spinal cord, resulting in deficits depending on the location as described above. Plain radiographs are usually more than adequate for diagnosing these issues. Unfortunately, euthanasia is the only realistic option. If you are a breeder, you should also consider the potential heritability, as this may have been inherited from a parent. Investigations into the offspring of one particular stud male in Australia with an abnormal tail found that 12 of 30 crias had abnormally deviated tails, and 5 had abnormally short tails.[1] The sire and nine of the offspring had their tails radiographed: the male had 5 abnormal vertebrae in his tail, and only one of his offspring was free of defects. While a crooked tail may not be a big deal for the animal, these defects can occur elsewhere in the spine, where they would cause neurological problems and be a welfare concern. Crooked tails are highly unlikely to be due to trauma, unlike small animals that are prone to door-trapping injuries. Owners are encouraged to investigate any crooked tails with radiography and avoid breeding affected animals in case these traits are passed on to their offspring.

Trauma

Traumatic injury to the head or spine can result in neurological signs. The clinical signs observed depend on the area of the nervous system that is damaged. Most commonly, cervical vertebral injuries result from incidents with fencing. From the owner's perspective, the primary consideration is whether recovery is likely, as this will help guide decisions about the level of time and financial investment to dedicate to these cases. Cervical vertebral injuries are well tolerated in adult animals, and they go unnoticed until shearing, when you notice that they have an abnormal bump or curvature of the neck. The reason they're well tolerated in adults is because the spinal canal is very wide in the neck region, so any curvature results in no or limited compression of the spinal cord. The pressure on the spinal cord causes the neurologic problems and deficits you might see. The lesions include luxation of the vertebrae, and fractures may also be associated with the articular facets that normally maintain alignment and limit excessive movement of the spine.

On the other hand, any neck trauma in crias is much more likely to result in neurological signs developing as they grow. This is because any fractures heal by fusing adjacent vertebrae, worsening the curvature as they grow, compressing the spinal cord and causing neuro deficits. The deficits will start with a lack of awareness of body position, so the affected individual will start to trip and fall or stand with the feet in an abnormal resting position. These will then develop into weakness, recumbency and eventual paralysis.

Radiographs are useful for distinguishing abnormalities from congenital malformations and vertebral infections. They will also help determine whether medical or surgical management would be more appropriate. For adult animals with cervical vertebral injuries, treatment usually involves rest and non-steroidal anti-inflammatory medications (NSAIDs); any initial neurological deficits will hopefully resolve. The prognosis is worse for crias due to the secondary issues that develop as they grow. Stabilisation of the neck with braces or casting is not well tolerated. Surgical fixation is also challenging but may be needed if the fractures are unstable. However, when adjacent vertebrae heal, they fuse, and the subsequent lack of neck mobility can cause the vertebrae on either side to also luxate. Surgical options are going to be costly and with an unknown prognosis, may be off-putting.

Spinal trauma at a location other than in the neck is uncommon compared with small animals. However, injuries may occur due to accidents with farm equipment or machinery. I have also seen crias with pathological fractures of the spine associated with rickets – essentially, their bones can thin and become so fragile that they may break their backs if they fall. This type of injury is more common in darker crias because rickets are likely to be more pronounced in darker animals due to pigment interfering with cutaneous vitamin D production. Supplementation prevents this.

Head trauma appears to be more common in crias. This may occur if they run headlong into fences or get their heads stuck during play or exploration. It may also occur if equipment accidentally falls on them. Head trauma may cause brain swelling that will cause dullness, depression and weakness or paralysis of the limbs. In contrast to spinal problems where crias tend to remain bright and alert, these crias will have neurological deficits associated with brain injury. Diagnosis involves careful assessment of the deficits. Imaging can be used to define the injury further. Treatment is aimed at minimising brain swelling using mannitol by slow IV infusion (via a catheter) and nursing care. Historically, steroids have commonly been used to treat traumatic brain injury, but a review of this practice in humans showed a significant increase in the rate of deaths in patients who received steroids. It is, therefore, no longer recommended.[2]

During my residency at Ohio State, there was an extremely memorable case of spinal trauma in a 4-year-old llama named Picalo. His owner called me after finding him down in a field under a fallen tree branch. She was unable to get a vet to visit him and was unable to move him due to his size and being on her own. She had no transportation to be able to bring him to us. Over the following month, his owner called me daily for advice and support. We spoke for an hour most days. She had him shorn and had rigged up a shelter for him, was doing lots of physio and moving him to reduce urine scald. The whole time, he remained bright and alert and ate well. Eventually, I convinced her to find someone to help her with transport, and she brought him in a truck to the university for us to evaluate. She'd rigged up a homemade shelter on the back of an open truck and accompanied him in the back on the 3-hour journey. After a month of recumbency, I was impressed at the condition he was in, given his size. His owner had worked tirelessly to keep him comfortable and clean.

Unfortunately, this is a story that doesn't end well. When we radiographed him, we found fractures of the lumbar spine as well as the left femur. The spinal fracture would have prevented him from feeling the pain associated with the other injuries over the previous month. He had no feeling in either of his hind legs, and we recommended euthanasia. After so long caring for him, his owner was clearly distraught but eventually understood that the prognosis was hopeless.

Infections

Infections in the Spine

Infections in the spine occur due to infection seeding there from elsewhere in the body. At some point, the affected animal likely experienced an infection that resulted in bacteria entering the bloodstream. Sometimes, it ends up causing a localised area of infection called discospondylitis. This is an infectious or inflammatory condition in the intervertebral disc that can extend into the adjacent vertebral endplates and vertebrae. The inflammation and swelling can extend towards the spinal cord, causing compression and associated neurological deficits. Subsequently, abscesses may form. In the early stages of the disease, you may notice subtle signs of neurological dysfunction, such as tripping, abnormal foot position and incoordination. Often, the first thing observed is that the animal is unable to get up, able to stand if assisted, but then can't walk or can't stand at all. What you see depends on the lesion's location and the damage's extent. Unfortunately, these lesions are often quite advanced when the affected individual shows any clinical signs, which can mean they are challenging to treat. However, careful examination to localise the lesion and its severity in conjunction with diagnostics helps determine whether treatment might be worth attempting.

Radiographs are useful as a preliminary diagnostic, but advanced imaging modalities such as CT and MRI are far more sensitive in providing assessment. The images shown in the case story here help to illustrate that. CT and MRI tend to be available at referral centres, although CT is now available more widely at larger clinics, with mobile services also available at practices. Both alpacas and llamas can fit in a standard CT machine for small animals and humans. Paralysed patients may be imaged without anaesthesia as they can be strapped onto the table and cannot move, but for imaging the cervical region, sedation may be required to reduce movement.

Some cases may be amenable to medical or surgical treatment. This is more likely if the patient still has some reflexes, such as a response to deep pain tests. One such case includes a female alpaca called Desi, whose story I present below. Another case was a valuable stud male who developed a low-head carriage and started tripping over his feet. He was also diagnosed with discospondylitis in the intervertebral discs low in his neck. In his case, the owners opted for surgical management to relieve the pressure. That was successful initially, allowing him to return to breeding 15 weeks post-operatively. He sired 10 crias over the

Desi was a 3-year-old black female alpaca who presented in winter for inability to rise. Initially, she'd become quieter than usual. The next day, she was walking in an uncoordinated manner but could still stand. The following day, she progressed to becoming recumbent: at that point, she could stand and walk if assisted but was knuckling over on her hindlimb fetlocks, dragging her back legs along. That day, her vet had started her on a course of non-steroidal anti-inflammatory medications, penicillin and oxytetracycline, but these were changed three days later to florphenicol. She was referred to us six days after the start of clinical signs.

She was seven months pregnant at the time of presentation and had been imported from Australia about five months earlier. At the time of her arrival, she could not bear weight on her hind limbs but could stand on her front limbs, and her reflexes were normal on the front limbs. She could not correct her hindlimb leg position when, for example, I flipped either of her feet over so that she was standing on the top surface of her feet. Her patellar reflexes were normal on both hind legs, meaning that when I knocked her patellar tendon with a reflex hammer, her lower leg jumped forward in a reflex reaction. When I squeezed the nail bed on her hind limb toes, she was able to respond by withdrawing her leg - this is what we call a "deep pain reflex response." One side was worse than the other, but I was able to elicit that withdrawal response on both sides, albeit reduced compared to normal. Deep pain is the last reflex to be lost in spinal cord damage because the nerves responsible for this reflex are the deepest ones in the spinal cord. By comparison, the nerves responsible for awareness of body position (proprioception) are the first to be damaged as they are the most superficial ones in the spinal cord. She had a good anal tone and reduced tail tone but was able to pee and poo normally. On palpation of her spine, an area in the upper lumbar area caused a pain response. Her lesion had to be located behind the nerve roots supplying the forelimbs, meaning it had to be after the second thoracic vertebra. Given the area of pain in the upper lumbar region, this is where we focused our imaging. The presence of reflexes on the hind limbs suggested cause for hope in this case, so the owner was willing to invest in the diagnostics.

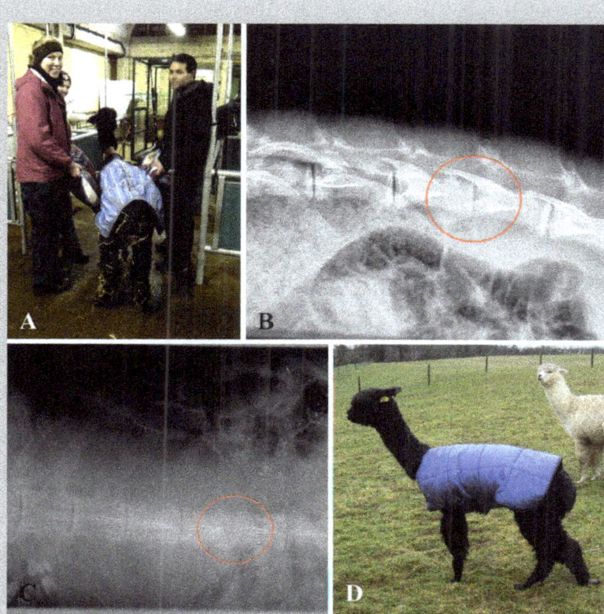

Figure 1. This image shows Desi soon after presentation, being assisted to stand and walk, and soon after discharge back home. Although ambulatory, she was still dragging her feet occasionally. The other two images show lateral (B) and dorsoventral (C) radiographs of her spine. The red circles highlight the narrowed space between the 2nd and 3rd lumbar vertebrae.

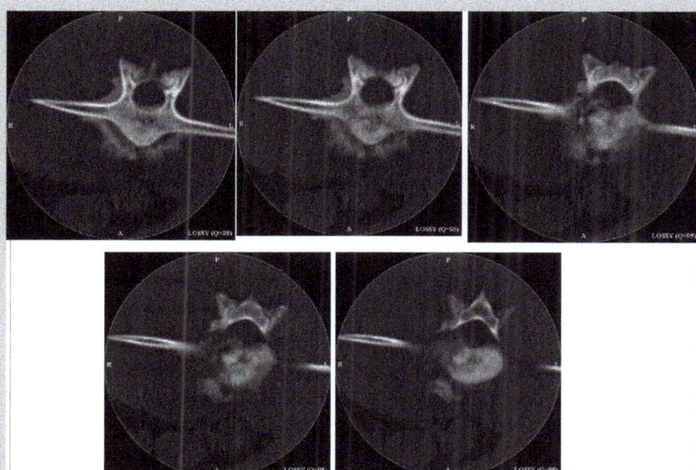

Figure 2. This image shows the CT images of sequential sections through the lumbar vertebrae affected with discospondylitis. You can see bony proliferation, loss of bone, as well as impingement into the spinal canal, which is the central black circle. The damage is quite extensive.

A spinal tap showed signs of inflammation with increased protein and increased white cells. We did plain radiographs first and could appreciate a narrowing of the intervertebral space between the 2nd and 3rd lumbar vertebrae. This was much more apparent in the view taken straight down from above her spine than in the side view. We then used the CT because it is much easier to see details in this area and give a more accurate prognosis. This showed that she had discospondylitis. This is an infectious or inflammatory condition in the intervertebral disc that can extend into the adjacent vertebral endplates and vertebrae. The inflammation can extend towards the spinal cord, causing compression and associated neurological deficits. Subsequently, abscesses may form.

It would have been ideal to have been able to obtain a culture from this lesion, but this would have required performing an MRI-guided aspirate. Given that she had received three different antibiotics the previous week, we decided this wasn't worth the additional cost. Since the owners were not willing to pay for surgical therapy, we opted for medical management that included ongoing antibiotics as well as anti-inflammatories and lots of nursing care. Nursing care was critical in this case. She needed to be moved regularly to keep her clean and avoid urine scalding. She was given physiotherapy three to four times daily to massage her inactive limbs, improve blood flow and provide passive extension and flexion exercises to keep her joints mobile. She was also lifted by a sling several times daily as she was unable to stand up herself, so she walked around the clinic with support. This allowed us to monitor her improvement in mobility. She had little booties put on her hind feet to keep them in the correct position and to prevent scuffing the tops of her feet.

Gradually, her strength returned, and she started to use her legs more and more. Soon, she began to improve the placement of her hind feet. Eventually, she was able to get herself into a standing position! She went home after about six weeks in the hospital, at which point she could rise and walk independently - although she was still turning over on her hind feet occasionally. The owner reported gradual, continuous improvement, and she gave birth to a healthy male cria a month or so later. In fact, she had another couple of crias after that, and her neurological problem resolved so well that it would only have been noticeable to those who knew what she'd been through.

following two seasons, but he was then euthanased due to progressive difficulty raising his head.[3]

Infections in the Brain

Infections in the brain are most likely due to meningitis in young crias, and this is normally an uncommon complication associated with failure of passive transfer of immunity. Occasionally, brain abscesses occur. This can occur at any age. The neurological signs observed depend on the location of the abscess and what structures it puts under pressure. A one-month-old cria presented with progressive neurological signs, including depression, lethargy, neck weakness and weakness in all four limbs.[4] Two brain abscesses were diagnosed on

MRI imaging, and the abscesses were successfully removed via craniotomy. The cria made a full recovery.

In another case, I was asked to evaluate an adult stud male for apparent infertility. The owners reported that he had lost interest in females and wasn't his usual self among the males, as he would normally be the top male and assert his dominance in the group. He'd recently had an abscess on one toe that had been dealt with. He was otherwise in good body condition and was eating well. On examination, he had increased lung sounds and became easily stressed and out of breath when handled. Abdominal and thoracic ultrasound was within normal limits. Bloodwork showed high total protein due to increased globulin concentrations and high liver enzymes, although a liver function test was normal. He also had a high white cell count and increased PCV. I thought he may have developed pneumonia following shearing and the miserable wet weather that had followed. I placed him on a course of antibiotics and anti-inflammatories, and chest x-rays a week later appeared normal. A couple of weeks later, he suddenly deteriorated, showing neurological signs that included incoordination of all four limbs and abnormalities of the cranial nerves. Despite treatment, he continued to deteriorate and was euthanased. A postmortem examination discovered that he had a pituitary abscess. Essentially, this had been causing him a monster headache until it eventually put pressure on other areas of the brain, causing more obvious neurological signs. So, I now have a new differential diagnosis for a male being "off his game"! Pituitary abscesses are not exactly common, but this was the first time it had been diagnosed in an alpaca, to my knowledge.

Infections in the Middle or Inner Ear

Infections in the middle or inner ear can cause neurological signs because they can affect the vestibular system that controls balance. These infections usually get into the middle and inner ear from the upper respiratory tract via the eustachian tubes. The infection gets trapped in the tympanic bulla, otherwise known as the eardrum, with nowhere to drain. In camelids, the tympanic bulla is filled with a network of very fine bone, a little bit like a honeycomb. Infection in the eardrum often results in abscess formation and pieces of bone can become sequestered such that the abscess won't resolve until the abscess ruptures out. This can occur externally, or the infection may extend into the brain. The inflammation and pressure within the eardrum cause lateralising clinical signs such as walking in circles, head tilt to one side, leaning or lying to one side only and a head tick that is slow in one direction and fast in the other. Sometimes, the facial nerve becomes affected because the facial nerve passes through the middle ear. This means we end up with a floppy ear, a lack of muscle tone in the face and potentially an inability to blink on the affected side. With these problems, CT is the only worthwhile diagnostic you can use, and CT-quality images are needed to aid in surgical planning. Radiographs are difficult to interpret due to all the overlying bone structures. Referral to a university clinic may be required where they have the diagnostic and surgical capability. Small animal surgeons are experienced with advanced ear surgeries, though the anatomy differs. University clinics typically have facilities for large animal hospitalisation along with skilled surgical and anaesthesia staff.

Listeriosis is a particular type of infection caused by the bacterium *Listeria monocytogenes.* This bacterium occurs in soil, and the disease listeriosis is often associated with silage feeding because *listeria* proliferates in spoiled silage and haylage bales. It can gain access to the neurological system via cuts in the mouth, from where it works its way to the brain. Listeriosis causes unilateral signs, so animals will have a head tilt, may lean or lie only to one side and may walk in unidirectional circles. Diagnosis is based on compatible clinical signs and a typical increase in a particular white cell type called monocytes on a spinal tap. The disease carries a very poor prognosis due to brain involvement unless treated aggressively and early with intravenous antibiotics, typically oxytetracycline or high-dose penicillin. Supportive care is also crucial, as affected animals often cannot eat or drink.

Space-Occupying Lesions in the Brain

Although rare, tumours or abscesses can occur in the brain. These are always differential diagnoses for animals displaying brain signs such as seizures, abnormal behaviour, circling, blindness, depression and cranial nerve deficits. These lesions are diagnosed premortem using CT or MRI. Reported tumours have included pituitary adenoma in a 12-year-old male llama and 14-year-old male alpaca[5 6], astrocytoma in a 1-month-old llama[7], teratoma in a 4-year-old alpaca[8] and an embryonal tumour in an 11-year-old female alpaca[9]. All cases were euthanased.

Brain abscesses are a possible sequel to the failure of passive transfer, which was the likely cause of two published cases in the literature.[4 10] In one of these cases, a one-month-old alpaca cria with signs of depression, lethargy, paralysis and neck weakness, they were able to surgically remove the two abscesses found on MRI imaging via craniotomy - impressive stuff! Another case in the literature involved a large brain abscess originating from an infection in the middle and inner ear.[11] This alpaca was not so lucky...

Although not caused by a discrete lesion like an abscess or tumour, hydrocephalus can sometimes arise when the drainage of CSF from the brain is obstructed and acts like a space-occupying lesion. I had one such case during my residency in a young cria that we had diagnosed with failure of passive transfer. While in the hospital, she started spending increased amounts of time sleeping until she was practically comatose. An electroencephalogram (EEG) showed that she had diffuse brain swelling, so we walked her down to CT. She didn't need anaesthesia at the time, which cut down our costs for the owner. The scan showed that she had an impressive amount of fluid, called hydrocephalus, that had built up in the ventricles of the brain. This was squashing the brain inside the skull. We assumed this came from meningitis secondary to FPT and the cellular debris obstructing drainage or inflammation impairing CSF absorption. Once the problem was diagnosed, we were able to treat the cria and reduce the swelling. The cria returned to normal, and was discharged home.

Polioencephalomalacia

Polioencephalomalacia (PEM), often "polio" for short (but not the same as polio in humans), is a neurological problem that is very common in camelids. It is also known as cerebrocortical necrosis (or CCN) and is associated with vitamin B1 or thiamine deficiency. The underlying cause is often unknown, but since the microbes normally produce thiamine in C1, deficiency most commonly occurs when the C1 microbes are disrupted. This is most likely when an animal ingests an excessive amount of rapidly fermentable carbohydrates. For example, if they are overfed grain (accidentally or intentionally), eat too many apples or provided uncontrolled access to a lush pasture when they've been used to a barren pasture. When the gut microbes are suddenly presented with an unfamiliar diet, they are sensitive to changes in pH and the thiamine-producing bacteria get killed off. Thiamine is incorporated in an enzyme that controls most glucose metabolism in the brain. When this enzyme is unavailable, in thiamine deficiency, glucose pre-cursors build up, and fluid management in the brain is impaired. This results in brain swelling, increased intracranial pressure and necrosis of the brain. Excessive sulphur intake has been associated with signs of PEM in other ruminants. Another way that signs of thiamine deficiency can occur is through an overdose of amprolium, which is an anticoccidial used in the US. Amprolium is a thiamine analogue, meaning that if too much amprolium is present, it can block thiamine receptors so that not enough thiamine is absorbed into circulation.

Clinical signs of PEM are consistent in that they typically include sudden onset blindness that can progress to depression. Very few other things will cause sudden onset blindness in animals. Differential diagnoses could include a space-occupying brain lesion like an abscess or a tumour but these would have to be very central to cause blindness that affects both eyes. Lead toxicity is the other main differential. Lead toxicity is usually associated with animals licking car batteries left lying around in fields or lead paint, but this is rare on a camelid farm.

In the early stages of disease, affected animals might still be walking around, appearing uncoordinated and staggering into things. If the disease progresses, they will become more depressed, recumbent and anorexic. Affected animals may fail to respond to irritating stimuli around the face. Typically, animals will react by pulling sharply away if you tickle the inside of a nostril, but if they've got PEM, this response is depressed. The depression and reduced sensation are indicative of brain swelling.

Occasionally, animals with thiamine deficiency will become hyper-excitable such that they react violently to minimal stimuli, sometimes running into walls. The self-trauma in these cases is a welfare issue, so I'm more likely to recommend euthanasia in these cases if they're not responding quickly to treatment.

Treatment must be aggressive and involve supplementation of vitamin B1 or thiamine. The required dose for thiamine deficiency is 15 mg/kg every 4 hours, either in IV fluids or IM, so the concentration of B1 in the product has to be quite high. A thiamine-only product is ideal for this, as the volume would be too high if multivitamin B products were used. If the thiamine is added to IV fluids that would be required if the patient isn't eating or drinking, it needs to be kept covered away from daylight to avoid deterioration. Thiamine supplementation should continue until several days after resolution of clinical signs and then be reduced gradually. Animals with CNS depression need something to reduce brain swelling as quickly as possible. Mannitol is a neuro-specific diuretic that will help to reduce brain swelling, and this needs to be given as early as possible before irreversible brain damage occurs. It is given as a slow IV infusion, usually over 20 minutes, necessitating IV catheter placement.

In terms of prognosis, where you have a recognised source of carbohydrate overload, in my experience, these cases tend to be much easier to treat than if we don't know the source of the problem. I have seen multiple animals affected in groups on lush pasture that are still ambulatory and eating. These cases recover purely with thiamine supplementation and management to feed and contain them safely until their eyesight returns. Otherwise, the prognosis is poor, particularly if they're intensely depressed, blind, and off food.

Degenerative Conditions

The main problem here to consider is arthritic changes that may occur between the spine's vertebrae, causing fusion. This is most likely at sites where most movement normally occurs, such as the neck and lumbar spine. If arthritic or degenerative changes occur in the neck, it may result in neck immobility, lowered head carriage and pain. Lumbar spine arthritis is more likely to occur in males. It may result in abnormal gait, reduced fertility due to discomfort during breeding and potentially neurological issues if there is impingement on the spinal cord. Surgical management of these cases may be possible if finances and location allow, but medical management with NSAIDs is more realistic for most owners due to the costs involved.

Parasitic Infections

Meningeal worm is a parasitic infection that causes neurological signs in camelids, sheep and goats. It is really a North American phenomenon and is due to the aberrant migration of *Parelaphostrongylus tenuis* larvae in the spinal cord and sometimes the brain of affected camelids. The natural definitive host of *P tenuis* is white-tailed deer, found anywhere east of the Mississippi in North America. The prevalence of meningeal worm in llamas and alpacas is much higher in hilly, forested areas, which provide an ideal habitat for white-tailed deer. Since the white-tailed deer is the animal host for which the parasite is adapted, in this species, the parasite still migrates through the CNS, which is a necessary part of its life cycle but rarely causes overt clinical signs.[12,13] A common misconception is that direct contact with the white-tailed deer causes alpacas and llamas to become infected. However, an intermediate host for the parasite is required. The intermediate hosts are small slugs and snails. First-stage larvae that hatch out of eggs excreted in the faeces of the deer are consumed by molluscs, and then L3 larvae are ingested by the white-tailed deer or inadvertently by llamas and alpacas. The parasitic larvae migrate to the CNS and since they are not within the definitive host, the parasites become "lost" and move about randomly in the CNS. The damage caused by this aberrant larval migration causes the neurological signs we see in llamas and alpacas. Since the migration is random, the clinical signs shown can vary from animal to animal.

An important note is that similar clinical signs have been reported in a llama in the UK that was affected by a different type of parasite called *Elaphostrongylus cervi*. *E cervi* is known to be found in red deer and is prevalent in some parts of the UK, Europe and New Zealand. I'm aware of other potential cases across European countries, so although rare in Europe, it is still worth considering as a differential diagnosis for neurological signs. Supposedly, this parasite is less pathogenic than *P tenuis.* [14]

Experimental infection of llamas with *P tenuis* resulted in clinical neurologic signs 45 to 53 days after infection.[15] This means that you will not see disease manifested in llamas and alpacas until nearly 2 months have passed since ingestion of the parasite. Most cases of meningeal worm occur during the autumn and winter months (October to March). In fact, 79% of 58 cases presented to The Ohio State University between 1993 and 2003 occurred during these months.[16] This can be explained by a knowledge of the parasite life cycle. During the spring and summer, slugs and snails are multiplying while white-tailed deer populations are moving around freely so that the number of infected molluscs accumulates. Susceptible animals ingest the molluscs while grazing, after which there is an incubation period until the development of clinical signs. Eventually, when the first frosts arrive, mollusc populations decline, and the infection rate mirrors this, although it may be up to 2 months before clinical cases are seen. Theoretically, then, there should be a disease-free window in the spring. However, this break in disease transmission may not occur in particularly wet years. For example, from winter to spring of 2004, despite good snowfall and freezing weather for 6 weeks in January and February in Ohio, PME cases were seen throughout this period. This was presumed to be due to a very wet summer and fall the previous year. This knowledge has implications as far as meningeal worm prevention strategies.

Adults are much more commonly infected with meningeal worm than younger animals. The youngest case of meningeal worm I have known was 5 months old. A few animals younger than this are expected to be affected since a certain amount of grazing behaviour is required to acquire the infection, and crias rarely graze significantly until they are at least 2 months old.

As previously mentioned, the clinical signs of meningeal worm can be varied depending on the extent of damage caused by the migrating *P tenuis* larvae. The signs may be sudden (acute) onset or a more gradual appearance of neurologic dysfunction. Typically, though, affected animals will primarily show problems with the hind limbs and often, the forelimbs appear to be spared. They may seem lame in one or both hind limbs and stand with a wide-based hind limb stance. They might stagger as if intoxicated (a condition known as ataxia), fall easily, walk on the tops of their fetlocks or be found lying down in the pasture. A down animal will often appear stronger in its front legs and may try to drag itself around by its front legs. Often, these animals will stand if assisted but need support at the back end to remain standing. Most of the time affected animals appear bright and alert, interested in their environment and have good appetites. However, if clinical signs are advanced or there is brain involvement, this may not be the case. In a small proportion of cases, parasitic migration extends into the brain, resulting in atypical signs of meningeal worm. In these cases, the animal appears depressed, and usually will not be interested in food and a rapid progression of clinical signs occurs. These signs may include vestibular signs (circling, leaning, head tilt) and/or seizures. In this situation, it can be hard to differentiate intracranial migration of *P tenuis* from another neurological disease called listeriosis. Once the brain is involved, the prognosis is extremely poor.

Blood work in animals affected by meningeal worm tends to be unremarkable, except that their muscle enzymes may be increased from lying down a lot more. A spinal tap is a useful diagnostic test in these cases. Out of 58 meningeal worm cases that presented to one teaching hospital, eosinophils were found to be increased in the CSF in 85% of cases having spinal cord signs only. Eosinophils are a type of white cell that is increased in response to parasite problems. The protein concentration was also increased in 73% of cases.[16]

Treatment includes high doses of fenbendazole, which comprises an oral dose of 50 mg/kg daily for 5 consecutive days, as well as NSAID medication. Vitamin B1 can be provided because it is neuro-supportive, and vitamin E can be provided for its antioxidant capability. Since most patients eat and drink normally, fluid therapy isn't required. Pantoprazole may be useful in preventing C3 ulcers, particularly in hospitalised camelids. Physiotherapy is key to keeping the muscles and joints in motion. This can include assistance with stand, slinging, massage and passive extension/flexion exercises, as required. It's important that flooring is non-slip because they are already struggling to stand. Since camelids use their hind legs to stand first, and these are often the most affected, they may sometimes need a bit of assistance to get into a standing position. Once upright, they can often maintain the position on their own for a while.

In my experience, the prognosis is favourable for spinal migration cases, which comprise the vast majority of cases. In one study, 76% of those cases were discharged home and recovered well.[16] By comparison, fewer than 10% of the ones with intracranial migration were discharged from the hospital. Clinical recovery for spinal migration cases is rapid at the beginning of treatment. Any continuing neurological deficits will show gradual improvement out to 6 months, and if any neurologic problems remain at that point, they may be permanent.

Thermoregulatory Problems

South American Camelids are not well adapted to hot and humid conditions. For welfare reasons, therefore, it is crucial to ensure that camelids are shorn before the onset of these hot conditions in summer. Heat stress becomes a risk when the heat stress index – the sum of the percentage humidity and the temperature in degrees Fahrenheit – exceeds 150. When conditions remain hot and humid for some time, the risk of heat stress will increase. Llamas appear to be at greater risk than alpacas, and this may be because they tend to be partially shorn, unlike alpacas that receive a whole-body shear. Also, llamas have a comparatively smaller cooling window. Camelids will sweat, and the most efficient cooling will be from evaporative cooling from the less hairy sites of the axilla, belly and inside hind legs. Fibre reduces that evaporative cooling effect, especially if it's excessively dirty or matted. Animals with limited or no access to shade or water will be at increased risk of heat stress. When the weather is hot, limiting any activity, such as breeding, to the cooler parts of the day is advised.

A camelid with heat stress may be found recumbent and unable to get up, so I have opted to include this under neurological problems. Interestingly, I have observed the forelimbs may be weaker than the hind limbs in heat stress cases. As a result, the camelid may attempt to rise, managing to stand on the hind legs while remaining down at the front. They may be open-mouth breathing and dehydrated. Rectal temperature may be very high, over 40.5°C (105°F) and heart and respiratory rates will be high. You may also want to look out for scrotal oedema in males, as this is an early indication of heat stress.

Checking for Dehydration

The easiest way to check for dehydration is to feel the gums with your fingertip. They should feel moist, like your own. If they feel tacky to the touch, you know that the animal is at least 8% dehydrated.

The first step should be removing the animal from direct sunlight and cooling it down. This can be achieved by shearing or hand-clipping if the animal is in fleece, as well as the provision of fans and ice packs. Intravenous fluid therapy may be necessary to address dehydration and correct electrolyte imbalances common in heat stress. However, animals affected by heat stress are particularly prone to pulmonary oedema if fluids are administered too rapidly. Anti-inflammatory therapy and physiotherapy are also required to treat heat stress cases. One thing we have observed is that these cases have difficulty regulating their body temperature for some time following an incident of heat stress.

Key Takeaways

In this chapter, I began by explaining what causes neurological dysfunction and how we, as veterinarians, can try and localise the problem. There are a number of congenital neurological problems that animals will be born with that may be evident at birth or may take a few months to become apparent. If these animals survive to breeding age, they should not be bred.

- Crooked tails should be investigated, as they are usually caused by deformed vertebrae. While these deformities may not affect the individual, they appear to be heritable and could be passed on to offspring, potentially leading to neurological problems.
- Neck injuries are common but are usually well tolerated in adults, while they may be life-limiting in crias.
- The main differential diagnoses to consider for an animal that cannot stand but remains bright and alert would be trauma, infections in the vertebrae and meningeal worm. Look out for subtle neurological signs in your animals because the damage is less severe and may be more treatable at an early stage.
- Infections that affect the brain generally carry a worse prognosis for recovery. Sudden onset blindness may be associated with thiamine deficiency and may occur following the ingestion of too many rapidly fermentable carbohydrates, which disrupts the ability of the gut microbes to produce thiamine. Supplementation with thiamine at sufficient doses for long enough is recommended. IV mannitol may also be required urgently in cases with depression to reduce brain swelling.
- Meningeal worm is common in eastern North America but is usually treatable - the earlier the treatment starts, the better.
- Heat-stressed animals can appear neurologic. If affected animals aren't too compromised, recovery is possible but may take a lot of nursing care, resulting in disrupted thermoregulation for the rest of the season.

13

Other Common Health Problems

In this chapter, I will present common health problems experienced by camelids. I will group these under the main clinical sign that you will recognise in your animals or by body system so that they are easier to find within the chapter. These are:

1. The "ADR" Camelid
2. Anaemia
3. Colic
4. C3 Ulcers
5. Dental problems
6. Gastrointestinal disease
7. Metabolic Syndrome
8. Orthopaedic Injuries
9. Weight loss
10. Eye Problems

The "ADR" Camelid

ADR is an expression I adopted when I was doing my residency in the US. When I arrived at the veterinary hospital, I kept seeing that the large animal office was recording the presenting complaints of cases we would see as "ADR." I didn't have the foggiest idea what this was, so I had to ask! The response I received was, "Ain't doin' right!" Clear enough! This is a catch-all term for an animal that is not behaving normally and would typically be off food, lethargic and possibly depressed – in other words, nothing specific. When the animal arrived, it could be anywhere on the spectrum of just a bit off to totally collapsed, and its status may have worsened in transit.

If you are faced with an alpaca or llama that isn't right, and there's nothing specific about it, you first need to consider whether it is eating and drinking. If the animal is not eating or drinking, taking action is more urgent because dehydration and negative energy balance are just around the corner, particularly if it's a late pregnant or lactating female. This means that you should not delay getting your veterinarian out to examine the animal. Most likely, you should look at bloodwork and a faecal test as a minimum database, as the underlying pathology is unlikely to be obvious from just a physical examination. If the patient is not eating or drinking, consideration should be given to providing IV fluid therapy until a diagnosis can be obtained. This will help to replace any fluid deficits that are already present while also helping to support normal organ perfusion and function.

I would usually like to see an abdominal ultrasound examination, too, as this can provide additional clues as to what might be happening in the abdomen. The physical examination of camelids is limited regarding what information you can gain from the abdomen. In small animals, we can palpate the abdomen, but in camelids, it is difficult to do this for two reasons: the space behind the rib cage is relatively short, and the whole left side is full of the C1 compartment. In larger animals like horses and cattle, we can palpate rectally to give further information of the organs within reach. This is not often useful in the smaller camelid species and may be difficult to achieve in the smaller patients.

Diagnostic testing can provide much more detailed information than what might be inferred from a physical examination and is often far more revealing than relying on the "veterinary imaginoscope." It can also be used to aid in treatment decisions. For example, electrolyte concentrations can indicate certain conditions, such as an upper gastrointestinal (GI) obstruction and guide fluid therapy. Low phosphorus can suggest the possibility of vitamin D deficiency. We can also see if there is any damage to the kidneys or liver, assess energy balance and evaluate for protein losses. Haematology results can reveal if an animal is dealing with an infection or inflammation, whether it is anaemic, and, if so, whether the body is responding appropriately. Additionally, the white cell count and differential counts can help identify the type of infection. Haematology results are much more revealing if your vet submits fresh samples along with fresh blood smears. The smears are essential in evaluating anaemia because the cells deteriorate quickly in a tube and because the camelid red-cell parasite *Mycoplasma haemolamae* is only found associated with the red cells on a fresh smear made at the time of collection. Diagnostic testing includes biochemistry, haematology, mineralysis, serology for infectious diseases and faecal testing, although other more specific tests are also available.

Diagnostic testing is key to finding a diagnosis in your ADR camelid and determining the correct course of action. The ADR camelid might be suffering from one of the issues outlined in this chapter, but it could also have other conditions, such as metabolic syndrome. In this case, a negative energy balance causes body fat to be mobilised from storage sites to the liver, where it is used as an alternative energy source. This is most common in late pregnant and lactating females with higher energy and protein demands. They can present with very vague signs of illness. Animals with tumours may also fall into this category and can be diagnosed following the diagnostic pathway, but are not discussed elsewhere in this chapter.

Anaemia

We have already discussed how to assess your camelids for evidence of anaemia in Chapter 3. With practice, you will be able to tell how anaemic your animal is. You can first detect anaemia once the PCV drops below about 15%. Lower than this, they will become progressively paler, down to 3%. I have never seen an alpaca or llama with a PCV of less than this, so I don't know if it's actually possible! With a PCV of 3 or 4%, the mucous membranes will literally be white as a sheet. These patients are unlikely to be standing when you find them or will rapidly become recumbent once caught for examination. They need veterinary attention fast!

The normal packed cell volume, or proportion of red blood cells in the blood, is 24–28% for adult camelids at sea level, while newborns tend to be slightly higher at 27–32%. Mild anaemia, characterised by a PCV of 20–24%, is typically not noticeable clinically. Moderate anaemia, with a PCV of 12–19%, is also usually not evident in terms of reduced activity levels but may be detectable through mucous membrane examination, particularly at the lower end of this range. Severe anaemia with PCV of 11% or less will become evident as lethargy, increased time lying down and quiet behaviour when caught. The pallor of the mucous membranes is very evident once a patient reaches about 8% PCV, and these patients will start to eat less and lie down considerably more.

Causes of Anaemia

By far and away, the most common cause of anaemia in camelids is parasitism, mainly due to *Haemonchus* (commonly known as the "Barber pole worm") and occasionally *trichuris.* Other causes of anaemia include the blood parasite *Mycoplasma haemolamae* and infestations with sucking lice. However, on its own, *M haemolamae* doesn't usually cause PCV to drop below about 10%. Other causes of mild to moderate anaemia include inactive bone marrow, iron deficiency, copper deficiency or toxicity, cancers, bleeding (internally or externally) and chronic disease.

What to Do If You Think Your Camelid Is Anaemic?

Anaemia is a condition that requires veterinary attention. Firstly, routine clinical evaluation of the patient is performed, and then diagnostics are done to determine the underlying problem. It's important to establish just how anaemic the patient is because this affects how the condition will be managed. If the PCV is less than 10% or even 12%, a blood transfusion is required in addition to addressing the underlying problem. This is because oxygen delivery to the tissues is impaired at values less than this. This can cause organ failure if the situation persists for too long. If the PCV is higher than 12%, then a blood transfusion isn't required, but appropriate management must be initiated to rectify the underlying problem and monitor the PCV to ensure recovery.

Camelids with a really low PCV of 3-5% may present collapsed (*Figures 1 and 2*). This is because they are very weak. The muscles that hold their head and neck up need oxygen, too, so when they don't have it, they collapse and can't even hold their heads up. These individuals' blood feels as thin as water when collecting a blood sample. Because they look so bad in this state, the temptation might be to think they are beyond help, but this is not normally the case. Once an IV catheter is placed and they receive a blood transfusion, it's phenomenal how dramatic a response you see as they will literally come back to life in front of your eyes. Giving them red blood cells returns the oxygen into their tissues, and they can start to function again. I have seen animals start eating during a transfusion and then walk off at the end. It is that quick!

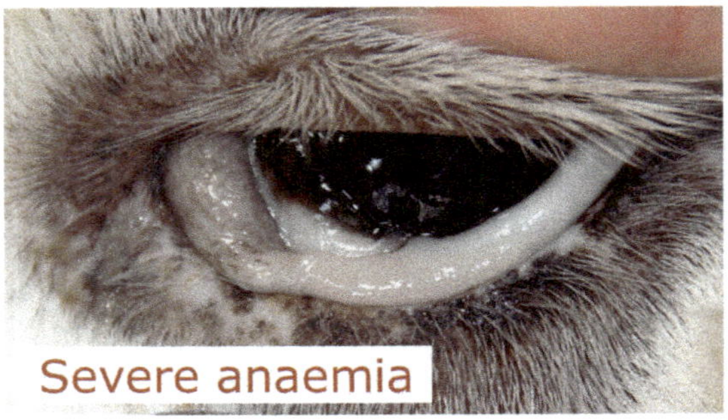

Figure 1. This alpaca has severe anaemia characterised by very pale mucous membranes. The patient will need a blood transfusion as soon as possible.

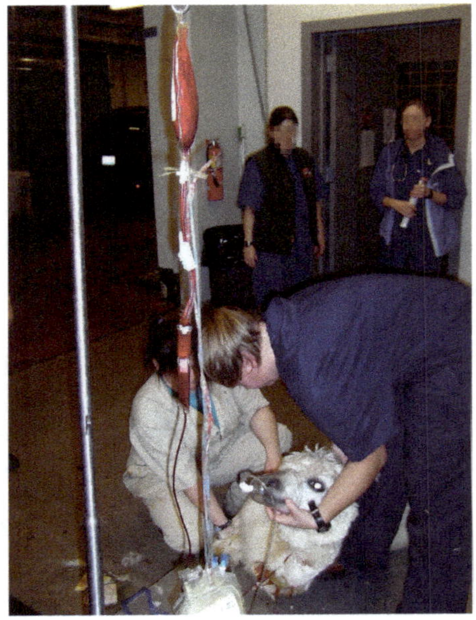

Figure 2. This alpaca has presented collapsed due to severe anaemia. She is being given a blood transfusion as well as oxygen for support.

Blood Transfusions

In the field, we can get a rough idea of what the PCV might be from a clinical examination and decide on that basis alone whether or not to perform a blood transfusion. However, a blood sample should be *collected* before any transfusion and submitted for biochemistry and haematology (to include evaluation of a fresh blood smear). At the very least, your vet should be able to check PCV and total protein even if they cannot perform other diagnostics in-house. A sample pre-transfusion is necessary because you want to determine what is happening in the patient rather than the donor. Also, following the transfusion, we can recheck the PCV a day or so later to assess improvement and determine the next steps. I would encourage your vet to come back and check on the animal the next day and re-assess.

For one of your animals to receive a blood transfusion, you will need a suitable donor. This will be one of your other animals. There is no commercial blood bank for camelids. The donor will need to be healthy, and ideally an adult male over three years of age. This is because these animals are big enough to tolerate the donation of a unit of blood, and they won't be pregnant or lactating. This is one very good reason to keep some males - or castrated males - around. You never know when you might need a donor! Donor matching is not required for camelids. We don't know anything about blood types in camelids, but transfusion reactions are extremely rare, so cross-matching is not normally done. The donor needs to be healthy, have good body condition, and have a healthy mucous membrane colour. I also recommend collecting a sample to check PCV and total protein from any donor. This can be done afterwards, but it provides reassurance about the donor's health and helps the vet establish where the recipient's PCV should get to following the transfusion.

We use 450 ml blood collection packs, the same size used for humans. It can be worth purchasing these yourself as an owner to stock on the farm in case of an emergency because most vets will not carry them in their vehicles and may need to order them in. That would be a suboptimal state of affairs in an emergency, as your anaemic camelid may die before the bags arrive! You can ask your vet to purchase them on your behalf. While the bags may go out of date, I think it is better to chuck an out-of-date blood pack worth no more than a couple of cups of coffee than lose an animal because you didn't have a collection pack. It is best practice to collect blood from a donor standing over a small bale of hay or straw (*Figure 3*). Donors will sometimes want to cush during the procedure, and if they do so, you will lose the benefit of gravity, and donation will slow down and sometimes clot in the line. I prefer to collect "off the needle" straight into the collection bag as this maintains a closed sterile system. This method is also quick, usually taking around 3.5–4 minutes to collect a unit. However, the donor's behaviour and the handlers' skills are crucial for this.

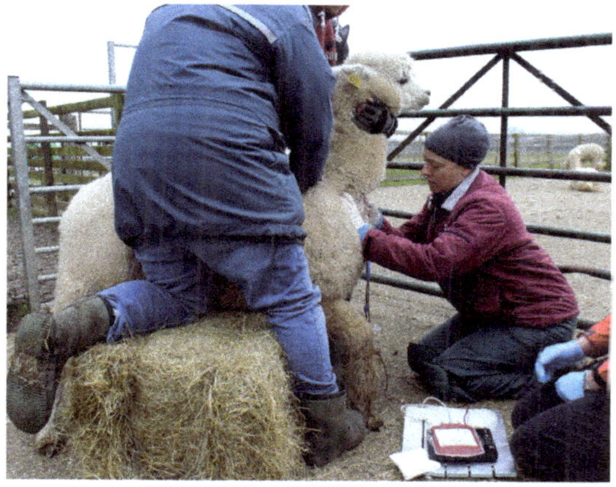

Figure 3. An adult male alpaca providing blood. Note that he is standing over a bale to facilitate the collection process.

Once you have the unit of blood, it can be transfused into the recipient over a period of about 45 to 60 minutes through an intravenous catheter that should already have been placed (so that you know the recipient is still alive before collecting blood). Blood must be administered through a blood products administration set rather than an ordinary fluid line because it has a filter to filter out clots. The patient is monitored throughout the transfusion. After the transfusion, I will typically leave the catheter in place, train owners on how to manage it and give IV treatments if needed. This maintains the IV access in case it is needed again over the next few days.

Don't forget that the underlying cause of anaemia must be diagnosed and treated simultaneously to remove the cause of red cell loss. In severe anaemia cases, I will collect a faecal sample for diagnostics, but I will not wait for the result to be known. This is due to the high prevalence of parasitism as a cause of anaemia and because an individual's egg count may not reveal a prepatent larval burden of *Haemonchus*. These larvae could quickly consume the blood cells you've just administered while waiting for a diagnosis. I still want to see the test result to confirm the diagnosis and to assess the rest of the group, as they may also be at risk.

Colic

Camelids exhibiting signs of colic can be extremely worrying. Unlike horses, camelids are generally not particularly demonstrative. They are more likely to separate themselves from the group, cush and avoid coming up to eat with the others. They might sit with their legs slightly out to the side, then stand up and later sit down in a different position. You may also notice nostril flaring, which indicates increased respiratory rate and depth due to pain. However, some causes of colic are more painful and more likely to cause severe signs, such as rolling, kicking and looking at the flanks. In these cases, the problem might be a lesion in the gastrointestinal system further down the intestinal tract. If there is an obstruction far down the small intestine or in the spiral colon, fluid will back up and stretch the intestinal walls, resulting in pain. In contrast, lesions in the upper intestine will be less painful because fluid can back up into the stomachs with a larger fluid-holding capacity.

Some of the most severe pain I've observed in alpacas was associated with spiral colon lesions. Another case was an alpaca that had a rectal tear that caused the intestines to come out of its anus. That, unsurprisingly, was the most distressingly painful colic case I have seen.

What Causes Colic in Camelids?

Colic can arise from several different causes. Essentially, colic means "abdominal pain." This may result from something as simple as inflammation in the gut (enteritis), hyperactivity of the intestinal tract that might occur following ingestion of lush spring grass (grass colic), and parasitic gastroenteritis, or it might be from ulcers, or a more severe intestinal problem such as an obstruction or perforation of the bowel. Intestinal ileus, which is when the intestines stop moving, is also painful. There may also be some non-gastrointestinal causes of colic relating to conditions of the intra-abdominal organs or pregnancy.

A spiral colon impaction is one of the most frequent causes of colic in my experience, other than simple enteritis, grass colic and ulcers. The spiral colon is where water gets reabsorbed in the gut. This is an especially well-developed portion of the gastrointestinal tract in camelids due to their adaptations to an arid climate. The spiral colon becomes progressively narrower and then changes direction at the apex, where impactions arise. Conditions that predispose an animal to drink less, such as when it is very cold and the water is icy, or when animals get a little dehydrated, such as when the weather is very hot, will make a spiral colon impaction more likely.

For this reason, some impactions can be dealt with by rehydrating the animal and, by default, the gut. In other words, just using IV fluid therapy in addition to pain medications can be helpful and sometimes therapeutic. However, some impactions will be bad enough to necessitate surgical resolution.

What to Do If You Have an Animal Showing Signs of Colic

This is an emergency, and you must get your veterinarian to evaluate these cases immediately. Our job is to understand the underlying problem by assessing the case history and the patient. We must pay particular attention to heart and respiratory rates, temperature, gut sounds, faecal output and its character and distension of regions of the gastrointestinal tract. It is an evaluation of all these systems that help us determine how best to manage the case. We must decide whether the underlying problem might be amenable to medical management or require surgery, which might necessitate referral.

Conditions with increased gut sounds tend to be something like enteritis or a grass colic, while decreased gut sounds are more concerning regarding the need for potential surgery. The absence of faecal output or faecal material in the rectum may increase concern about possible obstruction, but it can take an upper GI obstruction longer to get to the point of faecal output ceasing. Ultrasound can be employed to assess GI motility and see if any parts of the bowel are distended with fluid. We can also evaluate the abdominal organs. Blood work can help understand and assess the problem. Passing a stomach tube can be diagnostic because it's normally impossible to get fluid back up the tube. If we are able to collect fluid out of C1 via a stomach tube, this may indicate an intestinal lesion high up the intestines with fluid backing up into C1. This is actually quite rare: I can only recall a single case of this in an alpaca with a duodenal lesion – this is the first part of the small intestine, right after the stomachs. Finally, a belly tap is another diagnostic tool that may guide the decision about whether surgery is necessary. This is usually done in a hospital setting where there are instruments available to analyse the fluid.

Depending on what we find, we may try medications to manage pain or may decide that referral and/or potential surgery might be more appropriate. Non-steroidal anti-inflammatory medications are commonly used to control pain. Failure to respond to the administration of pain medications can be used as an indication that surgery may be required. Intravenous fluids may also be beneficial. One medication that I want to mention at this point is buscopan. This is an anticholinergic medication that reduces the motility of the bowel and is therefore *only* indicated where gut sounds are increased, for example, with a grass colic. It should *never* be used when gut sounds are normal or reduced, or where there may be a potential obstruction of the bowel. It can be hazardous to reduce intestinal motility in animals that ruminate, including camelids. My preference would be to use non-steroidal anti-inflammatories in a grass colic in addition to removing them from the lush grass initially and, after that, controlling access to it.

C3 Ulcers

One particular potential cause of abdominal pain in camelids is ulceration of C3. C3 ulcers are typically secondary to an underlying problem. This might be another disease condition, or it may be due to stress. We discussed the causes of stress in Chapter 2, and I also detailed a clinical case of C3 ulcers that I'd seen. Clinical signs of C3 ulcers might include drooling, teeth grinding, being off concentrates, hunched up abdominal appearance and signs of colic, as described above.

Confirming a diagnosis of C3 ulceration isn't easy because there is no definitive diagnostic test for this. Horses are also quite susceptible to stomach ulcers, but it is possible to pass an endoscope and confirm the diagnosis based on visual appearance. However, passing an endoscope in the third stomach compartment is impossible. Diagnosing a camelid patient relies upon having a compatible history of other underlying disease or stress and ruling out other problems based on diagnostic testing. The only abnormality on blood work will most often be an inflammatory white cell picture. Observing irregularities in the wall of C3 on ultrasound is also possible.

Treatment for C3 ulcers includes reducing acid secretion, protecting the damaged lining of the stomach and neutralising acid. Medicines that can reduce acid secretion in other species include cimetidine and ranitidine, which are ineffective in camelids.[1,2] Omeprazole can be used intravenously but needs administering four times a day to be effective and is not available everywhere. Oral omeprazole has been shown to have minimal effect on reducing C3 acid production.[2] Pantoprazole is the medication that has shown the best success for treating ulcers and can be used either intravenously or subcutaneously, only requiring once daily administration. Pantoprazole is marketed as Protium in the UK, Protonix in the US and Somac in Australia - there may be other trade names available. The dose is 2 mg/kg when given subcutaneously or 1 mg/kg intravenously. This treatment would normally be continued for a minimum of 5 days.

If pantoprazole isn't available, you could try gastric mucosal protectants such as sucralfate, given orally at a dose of 1–3 g two to three times daily. This can be purchased in liquid form, or tablets can be crushed and given in a suspension. This treatment would be continued for 7–10 days.

Dental Problems

In Chapter 4, I discussed dental care as one of the non-negotiable herd health activities. Retained incisors occur infrequently, but most of these will self-resolve in time. However, occasionally, they may need removal if they persist longer than usual or feed material packs around them and cause issues. This needs to be done under anaesthesia. Incisor overgrowth is much more common and is more apparent. It occurs due to poor dental conformation, so breeders should pay attention to this when making breeding decisions. Incisor trimming is often performed unnecessarily, sometimes with inappropriate tools, and often by untrained individuals with little care for the potential complications associated with unnecessary and excessive trimming. Trimming should never be done for cosmetic reasons and is not a "routine" ownership task. The decision to trim teeth should be made by a veterinarian, considering the effects on body condition and oral health. It may become necessary

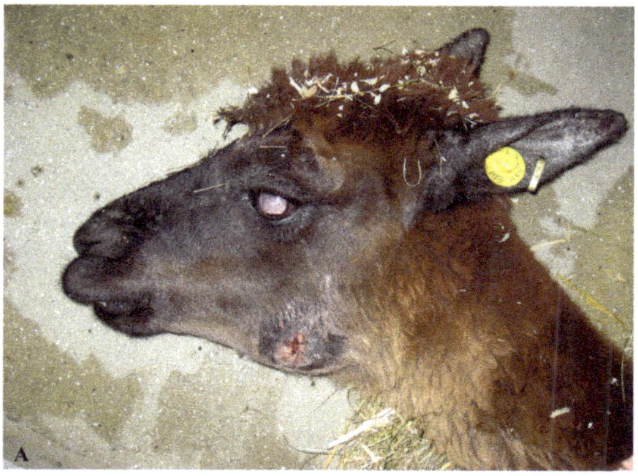

Figure 4a. An adult female alpaca that presented with a tooth root abscess that had ruptured out of the lower jaw, level with the middle molar teeth

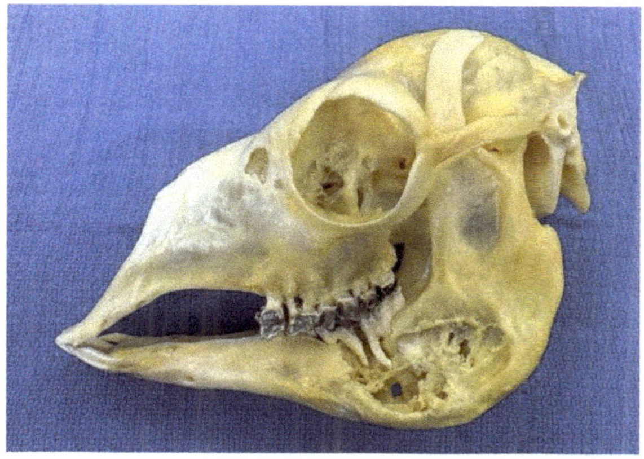

Figure 4b. The skull of the same adult female alpaca shows the extent of the infection within the mandibular bone. You can also see the large gap between the second and third molars that permitted the trapping of feed particles. They would have worked their way down into the tooth root from here.

if the overgrowth causes difficulty with grazing, material becomes stuck around the teeth or individuals are losing weight. Excessive trimming can result in exposure of the pulp cavity that contains nerves, making this extremely painful and can introduce infection into the tooth. Please refer to the section in Chapter 4 for more details.

Tooth root abscesses are relatively common in camelids. Any age of camelid can be affected by tooth root problems, but mostly, they tend to be between 2-8 years of age, around the age when the permanent molar tooth roots erupt. The mandibular molars are affected most commonly due to feed material working its way down inside the gums and into the roots, although rarely, the maxillary tooth roots (those in the upper jaw) can be similarly affected. The timing of many tooth root abscesses corresponds with when these teeth are erupting because the gums are soft and susceptible to scratchy, coarse forages. Often, the first thing you will be aware of is the sudden appearance of a lump on the jaw, but these may be difficult to appreciate in heavily fleeced animals until shearing – unless you feel the jawbones during handling. While some of the swelling is bony, extensive soft tissue inflammation can be overlying the bone, making the lump quite sensitive on palpation. You may have appreciated some weight loss, and affected animals may exhibit poor appetite due to pain. Sometimes, there may be smelly, purulent drainage from the lesion on the side or bottom of the jaw – you may notice scabs at first that are purulent underneath (*Figure 4a*). Affected individuals might be salivating excessively because of oral pain; they may be

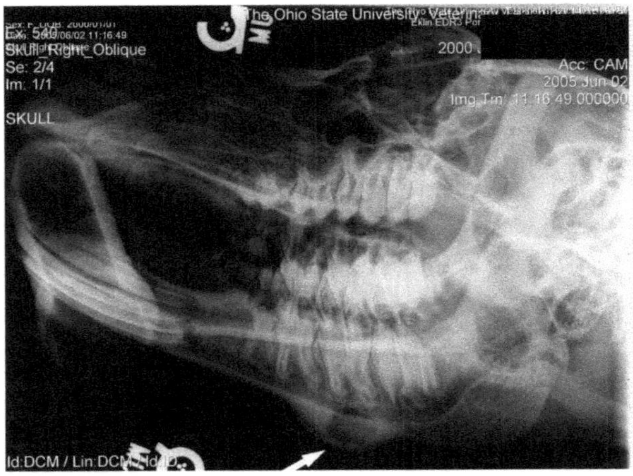

Figure 5. This skull radiograph shows a focal swelling in the mandibular bone (arrow) with an area of infection that can be seen to track back to the roots of the second molar tooth only.

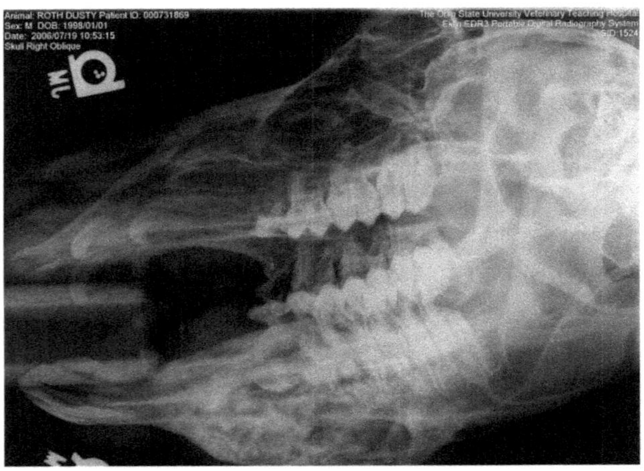

Figure 6. This skull radiograph shows much more extensive changes within the mandibular bone suggestive of osteomyelitis, together with involvement of the premolar and first molar tooth.

dropping feed out of their mouths or packing feed in their cheeks. They may also have breath that smells bad due to the infection. Maxillary tooth root abscesses are generally harder to spot because these often don't cause much visible swelling, and the abscesses invade the sinuses and nasal cavity from where any pus may be swallowed. Occasionally, a unilateral smelly nasal discharge may be evident.

It's important for us to perform x-rays in these cases to try and assess the extent and severity of infection in the jaw. Evaluating the radiographic changes helps us determine whether the infection will likely resolve with medical management using antibiotic and anti-inflammatory therapy or whether surgery will be more appropriate. A focally apparent abscess that hasn't spread to affect neighbouring roots or mandibular bone is more likely to be amenable to medical therapy (*Figure 5*) than one that has spread within the mandible (*Figure 6*). Medical therapy alone will often effect a visible change because the inflammation and swelling will subside, but the infection in the bone may remain and return later. Therefore, identifying which cases are likely amenable to medical therapy or require surgery at the start will result in more favourable outcomes for the patient, who will experience fewer problems and pain. Surgical management allows the removal of affected tooth roots (and teeth) and sequestered bone fragments, along with the debridement of infected bone, to aid in healing. It also allows for the sterile collection of purulent material and bone for culture and sensitivity testing to guide antimicrobial selection better.

Gastrointestinal Problems

Numerous conditions affect the gastrointestinal tract. Some of the more common causes and those to be aware of are included in Table 1. Some of these conditions have been dealt with elsewhere in detail, such as parasitic gastroenteritis and causes of colic and C3 ulceration, and won't be discussed again here.

Choke

Choke is a problem associated with rapid eating of concentrates and rarely may occur

Main Problem	Potential diagnoses
Obstruction	Choke Impaction of the forestomachs Spiral colon impaction Strangulation of the bowel
Diarrhoea	Clostridial enterotoxaemia Parasitic gastroenteritis Johnes Yersinia Inflammatory bowel Grain overload Disrupted microflora
Projectile vomiting	Rhododendron toxicity
Other	C3 ulceration Mega-oesophagus Cancerous growths

Table 1. Some common causes of gastrointestinal problems.

due to a congenital abnormality or tumour. Typically, there is a history of recent feeding and the affected individuals are often known to eat very enthusiastically! An episode of choke appears highly distressing for the animal. They tend to lower and extend their necks, open their mouth, and excessively breathe and salivate because they cannot swallow. You may observe a fluid wave at the bottom of the neck on the left side. These episodes usually last 15–20 minutes, and the choke will self-resolve. Gentle massage of the oesophagus, which runs down the left side of the neck next to the windpipe, can help pass the choke. If the episode does not self-resolve, you should call your veterinarian for assistance. Light sedation may help; occasionally, breaking up the obstructed material may be necessary using water flushed down a stomach tube. For this, the patient will need to be sedated more heavily and positioned with the head below the chest to enable any dislodged feed and fluid to drain out of the mouth and avoid aspiration.

Megaoesophagus

Megaoesophagus is a condition where the oesophagus becomes distended and is prone to filling with food material instead of food being pushed down into C1. The underlying cause is often unknown, but it has been associated with a vascular ring anomaly that forms a tight ring around the oesophagus, causing food to get stuck above the ring and distend the oesophagus.[3 4] Other causes have included organophosphate toxicity, degenerative disease of the oesophageal muscles, dysfunction of the nerve supply to the oesophagus, and, more recently, it was associated with *Trypanosoma cruzi* in a llama in the southern United States.[5 6] Neck trauma may also result in the development of megaoesophagus.

Megaoesophagus caused by a vascular ring anomaly typically results in clinical signs once crias begin eating solid food, as larger particles become stuck at the constricted ring, which limits the oesophagus's diameter during swallowing. If the condition is caused by something else, clinical signs will appear later in life. Affected animals generally present with repeated choke episodes and the appearance of a fluid wave at the bottom of the neck on the left side. Affected animals may also experience weight loss. Aspiration of feed material may result in pneumonia. The condition is diagnosed based on radiographs, sometimes with contrast, highlighting the distended oesophagus. Treatment involves small volume, frequent feeding from an elevated position to aid the gravity flow of digesta down into C1. The feed should be highly digestible and have small particle size; the challenge is maintaining their weight. Treatment of pneumonia may be needed periodically due to the increased risk of aspiration pneumonia.

Diarrhoea

Diarrhoea isn't particularly common in camelids but can result from various causes. There are many infectious causes of diarrhoea in young animals, and some of these are discussed in Chapter 9, namely coccidiosis, cryptosporidiosis and giardiasis. Neonates and crias are particularly vulnerable to fluid losses, so intravenous fluid therapy should always be considered for this age group. Viral causes of diarrhoea, including rotavirus and coronavirus, can worsen diarrhoea from other causes, especially the more common coccidiosis. These are a potential concern in crias under 60 days old. Diarrhoea testing panels allow you to test for cryptosporidiosis, giardiasis, rotavirus and coronavirus. If you don't seek a diagnosis, it is hard to treat specifically and know how to control the spread. Viruses, particularly rotavirus, can damage the intestinal epithelium, reducing the cells that produce the enzyme lactase required to break down milk. If crias can't digest milk it can perpetuate diarrhoea since the undigested milk will draw water with it as it passes down the bowel. There are no specific treatments for viruses, but one fairly benign treatment that *may* be useful in crias with a potential rotavirus diagnosis is lactase replacement using something like Lactaid. You can get Lactaid tablets over the counter in pharmacies – I suggest giving 1/4 to 1/3 tablet a couple of times a day for 7–10 days and see if it has a beneficial effect.

Diarrhoea in adults is less common than it is in crias. Changing diet can result in changes to the stool, particularly if it is a sudden change. For example, putting animals out on lush pasture may result in stool that is soft to liquid. This is primarily because of the disruption to the microflora in the forestomachs, which are unable to adapt quickly. Similarly, if animals are given too much rapidly fermentable carbohydrate (intentional or accidental overindulgence in concentrates, especially those that are grain-based, or too much fruit). In that case, the microbes are disrupted, shifting from producing volatile fatty acids to producing lactic acid. The lactic acid can be absorbed into the circulation, resulting in systemic acidosis and dehydration. In addition, clinical signs of polioencephalomalacia or thiamine deficiency may develop, including sudden onset blindness. In less severe cases, being fed too much concentrate, perhaps to try and gain weight, may cause periods of intermittent diarrhoea. Severe cases of grain overload will require IV fluid therapy to correct electrolyte imbalance and non-steroidal anti-inflammatory medications to treat any toxaemia. Antibiotics and thiamine may also be necessary for secondary complications. Transfaunation with rumen juice is extremely beneficial for re-populating the C1 microbes and stimulating appetite, though it is not always available. However, Dr Bob Van Saun has talked about collecting 5–10 ml of spit from an alpaca or llama to give orally, which can have a beneficial effect if repeated over a few days. Probiotics designed for ruminants would be the next best thing, but this needs to be a product for ruminants that doesn't contain Lactobacillus bacteria, which promote lactic acid production. Yeasts stabilise the ruminal microbes, so are useful in probiotics.

Clostridial enterotoxaemia is generally a fatal disease. It is caused by an overgrowth of Clostridium perfringens bacteria in the GI tract, and these produce toxins that are absorbed and cause collapse, signs of shock, colic, possible fever, abdominal distension and watery, sometimes haemorrhagic diarrhoea. The disease is sudden in onset and has a rapid course, and affected animals may die before the development of diarrhoea. Damage to the gut wall by nematodes, coccidia, viruses, ulceration or changes in microbial population can facilitate overgrowth of these bacteria that are typically present in the gut without causing problems. Aggressive treatment is required with IV fluids, antibiotics and anti-inflammatories. Plasma transfusions can be helpful. Post-mortem examination of any animals that die is crucial for diagnosis, and toxin assays can be done to determine the type of C perfringens involved. Type A is often involved, and sometimes type C. There are also types B, D and E. Clostridial vaccination is used to prevent clostridial enterotoxaemia, but the coverage varies depending on the vaccine.

Johnes disease is caused by infection with the bacterium *Mycobacterium avium* subsp *paratuberculosis.* This infection is usually acquired early in life via ingesting infected colostrum or faecal material. All ages may be affected, but being a mycobacterial disease, it may take some time to become apparent. You may not notice any clinical signs until the animal is older, when they may experience weight loss, diarrhoea and weakness.[7] These signs are due to the thickening of the intestinal wall so that the affected individual struggles to absorb digested nutrients from the gut. The thickened intestinal walls may be appreciated on abdominal ultrasound. The most reliable diagnostic test is faecal culture, but this takes up to three months, and false negatives are possible. It is even harder to detect carrier status. The conventional tests used in ruminants are not reliable, but faecal PCR may be more sensitive. Definitive diagnosis can be obtained at postmortem examination following submission of samples for histopathology. Animals confirmed to have Johnes should be euthanased because they remain a source of infection for other animals in the herd, particularly young animals. Treatment should not be attempted. In Australia, a market assurance programme was developed in the late 1990s in response to finding Johnes outbreaks in alpacas in Australia. The programme has now closed but was in place to provide evidence of a low risk of infection in zones considered low risk for Johnes infection in ruminants. It was based on a testing regime and implementation of biosecurity measures.

Metabolic Syndrome

Metabolic syndrome is a term that characterises the metabolic issues associated with negative energy balance that occur in camelids. It includes hyperlipaemia and ketoacidosis, and these can then lead to hepatic lipidosis, or "fatty liver." It is sometimes referred to as pregnancy toxaemia, but this is a term that is used in sheep with negative energy balance and doesn't properly reflect the syndrome that occurs in camelids.

Metabolic syndrome can occur at any age of animal experiencing a negative energy balance, but it can also occur in response to illness, extreme stress following transportation or changes in the weather. I often see it in females in late pregnancy or the first few months of lactation. In these cases, the energy and protein provided simply do not meet their demands. When this happens, they produce ketone bodies like beta-hydroxybutyrate (β-OHB), and non-esterified fatty acids (NEFAs) increase, a biomarker indicating a shortage of glucose. Production of ketones results in ketoacidosis, and this is similar to what happens in ruminants when they get into a negative energy balance. One key difference is that while sheep tend to have low blood glucose, camelids always have high blood glucose. However, camelids also get hyperlipaemic due to the mobilisation of fats from around the body for the liver to use as an alternative energy source. This is similar to horses when they get into negative energy balance and can detected as high triglycerides on bloodwork. Hyperlipaemia can also be recognised as milky (fatty) serum when a blood sample is spun down, but this may not be evident in milder cases. So camelids may get both ketoacidosis and hyperlipaemia at the same time, which can make them very sick metabolically.

If fat mobilisation is excessive, it can overwhelm the ability of the liver to process it, and this is when hepatic lipidosis occurs. This may become evident on bloodwork as a non-specific increase in liver enzymes. The liver can appear brighter on ultrasound due to the increased echogenicity of fat. Colic signs can occur due to the liver being painful.

In terms of treating this, the focus is on supportive care, including IV fluids initially, but these can then be changed to partial parenteral nutrition to provide amino acids. However, this needs to be provided via a continuous rate infusion that requires a pump and is only likely possible with hospitalisation. There is quite a lot of intensive management needed for these cases, including managing glucose levels using insulin and glucose monitoring. Heparin can also be used to help drive lipids into the cells. Appetite stimulation can include the presence of buddy animals, transfaunation with rumen juice (although this can be too stressful a procedure in these individuals), probiotics, B vitamins and even diazepam. For females in late pregnancy, my attention is focused on managing the metabolic syndrome and saving the mother. Often, the cria is already dead at the point of diagnosis. Providing cloprostenol to abort the cria may help accelerate the mother's recovery. However, it is not advisable to perform a C-section in camelids as the female will be unlikely to be able to tolerate the stress and may die. The only time a C-section would be worth considering is if the cria is known to be alive, is close enough to term to be viable and is more valuable than the mother. The owner would also have to be prepared to hand-rear the cria.

The prognosis depends on how far the state of metabolic disorder has progressed. In cases that occur earlier in the disease process, aggressive treatment may make recovery possible. However, obtaining accurate diagnostics is essential, as is identifying and aggressively addressing the underlying problem. A referral likely offers the best chance for success, as referral facilities can provide the intensive treatment and monitoring needed.

Finally, hepatic lipidosis is often reported on postmortem examinations. This is a significant finding as it indicates the animal was in a negative energy balance before death. However, it is relatively common in animals that experience a period of anorexia prior to death and is usually a secondary finding. The key is finding out the underlying reason for that negative energy balance.

Orthopaedic Injuries

In this section, we'll discuss fractures, luxation injuries and sequestra. All these types of injury will result in sudden onset lameness in the patient.

Fractures

Limb fractures are the most common type of fracture, although spinal fractures may also occur. Most limb fractures in camelids tend to be in the lower limb due to limbs getting caught in fencing or stuck in holes in the ground. These are more amenable to management. High limb fractures can also be treated, although they are harder to access and typically require internal surgical fixation methods such as plating. Fractures will have a better prognosis if the skin is not broken. Once the skin is broken, there is a risk of infection getting into the bone.

The first concern with any limb fracture is to immobilise it so it can't get any worse. Fractures have sharp bone fragments that could poke out holes through the skin, turning a closed fracture into an open fracture, while major vessel trauma is possible with upper limb fractures. You should avoid moving individuals until the limb has been stabilised with a heavy bandage and splint. Keeping the patient as calm as possible will also help to prevent further injury.

Radiographs will be required to assess these injuries and determine the best course of action. If your vet has a mobile X-ray unit, they can do this in the field. Otherwise, you may have to transport your animal to a veterinary facility that is able to do this. I suggest taking the animal somewhere that can also do surgery, which might mean taking it to a referral facility. With most fractures, we can use fixation methods similar to those used in dogs. Small animal orthopaedic surgeons will be very capable of dealing with camelid fractures and will likely have the right equipment. However, they will need to have an extended operating table to take the patient and someone able to manage camelid anaesthesia. In some places, equine surgeons may have orthopaedic expertise.

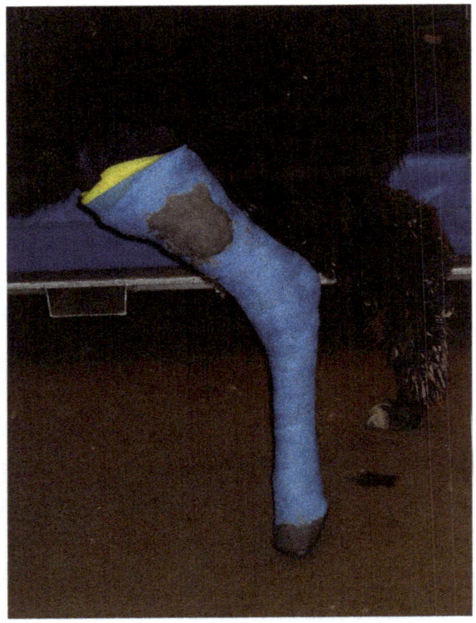

Figure 7. An alpaca with a hanging pin cast on the left hind limb. The fracture site here is in the lower part of the tibia, just above the hock. Pins have been placed in the healthy bone above the fracture site and then enclosed in the cast. The grey material on the outside of the cast helps to hold the pins in place.

A hanging pin cast is a nice and often

affordable way to fix a simple lower limb fracture where there is less overlying muscle. With this type of fracture fixation, if there is sufficient healthy bone above the fracture site, at least two pins are placed above the fracture site in the same bone, and then the leg is encased in a cast that incorporates the pins and the foot (*Figure 7*). Essentially, the healthy part of the leg is used to support the rest of the leg that hangs inside the cast. The cast immobilises the fragments, and they heal together. This type of cast is superior to a simple cast because the patient can still bear weight on the affected limb while it heals. Casts usually stay on for about six weeks before being re-radiographed and hopefully removed.

Shoulder Luxation

One orthopaedic problem that is really important to be aware of is shoulder luxation. If action is not taken immediately, there may be complications, and the affected individual may never regain soundness on the limb.

Shoulder luxation affects males most commonly, although females are occasionally affected. The injury usually occurs when the animal lands and twists on a forelimb. This causes the shoulder to dislocate, resulting in a sudden onset of non-weight-bearing forelimb lameness. Any animal exhibiting sudden onset severe lameness of a forelimb should be evaluated immediately for fractures, foot injuries and shoulder luxation. Do *not* just put them on NSAIDs and wait and see. Shoulder luxation must be ruled out. Careful palpation will reveal the shoulder blade to be shorter on one side than the other. The diagnosis can be confirmed with radiographs, which help rule out associated fractures. In the early

During my time at the Royal Veterinary College, a young two-year-old male was referred for non-weight-bearing lameness of six weeks' duration. The owner had been administering non-steroidal anti-inflammatory medications, but no improvement had occurred. The regular veterinarian referred him for radiographs. Shortening of the shoulder blade was appreciated on the right side, and the humeral head was palpable to the side of the shoulder blade. There had been quite a lot of muscle atrophy over the six weeks since the injury. Radiographs confirmed the diagnosis of shoulder luxation. However, there was also extensive osteoarthritis associated with the joint. Due to the severity of the arthritis, the prognosis for return to normal function with surgical management was extremely poor, and he was euthanased. Inspection of the shoulder joint at postmortem examination revealed that the shoulder had tried to form a false joint to regain some function. This male would have been in a lot of pain and would never have been breeding sound again. If only they had sought veterinary advice and diagnosed the shoulder luxation the day of the occurrence.

This is a precautionary tale to advise you not to delay seeking veterinary assistance in any sudden onset lameness. This injury is more common in camelids than other species, so it may not be high on your veterinarian's list of possible diagnoses. Therefore, please alert them to this possibility and ask them to check for shoulder luxation!

stages following the injury, the shoulder can be reduced back into the joint under heavy sedation, but this is usually only possible on the day of injury. After this, the muscles shorten and tighten, making it difficult to replace the shoulder manually. Then, surgical reduction will be required.

After putting the shoulder back into its socket, we apply a sling to keep it in the correct position and allow some fibrous tissue to form around the joint and support it better. The affected animal will also need to be stall-rested and will require NSAIDs. After a shoulder luxation, management adjustments are necessary. If a male is returned to a group with other males, the injury will likely recur due to fighting. These males will not be able to breed for a while, either. Sometimes, surgical reduction is required if the luxation recurs.

Cruciate Injury

The cruciate ligament provides rotational stability to the stifle joint. Twisting injuries can cause a rupture of the cruciate ligament, just as they can in humans and dogs. Camelids with a ruptured cruciate will present with sudden lameness on a hind limb. They will probably be toe-touching, and the knee will be turned out when they walk. There will be heat and swelling associated with the stifle joint. These can be managed with icing in the early stages, NSAIDs and stall rest. But occasionally, surgery may be necessary to stabilise the joint.

Patella luxation

Patella luxation is a differential diagnosis for stifle problems. This can be unilateral or bilateral. Bilateral patella luxation may be a congenital problem, meaning that they were born with it due to abnormal conformation of the knee structures. However, it may not be apparent from birth; rather, it develops as they grow. Unilateral luxation may be traumatic in origin and amenable to medical (or surgical) treatment. Diagnosis is best achieved with the patient standing. The patella may be locked out to one side or be easily pushed out.

Bone Sequestra

Bone sequestra are little pockets of avascular or infected bone. They may occur because of trauma that damages the circulation to an area of bone or because an infection sets up in the bone at that location. They are often sterile, meaning that bacteria can't be grown from material collected from them. Most of the time, you will find that an individual becomes suddenly lame. There may be a discharging wound, but this usually occurs much later in the disease if it remains untreated.

Carefully examining these patients is important, first ruling out joint issues and then palpating all over the long bones with digital pressure. With bone sequestra, there will be a painful focus that might feel hotter than the surrounding skin. X-rays at this early stage may reveal nothing diagnostically because radiographic changes lag behind the bony change. These patients require stall rest and non-steroidal anti-inflammatories for 10–14 days, at which point they can be re-radiographed. Sequestra will usually become evident within the bone after this time (*Figure 8*). Treatment is the surgical removal of the sequestrum, a relatively quick and easy surgery.

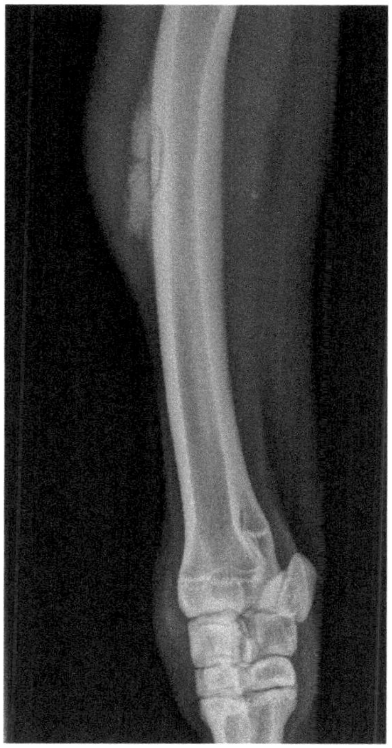

Figure 8. This radiograph shows a bone sequestrum on the front of the upper radius (forelimb). The sequestered piece of bone is clearly visible as a piece of bone surrounded by a zone of lysis (blacker area), and there is a lot of bony reaction and soft tissue swelling around it.

Weight Loss

Weight loss is a common problem in camelids and has many potential causes. The main categories leading to weight loss are listed in *Table 2*. A detailed clinical examination, diagnostic testing and imaging will help define the diagnosis in these cases. Common things are common, so it is always worth ruling out the most common problems first, such as the nutritional provision not matching requirements, dental issues and parasites. As an owner, you can do preliminary checks before calling your veterinarian. Do not waste time calling for assistance if the weight loss is more dramatic or concerning or the affected individual is not eating.

Firstly, when you're body condition scoring, check both jaws for evidence of swellings that could suggest a tooth root abscess. Also, check the incisor teeth to ensure there is no apparent overgrowth that could be causing issues with grazing. Second, a faecal sample should be collected to rule out intestinal parasitism. Don't forget to request fluke testing if this is a potential concern in your area. Observe feeding behaviour, noting if the animal is coming in to feed with everyone else, if they can access the feed or if dominant animals are forcing them out. If you can rule out social interactions, consider the quality of the forage you are feeding, particularly for animals with higher requirements such as growing animals, females in the last few months of pregnancy or lactating. These animals will be susceptible to inadequacies of protein and energy in the forage and more dependent on supplements if your forage isn't good enough. Feeding too much concentrate can, in turn, negatively affect the gut microbial population, resulting in inefficient digestion and other concerns. Do you even know the quality of your forage and grass?

Problem Resulting in Weight Loss	Specific Causes
Poor nutrition	Nutrition inadequate to suit needs Social interaction limiting access Vitamin D deficiency, especially in growing animals
Dental Problems	Tooth root abscess Sharp points on cheek teeth causing oral pain Overgrown incisors
Parasites	Worms Coccidia, especially *E mac* Fluke
Infections	Abscessation - dental, thoracic, intraabdominal Tuberculosis Johnes disease
Neoplasia (cancer, tumours	Lymphoma or lymphosarcoma Squamous cell carcinoma Other
Chronic disease	Inflammatory bowel disease Kidney problems Arthritis
Stress	Social stress Ulcers Poor weather conditions

Table 2. Most common causes of weight loss in camelids.

Taking some time to perform basic observations and tests can save time when your veterinarian arrives. This allows them to focus on a thorough examination and proceed with more advanced diagnostics, such as bloodwork and abdominal ultrasound imaging. Bloodwork can clarify whether systemic disease may be present. Try to get as comprehensive a panel as possible to include haematology, biochemistry (liver and kidney values, measures of negative energy balance, electrolytes) and minerals. I am regularly sent bloodwork from vets wanting my opinion on a partial set of bloodwork. Without a full panel, it's difficult to rule out problems. Some problems will provide clues in haematology, while others are easier to differentiate based on chemistry results. Fibrinogen testing can be a useful measure of chronic inflammation. Globulin concentrations provide similar information, but many profiles fail to provide these values.

I use ultrasound as an extension of my physical examination as this allows me to look for abnormalities associated with the intra-abdominal organs. It allows me to find lesions that may indicate inflammation, tumours or abscesses and direct further diagnostics. Once, I found an abscess that was taking up a significant portion of the abdomen and was associated with C3. Once we were able to drain this, remove that source of inflammation in the body and create space for food, this female was able to start gaining weight again. You may occasionally detect organ enlargement, free fluid in the abdomen, or both. On one occasion, I found an adult female alpaca with a liver so large it was visible on the left side of the abdomen in front of C1 and directly behind the heart. There was also free fluid in the abdomen. I took an aspirate from the liver and sampled the peritoneal fluid. I was in a teaching hospital at the time, so I was able to get slides viewed straight away by a pathologist who diagnosed lymphosarcoma. On that basis, the alpaca was euthanased without wasting any further funds. I have also found ultrasound to be an extremely sensitive tool for diagnosing tuberculosis in camelids exhibiting clinical signs of weight loss and respiratory issues. Since camelids with TB have lung lesions throughout the lung fields, including the edges of the lungs and the membrane that encases them, known as the pleural membranes, I have found that thoracic ultrasonography is useful for finding lesions consistent with TB.

Regardless of the underlying problem, and assuming that it is treatable, you will need to try to reverse the weight loss by providing extra nutrition to help these animals gain weight. One should aim to provide good quality forage as forage should provide the majority of the nutrient requirements. If you don't know the quality of your forage, it can be hard to know what you are providing. Therefore, one recommendation I often give, because so many people are clueless about their homemade or bought-in hay, is to provide chopped dried grass. This product comes bagged with a nutritional analysis printed on the side of the package, so it provides a forage of consistent and high quality, typically around 16% protein. Next, we look at the concentrates that you provide. We don't usually want to increase cereal grains, but adding sugar beet (or beet pulp) is a great energy source, while alfalfa/ lucerne, chopped or pelleted, provides protein. You want to add energy and protein to ensure efficient utilisation. Any additional feed should be introduced gradually, over 7-10 days, to allow the gut microbes time to adjust.

Eye Problems

Camelids have lovely big eyes, making them slightly susceptible to trauma. This can include scratches or severe perforations from foreign bodies. Any eye injuries must be assessed by your veterinarian without delay. Ulcers on the eyes usually result from some sort of injury. You will notice an animal blinking excessively or holding its eyes closed. There may also be discharge from the eye, swelling of the eyelids or cloudiness of the cornea, which is the eye's outer surface. Any cultures are best obtained prior to using any dye to highlight ulcers or the use of any ophthalmic ointments and can help direct antimicrobial therapy if initial treatment fails. Systemic NSAIDs can be used to manage pain. For deeper

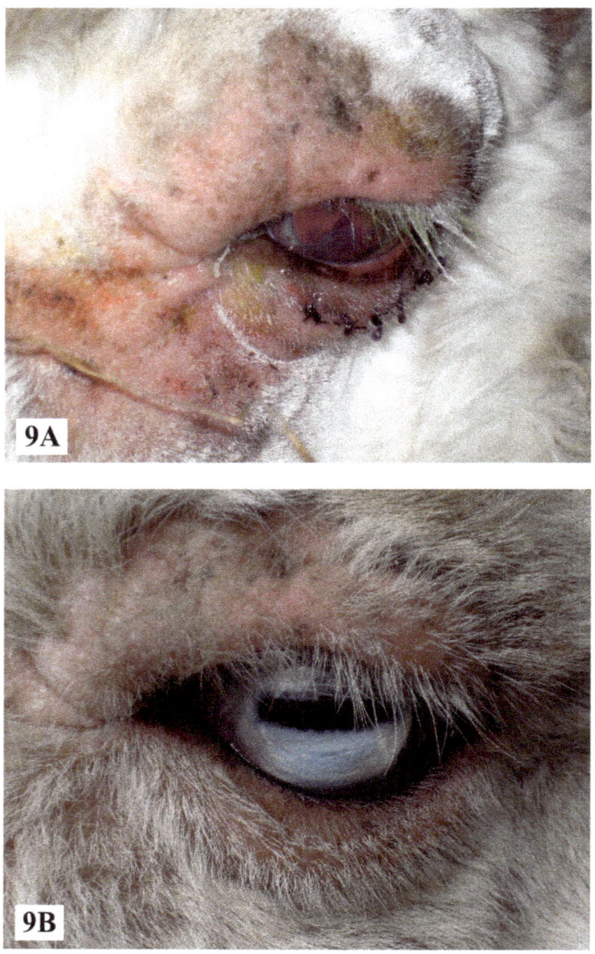

Figure 9. These images show an adult female alpaca with excessive skin in her lower lid due to mange-associated inflammation. Fig 9a shows her immediately post-operatively having had entropian surgery to remove the excess skin. In this photo, you can also see the blood vessels on the surface of the eye that occur due to long-term ulceration from hairs touching the cornea. Fig 9b shows her two months later, following treatment for mange as well as treatment for her eye changes

ulcers, more aggressive treatment may be required. Camelids have an impressive ability to heal even melting ulcers, so don't be afraid to let your veterinarian try and persist with what may seem like a lot of daily treatments in these cases, even if it might appear hopeless. You can always remove an eye later, but you can't put one back!

Ulcers may sometimes occur due to exposure if the animal is unable to blink due to nerve damage or anaesthesia or secondary to hairs from the eyelid touching the surface of the eye. These are treated the same way as traumatic ulcers, but it is important to remove the underlying problem. If the eyelids are rolling inward due to congenital malformation or excessive skin production around the eyes due to mange, then a cosmetic procedure can be done to remove a thin sliver of eyelid skin. This results in the eyelid rolling back out so that the hairs of the eyelid no

Figure 10. This four-month-old cria has had tear staining and purulent discharge down his face for some time, making his facial hair all sticky. He has normal tear ducts, but they have become blocked and need to be flushed clear.

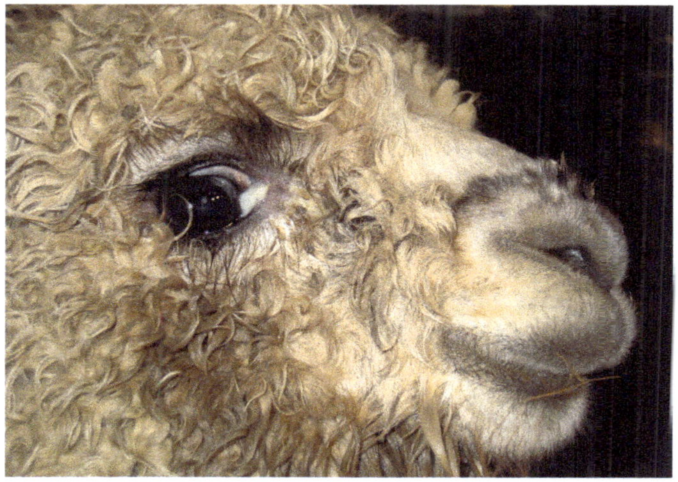

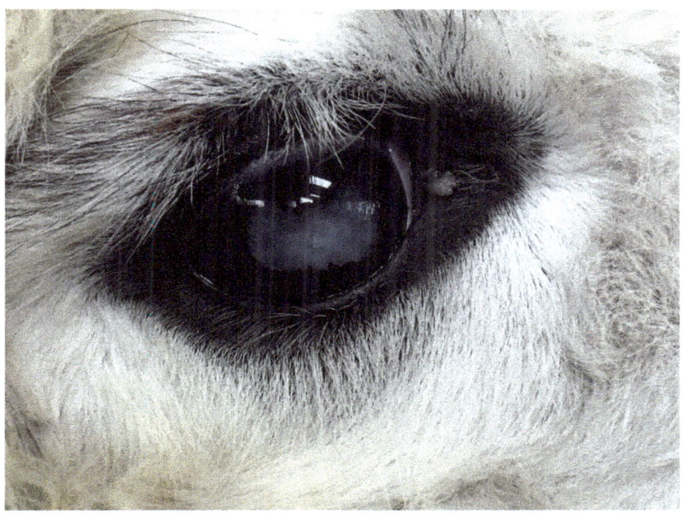

Figure 11. Congenital cataract in the lens of an alpaca. These are thought to be heritable.

longer touch the surface of the eye (*Figures 9a and 9b*).

Episodes of conjunctivitis in crias can result in blockage of the tear ducts. Tear ducts are quite narrow in youngsters, and cellular debris from conjunctivitis can clog them up (Figure 10). This may result in a cria that appears to have repeated episodes of conjunctivitis and tear staining down the face. The only way to resolve this is to flush them out under sedation. Occasionally, the tear ducts are blocked because of a congenital malformation known as nasolacrimal duct atresia. In these cases, the duct opening has failed to form during foetal development. It's usually the bottom end of the duct that is closed, and this is found inside the nostrils. The solution is to create a new opening to fully open the tear duct. This can be tricky, and your veterinarian may need some training to learn this technique.

You may sometimes see lens cataracts in camelids (*Figure 11*). These are known to be heritable in small animals, and I have seen this carried through to offspring in camelids, too, suggesting that heritability is also an issue in camelids. These often start smaller, but the lens can become quite white in colour over time. Occasionally, lenses affected by cataracts can luxate because they become hard and inflexible. This can result in glaucoma, because the drainage from the eye becomes blocked. Enucleation would be required in these cases.

Key Takeaways

We have looked at some of the most common problems in their own chapter, namely parasites, skin and neurological problems. In this chapter, we have covered the ten most common *other* health problems experienced by camelids. It is not a comprehensive list of what may go wrong with your animals but it should provide a starting point covering most of the potential issues seen. Each problem is addressed under the heading of the clinical problem that you might observe in your animals so that you can go straight to the relevant section.

The key things to remember are:

- If one of your animals doesn't seem right, trust your instinct and get it examined. Don't let the vet leave the farm without doing some diagnostics if they haven't found something because they may continue to deteriorate.
- Animals that are not eating and drinking can get sicker quite fast, so do not delay in seeking help.
- Anaemia can be very severe in camelids, but blood transfusions along with correction of the underlying problem work wonders!
- Some problems are unique to camelids or manifest differently in these species. Be aware of what these are in case your veterinarian is not as familiar with camelids. These include, but are not limited to: bone sequestra, shoulder luxation, choke, metabolic syndrome and ulcers. Don't be afraid to share your knowledge and ask your veterinarian to seek help from colleagues who may have more experience.

The next chapter will discuss your approach to dealing with emergencies.

14

Dealing With Emergencies

When faced with a sick animal, it's useful to have a plan for the actions you should take. First, you need to get them to a safe area and get them comfortable, and then follow up with actions you can achieve either on your own or before calling your veterinarian out to assist. In this chapter, we will also discuss the array of diagnostic tests available to help your vet make a diagnosis. It is helpful to know what tests are available because, if not available with your regular vet, you can ask for a referral to a specialist facility or consult a specialist veterinarian who may help your vet manage the case in the field.

We will also cover field therapeutics, medicines we can use in camelids (and those to avoid) and IV fluid therapy, which is extremely important when treating camelids.

The Sick Camelid

Camelids are prey species. This makes them really good at masking clinical signs of illness because it's not advantageous to telegraph to predators that they are vulnerable. So, to an untrained observer, they may appear completely fine. With experience, you will recognise that they're not. It's always surprising to me how a camelid can appear comparatively well but massively worse on paper, or rather on biochemistry and haematology. So, whenever you have a sick camelid, if the physical examination that your veterinarian performs doesn't yield a clear diagnosis, trust your instinct – it is always worth investing in further diagnostics.

The physical examination that we're able to achieve in these animals is somewhat limited. We can get our stethoscopes out, listen to heart and lung sounds, listen to gut sounds and look at the head, the mucous membranes, eyes and so on. However, we're not able to effectively and fully evaluate the abdomen, which leaves a big gap in our physical exam findings. In small animal patients, we can palpate the abdomen very easily, while in larger animals, we can discover quite a lot of information via rectal palpation. Camelids are somewhere in between. It's difficult to palpate the abdomen externally because the large fermentation vat of C1 gets in the way, while their physical size makes rectal palpation challenging. This, therefore, makes us more reliant on other diagnostics, such as bloodwork and abdominal ultrasound. If you know something's wrong with your animal, but an initial examination hasn't revealed anything obvious, trust your instinct. You need those other diagnostic tests to look a bit deeper. Bloodwork can include biochemistry, haematology and mineral tests – the more complete the panel, the better. A faecal test is always a useful addition to any case workup. You can always get that submitted as an initial test before calling the vet if you don't think the problem is serious. For animals not eating, delaying these diagnostics is not worth it as the clinical condition could worsen the next day, and you'll have lost time. Remember that a second vet visit is also costly.

Ultrasound is my next most valuable asset in the diagnostic toolbox. If I'm presented with a sick camelid, I'll always check bloodwork, run a faecal test and perform an abdominal ultrasound. I consider it an extension of my physical examination. Ultrasound allows me to evaluate the gastrointestinal tract and all the other intra-abdominal structures. It provides a window into the abdomen of a camelid. We also perform the above to evaluate the foetus in pregnant females. Knowing that the animal is pregnant and what stage of pregnancy they're in may influence our diagnosis, and we can also discover if the foetus is distressed as it passes meconium in the foetal fluids.

What Can You Do As an Owner?

Firstly, if you find an animal cushed down in the field, you should establish whether it has any broken limbs. An animal with fractures shouldn't be moved if it's quiet. Any movement without prior stabilisation of a fracture could worsen the fracture. Once you've established that the animal hasn't broken anything, you can try and get it to stand up. A weak animal will struggle to get up because getting up requires more energy than just standing. You can assist them in standing by lifting gently at the base of the tail. They may hop up at the front end, but this will not work if people are crowded around the front. Make sure other people stand back to give them room and preferably remain behind their shoulder so the animal can see the exit route clearly. Once they're up, hopefully, they will be able to walk. If not, that may be useful from a diagnostic perspective.

When an animal is unwell, especially outside in cold or wet weather, you should bring it indoors. If an individual animal is unwell, consider bringing in a friend to keep it company. For females with a cria, bring in its cria. The companion animal will help minimise their stress, as camelids become stressed if they're contained on their own.

Bed sick animals on straw because straw is the most insulating material on a cold floor. If they're recumbent and on their sides, you should try to get them sat up into a normal cushed position. If they stay lying on their sides, the lungs can become congested on one side. If they're weak and cannot maintain a normal cush position, you can use bales of hay or straw on either side to stop them from falling over.

Once the animal is inside in a well-bedded sick pen, and you've got them upright if they're recumbent, ensure they've got some good quality dry hay and fresh water. If it's very cold outside, they won't want to drink icy cold water, so provide warm water that might encourage them to drink. You want to see if they'll eat, so offer them their normal food. If they're not interested in that, try something else. Food such as sugar beet might be more palatable for them. Sometimes, they like chopped, dried grass. You may have your own special feeds and snacks to tempt them with.

The Owner Health Check

As an owner, you can perform a rudimentary examination, perhaps even before you call the vet, and relay the information you've found on the phone. I have included a quick checklist in *Table 1*, giving you questions to ask and things you can check easily.

Check their body condition score. If you haven't already done so, try to get them standing to differentiate whether they might be weak or neurological. There are some simple tests that you can do at this point. If they're standing, you can flip their feet onto the tops of their fetlocks. I usually try the front feet first and then the back feet. They should normally right them and put them the right way up. If they don't put them back in the correct position, this may indicate a lack of awareness of normal body position.

You can check teeth in any animal. Look at their incisors and feel along both jawlines for lumps and bumps that might indicate tooth root abscesses. Sometimes, these abscesses rupture, and you may feel a scab. While at the mouth, peel back the upper lip and check if the mucous membranes feel moist or tacky – tackiness indicates dehydration and a need for IV fluids. Also, at the head, you can check the mucous membrane colour around the eyes to assess for evidence of anaemia. To do this, you will place your thumb over the top eyelid over the eye and press gently over the eye while pressing the lower lid. This allows the mucus membranes to protrude out from underneath the lower eyelid. The membranes should be a healthy pink, similar to your own mucous membranes in the mirror. If you're ever unsure what is normal, check a healthy animal. You're always going to have another animal nearby that you can check and compare. If you find anaemia, go ahead and collect a faecal sample. Check for lice in the fleece over the body, too. These checks will help provide clues about the underlying cause.

You can also take a rectal temperature using a veterinary thermometer. I usually put a little blob of lubricating gel on the tip and then pop this in through the anus. You do not have to insert the thermometer very far, just about an inch or two is adequate. A normal rectal temperature should be 37.5 to 38.9°C (99.5 to 102°F).

If you've got an animal showing signs of colic, one question you should ask is whether or not the animal is passing faeces. If they're cushed, is there a pile of poop behind them? If not, or you're unsure because the animal hasn't been stationary, I suggest you put on a medical examination glove, put a little lube on your index and middle fingers and stick a finger or two in through the anus gently feeling for faeces. If you feel faeces, collect a sample to put in a pot for your vet or to send to the lab.

It is useful to know the quality of the faeces. Are they normal beans? Or are they very dried and dehydrated-looking or soft and liquid? If no faeces are present at all, note that down as it is also useful information.

Checklist	Considered?
Body condition Score	
Check mucous membrane colour • *If anaemic, collect a faecal sample and check for lice in the hair coat.*	
Can the animal stand?	
If they can stand, are they able to walk? • *Does the movement look normal?*	
Check teeth, including the incisors, for overgrowth and check the jaws for any swellings.	
Check rectal temperature	
Colic? Are they passing faeces and urinating? • *What is the quality of the faeces?* • *Are they in the last few months of pregnancy?*	
Are they pregnant or lactating? • *Are you feeding enough?*	
Has anything changed recently in this animal's environment or social structure?	

Table 1. Quick checklist for the owner. These are things to check and questions to ask yourself when you find a sick animal. These will be useful for your vet to know the answers to.

If you have a female alpaca or llama, consider whether she is pregnant or lactating. Most of the time, alpacas will be either pregnant, lactating or both. In late gestation, we need to think about the metabolic demands of the rapidly growing foetus and whether the mother is being fed enough or if she is potentially getting into a negative energy balance. Are there other demands on her energy, such as parasites, that might create a negative energy balance? Another potential issue during late pregnancy is uterine torsion, which can cause signs of colic. In a full-term female, uterine torsion is still a consideration, as is dystocia or difficult birth. Females with uterine torsion typically separate themselves from the rest of the herd, don't come up to eat, sit with their legs out to one side, then switch sides and stand up and down regularly. Their respiratory rate and effort will be increased due to pain. Lactating females also have high metabolic demands, with peak milk production expected once crias are around 4–8 weeks old. Other postpartum complications may be a concern in lactating females, such as mastitis or a uterine infection (metritis) that occurs within a few weeks of birth.

If you've got a sick newborn cria, consider whether it could be hypothermic. You can check the rectal temperature for this. If it is hypothermic, you will need to take steps to warm it up. For newborns that haven't nursed and are weak, hypoglycaemia may be an issue. If they've not yet fed, get some honey or syrup that you can smear inside their mouth, as this will be rapidly absorbed and give them a little energy to keep them going until your vet arrives. Alternatively, you could transport the cria to the vet for an IV catheter and care as appropriate. If they can nurse, get them nursing from their dam or bottle feed them.

Finally, think about whether you changed something recently that potentially resulted in the problem you're seeing. For example, have you made any dietary changes, and if so, what did you do? Did you make those changes sufficiently? Did the gut have time to adapt? Have there been any recent stresses in this animal's life, such as recent weaning, or is the animal new to the herd or has social stress from being moved to a different group? Remember that stress can leave them more susceptible to other problems.

What's Next?

Once you've done your initial checks on the animal, decide whether to call the vet. If it's really an emergency – for example, if you know an animal has broken a leg – call the vet first! Then, you can take the steps above to stabilise the animal.

Once your vet gets to the farm, they will want to hear as much information about the case as possible and will want answers to all the questions I posed above. They will also perform a thorough examination. The problem is that many sick alpacas appear the same. They're lethargic, they're anorexic, depressed, recumbent and so on. Physical exam findings might be unremarkable or just not specific enough to point to one particular diagnosis. Remember that we can't evaluate the abdomen particularly well in camelids because of their size. If the animal is not eating, you don't want to wait around for 24 hours and see what happens, as that can be costly. Discuss the options with the vet for further diagnostics, such as blood work, ultrasound and faecal testing. Consider asking for assistance from a specialist camelid vet or referring the case to a referral facility if necessary.

Options for Further Diagnostics

There are many different options for further diagnostics. Below, I have outlined the most important ones so you can get an idea of what is available and request them. Remember that these will cost money, but expecting your vet to work miracles with their "imaginoscope" to save money is somewhat unreasonable!

Lab Work

As I indicated earlier, camelids can look sicker on paper than they appear in front of you. They are good at masking the clinical signs of illness to avoid predation. So, if you know there's something wrong with an animal and the cause is not obvious on clinical examination, your vet is working in the dark until they get more information. Blood work and other tests can be hugely illuminating. If you "wait and see what happens," the animal *may* improve. But if it doesn't, it could get considerably worse in the following 24 hours, and you'll have no data suggesting what might be happening. On top of that, you've also delayed getting that data, which can entail a much worse outcome for the patient. So, although there is a cost implication in getting those lab results, you may need an additional, more costly vet visit. Remember that most first-opinion vets will need to send blood to a lab to get results, so there is already a 24-hour delay built in. And if it's a Thursday, there's another reason not to delay: Lab services may not be available on the weekend, so you don't necessarily even have a day in hand. The situation always carries more urgency if you have an alpaca or llama not eating or drinking. We can always do things to support the patient while waiting to get further information, but treatment can be more effectively targeted when the lab results are known.

Now, there are various types of lab work that we can do.

1. **Complete Biochemistry and Haematology**
   In an ideal world, I would always like to run this because it provides the most detailed information. However, it is not always available, particularly in emergencies that occur out of hours, on the weekends and in the field. In referral facilities, this is one major advantage they have: They can often run full panels at any time of day or night, giving very rapid access to the patient's clinical status. At Ohio State, we were always able to get this within 30 minutes overnight from the student extern who assisted us out of hours.

   With a complete panel, we can see what is going on with the red and white cell populations, whether there is an infection and how the body responds. We can also see protein concentrations and the balance of proteins, evaluate the liver and kidneys, and assess the balance of the key electrolytes responsible for the body's homeostasis. We can also see glucose and indicators of energy balance. Finally, a full panel can also include an indication of acid-base balance with a bicarbonate concentration.

Check the supplementary PDF for the ideal bloodwork panel and reference ranges that may help you and your veterinarian.

2. **Emergency Lab Work**

Some vets may have access to emergency lab work using special equipment. This equipment won't provide as comprehensive a panel as the complete biochemistry and haematology, but it enables us to stabilise a patient out of hours until we can run the full panel. Examples of this equipment include the EPOC and iSTAT machines. The EPOC is an excellent tool for large animal practitioners because the cartridges do not require refrigeration, unlike the iSTAT ones. It can save time and extra visits in emergency cases.

This equipment will check kidney parameters, which is important for assessing fluid balance since these values often rise when camelids are dehydrated. It will also assess kidney disease and conditions that lead to urine retention. The equipment will also assess key electrolytes, such as glucose, lactate and acid-base balances, which are important in managing fluid balance.

3. **Packed Cell Volume and Total Protein Concentration (PCV/TP)**

These are key parameters to evaluate in sick camelids. Along with the fresh blood smear, faecal test and perhaps glucose concentration, PCV and TP constitute the *minimum* database in an emergency without access to the other labs mentioned above or where funds are limited.

We instantly get so much information about our patients with just these two critical indicators. If both are increased, it might suggest dehydration. If they are decreased, it could indicate conditions that cause loss of protein or red cells, such as parasitism or chronic disease. If PCV alone is decreased, I'd think more about causes of anaemia such as *Haemonchus, Mycoplasma haemolamae,* lice infestation or blood loss. If the TP is decreased but PCV isn't, I'd think about conditions that cause protein loss, such as *E mac* infestations or other protein-losing disorders.

While these are simplifications and certainly do not provide the whole picture, they can provide us with some key and early information using basic lab equipment. All we need is a centrifuge, microhaematocrit tubes and reader, and a refractometer. Most vets should have this equipment in-house.

4. **Fresh Blood Smear Evaluation**

Blood smears are crucial for evaluating haematology. While a machine can give you the total red and white cell counts, they may not be accurate for doing differential white cell counts. This is because they need to be calibrated correctly for camelid cells, which are different. The blood smear allows you to count the proportions of cells of each type on a slide. A good lab will always read this manually to confirm the results. This can be important to determine whether there's an infection or a parasite problem, for example. You can also look for *Mycoplasma haemolamae* on the red cells and determine whether an anaemic animal is trying to replace its lost red cells.

The blood smear needs to be made *fresh* immediately after the sample is collected to obtain accurate information. If it's not fresh, *Mycoplasma haemolamae* may fail to be diagnosed as it drops off the red cells, while the white cell morphology deteriorates, so not as much information is acquired. This is important whether performing the analysis in-house or sending the sample to a lab. An expensive lab can only provide valuable information if you provide it with a quality sample. Another example of "you get out what you put in"!

I don't have a machine, but I can get a crude idea of the total white cell count on a slide and perform a differential white cell count in about 10 minutes, while the centrifuge runs to give me the PCV/TP. Recognising what is normal and abnormal takes a little practice, but it is relatively simple.

5. **Glucose Concentration**

Many sick and stressed camelids have high glucose concentrations. If they are particularly high or remain high despite treatment of the underlying problem, insulin therapy may be required to return them to normal.

Hypoglycaemia is rarely a problem except in neonates that have yet to nurse. In these cases, blood glucose levels can be extremely low and necessitate immediate glucose administration.

Glucose is really easy to measure, and a handheld glucometer is a worthwhile investment. Although expensive veterinary glucometers are available now, these are calibrated for dogs and cats and have not been tested in camelids. Human glucometers are cheap and readily available through your local pharmacy. Given the usually significant abnormalities in camelid blood glucose measurements we monitor, I believe they are perfectly adequate for managing sick camelids. Additionally, you can check a blood glucose concentration without needing to be able to collect a jugular blood sample – you can do this yourself by clipping the hair away from the inside edge base of the ear and using a lancet or hypodermic needle to draw a small bleb of blood, which is all that is required.

The glucometer is a really useful tool for your first aid kit to use on sick animals, particularly crias! However, remember to replace the strips when they go out of date because the machines won't work with out-of-date strips.

6. **Minerals**

Depending on a patient's clinical signs, these can be added to the complete biochemistry and haematology profile as needed. They can also be used as stand-alone tests to monitor the trace element status that your nutrition is providing. The most common minerals tested include copper, selenium, cobalt, zinc and iron.

Faecal Testing

A key diagnostic test that should always be included to evaluate any sick camelid is a faecal test. The incidence of parasite problems is so high wherever you are in the world that it must be ruled out. Important facts to remember:

- Camelids can have very significant parasite burdens with perfectly normal-looking stools.
- The type of test performed is important. Some tests will not detect potentially significant burdens of heavier or denser eggs and oocysts, such as *Nematodirus, Trichuris* and *E mac.* Check with your lab to find out what test they do. The Modified Stolls test is the ideal choice for doing camelid faecal testing. For more information on this, please refer to Chapter 10.

Abdominal Ultrasound

The diagnostic importance of ultrasonography in camelid medicine cannot be emphasised enough. In my practice, abdominal ultrasound is an extension of the physical examination of all sick camelids, especially in adult animals. It enables me to evaluate the gastrointestinal tract and all the other intra-abdominal structures. It provides a "window" into the abdomen of a camelid. Ultrasonography may also be used in the evaluation of externally palpable masses prior to taking aspirates, as a guide for taking fluid samples from the abdominal or thoracic cavities, or to guide biopsy of internal organs, as well as for evaluation of the chest in some instances and for echocardiography. Evaluation of the foetus in pregnant females can also be valuable.

Portable ultrasound quality is now excellent and much more affordable. However, many large animal vets have ultrasound machines focused purely on cattle reproduction, which may not be the best for abdominal ultrasound. The good news for owners is that clipping the fleece is not normally required for ultrasound. I just part the fleece and use alcohol/spirit as my contact medium. I avoid using gel, which requires clipping and leaves a sticky residue that can't be adequately removed. In contrast, alcohol just dries out. The only time I need to clip is for specific indications, such as if there is a particular need to follow a structure like the bile duct or if I want to aspirate a lesion.

Radiography

Radiography will be useful for investigating fractures or lameness of unknown origin. It can also evaluate mandibular swellings or examine the animal's chest or abdomen. The main barrier to using radiography is that many farm animal veterinarians do not have access to a machine because this equipment is expensive, and they don't use it enough. If your vet belongs to a practice that also works with horses or small animals, they will almost certainly have access to a machine, but if they are farm animals only, they may need to refer you for radiography.

Consultation With or Referral to a Specialist

If your veterinarian is struggling to diagnose a case, it may be worth asking them to consult with a specialist or to consider referring your animal to a specialist. This should never be seen as a failure on their part. Rather, it recognises that specialists have knowledge and skills in a particular area that are a valuable adjunct to the care that a generalist can provide in the field. General practice vets have a vast amount of knowledge and skill across various topics, but it is unfair to expect them to know everything. For the same reason, if we have a particular health problem, our doctor will refer us to a specialist in that area of human medicine or surgery, and the same system exists in veterinary medicine to support general practice vets.

When progressing to this next step, if I am asked to provide a remote consultation, it works best if I can involve both the owner and vet at this stage to get a complete picture. I get detailed veterinary clinical exam findings from the veterinarian, but owners can often give me historical information that perhaps the vet hasn't already discovered. If everyone is included, it is easier to provide the right advice and everyone is on the same page. The animal's primary care veterinarian must be included because they will provide ongoing care for the patient and need to know what I may have shared with the owner or what I recommended. I call this the "veterinary care triad."

With modern video-calling technology, I have been able to assist general practice vets in their examinations. This works quite well in neuro and dermatology cases, as I get the vet to do some diagnostic testing while the owner holds the phone for me to see what's going on and talk them through the examination. This works well for helping with neurological localisation, such as directing the vet to the region of concern.

Field Therapeutics

It's important to realise that wherever you are in the world, almost all drugs used in camelids are used off-label, meaning that they're neither licensed for use in camelids nor tested for safety and efficacy, and they are never likely to be. Why is that? The reason is simply that there is no money in camelids for the pharmaceutical companies. It's incredibly costly to license a drug in each species, and this would have to be repeated in every jurisdiction around the world. For perspective, there are only about 4 million alpacas globally. Compare this to global numbers of 1.4 billion cattle, 1 billion sheep and 0.5 billion goats. Given that very few medicines are licensed for goats either, and there are more than 100 times the number of goats in the world, you can see that the financial incentive just doesn't exist. While there isn't a financial incentive for big pharma, fortunately, many research studies on the use of various medicines in camelids have been conducted by interested specialists within academia. These are only ever going to be small in scale, but they help us understand what medicines can and cannot be used, whether or not they are safe and what doses we should use them at.

Medicine Use

There are three main issues to address when we decide what medicines to use. Firstly, we need to know that a particular medicine is safe. Then, we need to see if it's effective and at what dose it needs to be used to be effective. The route of administration is also important. In most cases, the medicines we use in camelids will need to be administered by some route other than orally because most drugs cannot get past the first stomach compartment in sufficient concentrations to be absorbed as an effective dose. Mostly, these will be injectable medicines. The big exception to this rule is the wormers, which are effective orally. The need for injectable medicines limits our potential medicine chest contents because many veterinary medicines developed for use in small animal patients are only available in tablet form. For example, our options are extremely limited for treating camelids with heart failure. We only have diuretics and none of the beta-blockers, ACE inhibitors or calcium channel blockers.

We'll discuss each of the three main issues below, concerning camelids specifically.

Safety

It is not safe to assume that because a medicine is used for a certain indication in another ruminant species, it must be okay in camelids. When new medicines come onto the market, wait for information before jumping in. We know that some drugs are toxic to camelids.

Lutalyse (Zoetis) is a medicine with known toxicity in camelids.[1] Lutalyse contains dinoprost and is a natural prostaglandin used to treat retained corpora lutea or control reproduction. It has caused severe reactions in camelids, including respiratory distress and death. Therefore, it is best avoided. Instead, we normally use cloprostenol, which is a synthetic form of prostaglandin.

Some antibiotics are also best avoided. Tilmicosin is the active ingredient in Micotil (Elanco) and is an antibiotic used for treating pneumonia in cattle but has caused deaths in treated alpacas. The datasheet is quite scary: there are dire warnings about self-injection causing fatalities in humans and contraindications for use in pigs, equines and goats, which does not usually offer an invitation for off-label usage. The toxicity may be due to cardiovascular issues associated with its calcium channel-blocking effect, a feature of the class of antibiotics. Therefore, I recommend avoiding Micotil or any closely related macrolide antibiotics such as tulathromycin (Draxxin, Zoetis) and gamithromycin (Zactran, Boehringer Ingelheim). These all work in the same way by blocking calcium channels.

I am aware of anecdotal reports of fatalities in alpacas administered tulathromycin but not specifically for gamithromycin. A recent study showed that gamithromycin concentrated well into the lung and white blood cells, making it useful in treating pneumonia, which camelids don't often get compared with cattle. However, one of the six treated alpacas developed colic.[2] The authors of the study recommended only using it with caution until further investigations could be done concerning potential side effects. However, it would be sensible to avoid it until reliable safety data is obtained. Fortunately, alternative antibiotics are available that we do know are safe and effective.

Medicines to Avoid Due to Known Toxicity

- **Lutalyse.** A natural prostaglandin used to induce luteolysis and treat retained CL. Has caused severe reactions in camelids, including respiratory distress and death. Synthetic prostaglandins are safer.
- **Tilmicosin (Micotil) and the related macrolide antibiotics: tulathromycin (Draxxin) and gamithromycin (Zactran).** Tilmicosin is known to cause deaths, while there is anecdotal evidence of tulathromycin. Gamithromycin has not caused deaths that I am aware of, but one animal in a study displayed colic signs. I urge caution since all act via the same mechanism. Select something less risky.
- **Multimin (Virbac).** This has been associated with multiple deaths due to selenium toxicity.

Efficacy

Some medicines are known to be effective in camelids, while others are not.

There are many different non-steroidal anti-inflammatory drugs (NSAIDs), and we know that the pharmacokinetics of these drugs differ significantly across different species. Some of these have been tested in camelid species. We can use flunixin and meloxicam, for instance, but not phenylbutazone. Phenylbutazone, readily available in powder form for oral administration to horses, is not adequately absorbed in camelids. It can be given intravenously but has a short half-life.[3] Both flunixin and meloxicam are available in injectable and oral formulations for large animals. We know we can use flunixin as an injectable, but it is not absorbed reliably when given orally.[4] However, meloxicam can be used both orally and as an injectable.[5] Flunixin is recommended only for short-term use (normally 5 days), while meloxicam has fewer expected adverse effects on the kidneys and stomach lining, so it is used for longer-term therapy.

Likewise, we have pharmacokinetic data for several antibiotics. People always like to grab long-acting medicines because it means less dosing is required. One such antibiotic is a long-acting ceftiofur, known as Excede (Zoetis) in the US but as Naxcel (Zoetis) in the UK, which is a little confusing because Naxcel is the name of a shorter-acting ceftiofur in the US. The long-acting formulation has a 7-day effect in cattle. However, to achieve reasonably high concentrations in camelids, it has to be used every 2-3 days. It is only recommended for use for highly susceptible bacteria based on culture and susceptibility testing results. I do not recommend using this drug empirically purely for ease of use as it may be ineffective and may contribute to resistance in this critically important antibiotic class.

An important point concerning efficacy is that you should not keep open bottles of antibiotics. Write the date of opening on the bottle or box and throw it away after 28 days. Medicines are not tested beyond that point for safety or efficacy. Knowing that an antibiotic will be effective in a sick animal is vital when you want to use it. Make sure you store antibiotics according to their label directions, as some need to be kept in the fridge.

Dose

The dose of medicine you use should be effective, so the points on efficacy and dosage are intimately related. It is worth waiting for information to be published regarding safe and effective dosing regimes for medicine use in camelids because camelids metabolise and eliminate drugs differently than other species, so direct extrapolation from a label can be potentially harmful. The dose, dosing interval and recommended duration of treatment should be followed. Here are some examples:

- If your vet wants to prescribe ceftiofur, I suggest using the shorter-acting formulations at 2.2 mg/kg, which is the dose used in horses but twice the dose used in cattle.[6]
- Penicillin is best used at 22,000 IU/kg (or 13.2 mg/kg), while label recommendations are 10 mg/kg.
- Amoxicillin trihydrate (e.g., Synulox or Clamoxyl, Zoetis) needs to be used at 15 mg/kg, though the label dose for all species it is licensed for is 7 mg/kg. It can be used once daily for highly susceptible organisms or twice daily for less susceptible organisms. The dose should be differentiated based on culture and sensitivity results.
- We use wormer medications at doses that are vastly different from the label doses for other species, with the exception of levamisole, which has quite a narrow safety index. For example, monepantel is used three times the label dose, moxidectin is used two times the label dose for the oral formulation and fenbendazole is used two to four times the label dose.

I provide an owners' drug formulary in the book's supplementary PDF.

While I will deal with the responsible use of medicines in Chapter 15, it is worth mentioning the responsible use of antibiotics here. Remember that all antibiotics are prescription-only medicines wherever you are in the world. That means that a vet must prescribe them, and in certain parts of the world, a vet is required to inject them as well. It is essential for us all to have a responsible mindset around the use of antibiotics because we need to try and avoid the development of drug-resistant bacteria when antibiotics are misused. Do not self-prescribe antibiotics (or recommend them to other owners online!) because, as an owner, you have not been trained to know which antibiotic is appropriate for which problem, which drugs are toxic under which conditions or interactions between medicines that could be harmful. Also, for non-urgent problems, it's really important to get a culture and sensitivity and then medicate accordingly. For example, if I think a female has an infection in the uterus, I will never use antibiotics without doing culture and sensitivity first. I want to use the antibiotic that will have the best effect, and it's not always the first choice I might have initially guessed.

Intravenous Fluid Therapy

Intravenous (IV) fluid therapy is a life-saving intervention and one that is very possible to do in the field. There is sometimes a reluctance for vets to do this, either because they need to get used to IV fluid therapy in other species or because they're worried about placing IV catheters. However, encourage them to train on this because it can be the difference between survival and non-survival. In the box below, you will find a case story of just one case where IV fluids made the difference. I have run multiple free webinars for vets on this exact topic and offer an online Intensive Camelid Veterinary Care Course for those who want to learn more, so put them in touch so I can help. They can learn from anywhere in the world.

Farm animal vets have often relied on oral fluid administration for rehydration therapy. In larger animals that are severely compromised or septic from conditions such as toxic metritis or mastitis, provided this follows intravenous hypertonic saline administration it can sometimes be sufficient. However, if not used in this way, it can be a waste of time. In shock, the blood supply to "non-essential" organs such as the gastrointestinal tract is reduced, so absorption of fluids is likely to be much reduced. In addition, fluid dynamics across membranes may be altered and compromised if sepsis is involved. Camelids like sheep, particularly alpacas, are not much bigger than a large dog, so the required fluid volumes are quite manageable. Collapsed camelids in shock (high heart rate, poor peripheral perfusion, weak/thready pulses, evidence of dehydration) require emergency intravenous fluid therapy to provide cardiovascular support. Fluids should be administered via an indwelling catheter placed in the jugular vein rather than "off the needle" as it is difficult to remain in the vein, and this doesn't facilitate any further IV fluids. This can be an initial bolus that can be repeated periodically over the first 24 hours and tapered depending on the clinical response to treatment. I typically calculate the volume of fluids needed over the first 24 hours and divide this volume into boluses administered every 2–4 hours. I find bolus therapy easier to manage in the field than a drip because there are no lines for animals to get tangled in. I also find that most owners are open to being trained on giving those boluses themselves since no one is usually more motivated to help their alpaca or llama than its owner! I advise the vet to revisit the farm the next day to reassess the patient, the catheter and the ongoing management needs.

Here is an example of a case where IV fluid therapy was a key factor in her survival.

Figure 1 is a photo of an adult female huacaya alpaca I once saw in the field. She had been down for about 36 hours before I saw her. The owner kept thinking she was going to die and that it wasn't worth calling the vet. So they waited and waited, but she didn't die... Eventually, I was called to come and see her. The photo shows what she looked like on my arrival at the farm.

Her heart rate was high at 108 beats per minute – again, this would be consistent with shock. Her respiratory rate was okay. She had quiet gutsounds. She did have some faeces present in the rectum, but they were soft.

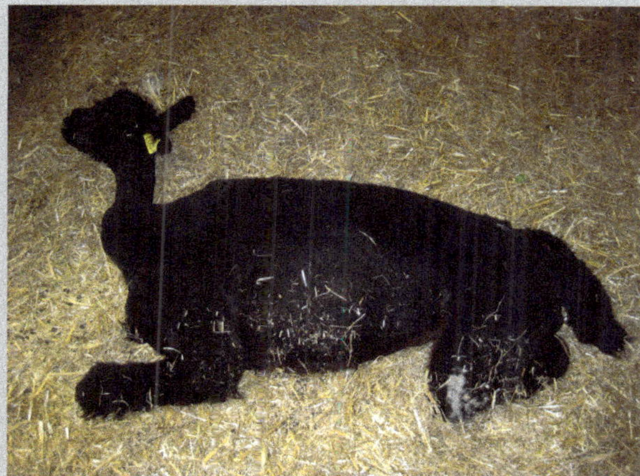

Figure 1. A collapsed adult female alpaca.
She was unable to stand or even hold her head up.

I collected a sample for analysis. She had red mucous membranes that were moist. Therefore, she didn't seem that dehydrated, but her capillary refill time – which is when you press on the mucous membranes to blanche the blood out of the area and see how quickly the blood reperfuses – was starting to prolong. She was very weak, as you could tell from the photo, unable to stand and had absolutely no neck strength whatsoever. These symptoms are quite common for sick camelids. If they're dehydrated or stop eating and their potassium levels get low, they don't have any neck strength.

On this particular day, I didn't have my ultrasound machine because it was away for servicing, which made me very unhappy. Thus, I often use this case for teaching because I managed it without any specialised diagnostic tools, similar to how many field veterinarians would have to operate. Based on my examination, I decided that she was in shock, and I placed an IV catheter so that I could provide IV fluid support. While I was placing the catheter, she sounded like she was trying to die! A sick alpaca is a stressed alpaca, and when you add more stress in placing a catheter, this can potentially tip them over the edge – but they will surely die without the catheter and IV fluid support! So, if you observe this, please do not panic! Let your vet work!

I gave her a litre of a balanced electrolyte solution. I started her on IV antibiotics because her bright red mucous membranes suggested she was septic, and I also gave her IV flunixin as an anti-inflammatory. I collected a blood sample, made a fresh blood smear and took these along with the faecal sample back to my shed. At the time, I was working out of my shed at home, where I had some basic lab facilities and stored my veterinary equipment.

When I looked at the blood smear, I found that she had a massively increased white cell count with a left shift, which meant she was septic, so I felt justified in having given her the antibiotics. The faecal was negative – no eggs or oocysts were seen. It had been about one o'clock when I left the farm, and I went back a couple of hours later to provide another IV fluid bolus and to set the plan for the next 24 hours. I ensured the caretakers were happy with their instructions on checking the catheter and providing the bolus of fluids. At about five o'clock, I called the farm and asked how she was. They said she was standing and eating, so they were happy. They gave her IV fluids every two hours until midnight and then again at four, six, and eight o'clock. The following day, she looked great! We made a plan to taper her fluids over the next 24 hours. The photo in Figure 2 shows how she looked just 18 hours after I arrived on the farm to examine her.

Now, you're probably wondering what caused this alpaca to be so unwell in the first place. Well, what I had thought had happened was that it was a warm summer day, she was a black animal and there didn't happen to be any shelter in the field she was in. I think she went sunbathing, and then, because she had a six-week-old cria that she was feeding, the water demand increased and her body couldn't keep up. She got herself a little bit dehydrated and perhaps heat-stressed. At six weeks of lactation, this is around the time that they have the highest milk yield. Ultimately, I think she got a little stressed and developed some erosions or ulcers in her third stomach compartment, developed erosions or ulcers in her third stomach compartment, allowing bacteria to enter her bloodstream and causing sepsis. She needed the fluid therapy to support her cardiovascular system, and the IV antibiotics were also obviously vital as well. However, I believe the IV fluid therapy saved this animal. If I'd just gone with IV antibiotics and NSAIDs, I'm confident that she would have died. This case demonstrates how rapid recovery can be for a relatively simple case with the correct level of care. It would have been easy to have assumed she was beyond help. And all that was achieved without hospital-level diagnostics access or equipment - just simple tools and skills.

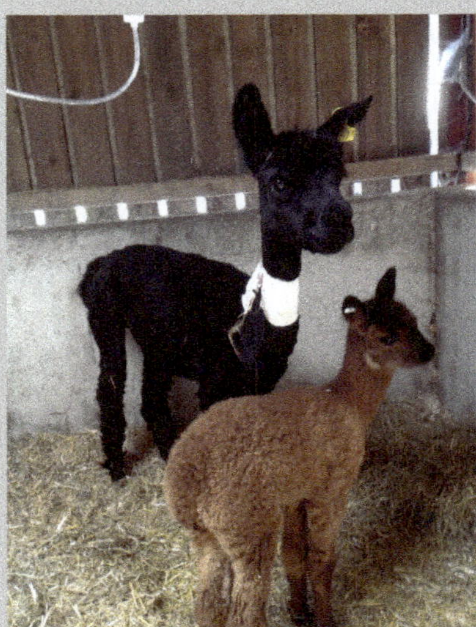

Figure 2. The same alpaca as in Figure 1, but 18 hours later.

Wound Care

Most cuts and abrasions will heal well, especially those that have not gone through the skin (full thickness). It is helpful to clean the wound to remove any visible and microscopic contamination and reduce bacterial load that may cause wound infection. Cleaning allows you to inspect the wound more closely. Full-thickness lacerations that have cut through the layers of the skin will heal more quickly and with less scarring or secondary complications if your veterinarian sutures them. Fresh wounds, such as those that occur at shearing when the blades cut the skin, can be cleaned and the edges apposed using veterinary tissue glue. Tissue glue is medical glue developed specifically for use on skin wounds, rather than "superglue," which is toxic to tissues due to the heat it produces. Note that wounds over 8 hours old should not be glued or sutured since infection may be sealed inside. Instead, they should be managed with cleaning and allowed to heal themselves. Puncture wounds such as dog bites can cause extensive tissue damage under the skin and should always be assessed by a vet.

Here are some step-by-step instructions to help you deal with wounds:

1. If the wound is actively bleeding, apply pressure using gauze swabs directly over the wound until bleeding stops.

2. Clipping around the wound's edges helps remove excessive hair and allows for effective cleaning.

3. Wash the wound using diluted iodine solution to the colour of weak tea, or use salt water. Use a large syringe to flush the wound (under a little bit of pressure) to remove contamination until you're satisfied that the wound is clean. Soak gauze swabs in the diluted iodine solution (or salt water) to aid in cleaning. These can help remove debris and any dead tissue. When satisfied, dab the wound with a clean, dry swab to remove excess solution. Avoid using cotton wool to clean wounds as it leaves little white fibres in the wound.

4. Minor wounds can be left uncovered to heal, while more serious wounds on the limbs can be covered. First, cut a non-adhesive dressing, such as melolin, to fit the wound. Then, secure it in place using a conforming bandage, cohesive bandage (such as Vetrap) and elasticated adhesive bandage, as required, to secure the bandage by sticking to the surrounding haircoat. These dressings must be changed daily to allow for the inspection of wounds and further cleaning as required. Sutured wounds do not normally require a dressing, but your vet will advise you.

5. Inspect the wound twice daily and repeat cleaning as required.

6. Antibiotic spray (often called "purple spray" because of its colour and usually containing oxytetracycline antibiotic) is often used and can be helpful to highlight a wound. However, it can make a mess on white animals and doesn't achieve much beyond daily cleaning using antibacterial solutions (iodine or

salt water). Alternative options include aluminium or silver wound sprays.

7. A fly spray may be needed to dab *around* a wound when flies are present to prevent them from laying eggs, which could result in a fly strike.

You should call your vet to help you with any of the following wounds:

- Full-thickness lacerations that require suturing, including lacerations from shearing clippers. Get these sutured as soon as possible while they are clean and fresh. You can't normally suture anything older than 8 hours because an infection may be sealed inside the wound.
- Any wounds with dead tissue or skin need debriding to aid healing.
- Anything that you are not comfortable dealing with.

Puncture wounds from animal bites.

If you find a bleeding wound, the first goal is to stop the bleeding by applying pressure. For minor wounds, use gauze swabs. Place several of these directly over the bleeding wound and apply pressure until it stops bleeding. This may take a few minutes. If it bleeds through, add more swabs. For more significant wounds, apply pressure directly using larger, clean towels.

Management of Recumbent Camelids

In this final section of the chapter, I would like to discuss how to manage recumbent animals, as they are not uncommon, and there are some important things you need to be aware of that will help you care for them.

Firstly, maintain them in a normal cushed position rather than letting them lie on their sides. This position is better for their lungs. When animals lie on their sides for long, the lung closest to the ground can become congested with fluid. If they don't want to stay upright, try propping them up using small hay or straw bales. If that doesn't work, then at least try to turn them from one side to the other every few hours to try and avoid that lung congestion. There are some conditions, though, like listeriosis, where animals cannot physically remain on one side and will only lie on the other. If so, deep bedding with straw will be needed to ensure comfort and reduce pressure sores.

Since recumbent animals cannot move themselves to defecate or urinate, you will need to move them around regularly so that they are sitting on clean straw. If they sit in their urine, their skin may get urine scalded. This is particularly a problem with recumbent males as they are literally sitting on top of the urine that they pass. If you find that they get urine staining on the fleece, and you will know this because the smell of urine will be very strong when you turn them to the side, then you should clean them with warm, soapy water and apply a barrier cream like Sudocrem to protect the skin.

If your patient cannot stand by themselves, I would assist them to stand several times a day because it's good for their muscles to move around. Some animals just require assistance to stand up, but once they're standing, they can remain standing and walk around for a little while.

Performing physiotherapy with recumbent animals is useful. This can include massaging the leg muscles, particularly those of the upper limb, and passive flexion and extension exercises to get the joints moving because recumbent animals can become stiff and lose mobility. Slinging can also be used to try to rest their legs. Slings can be challenging to manage. You have to have a sling to support the patient, and it must be positioned in such a way that it doesn't hurt the belly or cover the penis of a male but still help in holding the animal up. Hoists with ropes and pulleys can be used, and specially designed slings with frames made for calves also work well for camelid patients. Overall, camelids tend to tolerate these devices quite well. However, I had one llama patient who would only swing when we tried to elevate him in a sling, which was quite frustrating. I also had an alpaca patient who wanted to keep walking on just the forelimbs when you lifted her. She didn't appreciate a fixed sling but was very happy to walk around with a team of students supporting her weight in a sleeping bag slung under her belly!

Key Takeaways

In this chapter, I emphasised the importance of learning your animals' behaviour and trusting your instinct if you think something is wrong. Further diagnostics are worth investing in because a physical examination may only provide limited information, and camelids are experts at hiding signs of illness. Always consider performing lab work, getting a faecal sample tested and, if available, an abdominal ultrasound. Do not hesitate to ask your vet for a second opinion or a referral.

I've provided valuable tips on approaching a sick animal and what actions to take. I've also included a list of things to consider and check that may provide important clues about the problem at hand.

When deciding to use a particular medicine, you need to know whether it is safe and effective and what dose to use. Don't be tempted to use medicines we don't know anything about in camelids because there can be problems with safety and dosing. We know to avoid Lutalyse, tilmicosin, related macrolide antibiotics, and Multimin.

Intravenous (IV) fluid therapy is a life-saving intervention and one that is very possible to do in the field. It should be considered for any collapsed camelid or one not eating or drinking while awaiting diagnostic testing results.

15

Responsible Camelid Ownership

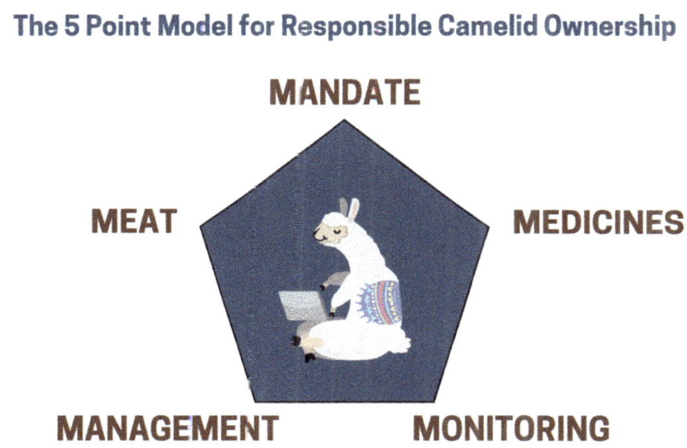

Figure 1. The 5-point model for Responsible Camelid Ownership covers the 5 areas of responsibility.

There are a number of responsibilities you have to be aware of to meet your legal, ethical and animal health obligations for keeping camelids. To make these memorable, I have developed a 5-point model to help you remember them. There are five components to the model, each one starting with the letter M.

The five areas of responsibility are highlighted at the points of the pentagon in *Figure 1*:

1. **MANDATE** – The legal obligations you must meet
2. **MEDICINES** – The responsible use of medicines
3. **MONITORING** – Regular observations to spot signs of illness
4. **MANAGEMENT** – Day-to-day care practices that keep your animals healthy
5. **MEAT** – For those owners who put camelids into the food chain, you have specific legal obligations to ensure meat is safe for human consumption.

We'll now work through each of the five areas of responsibility, starting with your legal obligations.

MANDATE

If you own animals, you have a legal and ethical responsibility to look after those animals. Although there are different legal definitions around your specific responsibilities depending on the country within which you abide, the Animal Welfare Act 2006 (UK legislation) provides regulations that specify some basic elements of the duty of care that provide a good model for camelid owners anywhere in the world. These elements require that, as owners and caretakers, you have a duty of care to your animals. You must provide them with a suitable living environment, an appropriate diet, opportunities to exhibit normal behaviour, companionship with other animals if applicable for the species, and protection from pain, injury, suffering and disease.

You could be prosecuted for not providing acceptable animal welfare standards in your country. The guidelines of the Animal Welfare Act are closely related to "the 5 Freedoms." The freedoms were developed in 1965 in response to a UK government investigation into farmed animal welfare and have been adopted internationally. The five freedoms are:

1. **Freedom from hunger and thirst.** Animals must have access to fresh water and a proper diet that maintains their health.
2. **Freedom from discomfort.** Animals must be provided with an appropriate environment, including shelter and somewhere to rest.
3. **Freedom from pain, injury or disease.** This is assured by prevention strategies, including herd health planning and ensuring that the animal areas are clear of dangerous features. Provision of rapid diagnosis and treatment in the event of an injury or illness is also required and will involve having a relationship with a local veterinary care provider.
4. **Freedom to express normal behaviour.** Animals need to have sufficient space in which to express normal behaviours. Assuring this freedom includes providing the proper facilities and ensuring they have their own kind for company. This is also why having a solitary camelid is not considered good welfare. It may be that some individuals need to be kept on their own in a paddock or holding area due to injury or to prevent injury or for quarantine purposes, but they should be close enough to other camelids to be able to see and "engage" with them.
5. **Freedom from fear and distress.** This is interesting because it covers ensuring the mental well-being of your animals. You should do what you can to minimise stress.

Most of these freedoms are rooted in common sense. However, they emphasise the responsibility to learn what constitutes an appropriate diet for camelids, what a suitable living environment looks like and what kind of shelter is necessary based on your location and weather conditions. They also require you to understand normal behaviour in camelids and to recognise any issues with your animals, taking appropriate action to ensure their welfare. Having read most of this book up to this point, you are likely already aware of these requirements, but if you are selling animals, you should also feel obliged to ensure that any new owners know what is expected of them. Make sure that they take steps to learn or take some courses – feel free to provide them with a copy of this book! If you don't think that they are appropriate owners or that their incentives for keeping camelids are not honourable, you have an ethical responsibility to those animals to deny the sale.

Be sure to familiarise yourself with any additional responsibilities in your country, such as registering your animals or the property where they are kept and whether animal identification is required. Pay close attention to regulations regarding which procedures can or cannot be performed on your animals, who are authorised to perform them, and any age restrictions that may apply. Additionally, familiarise yourself with rules for transporting animals, using them in paid or unpaid activities involving the public, and disposing of deceased animals. In most countries, certain diseases will be considered "notifiable," meaning that if you suspect an animal might have a particular disease, you are legally obliged to report it to the authorities. For example, some notifiable diseases in the UK include bovine TB, brucellosis, anthrax, bluetongue, foot and mouth disease, bird flu and rabies.

The following section will discuss the responsible use of medicines in camelids. This topic is very important because we want to ensure that medicines are available when needed. This is to ensure animal welfare and the right medicines are used.

MEDICINES

To my knowledge, no medicines are licensed outside of South America for use in camelids. This means that labels do not contain any information about dosing recommendations either. When vets prescribe medicines for camelids in the UK, we do so under a system called the "cascade," which permits the use of medicines licensed for similar uses in other species.

Other countries have their own regulations for "off-label" use, that is, using a medicine in a species it is not licensed in or for a use it is not licensed for. You must be aware of these regulations.

Ask your regular veterinarian for information relevant to you, wherever you are in the world. There are various sources of information about how these drugs are dosed, but probably the most comprehensive recent resource is within the pages of *Llama & Alpaca Care* (Elsevier 2014, editors Cebra, Anderson, Tibary, van Saun and Johnson). Within this text, the doses of various medicines are provided based on pharmacological studies or sound clinical experience. I often hear people say, "We don't know anything about camelids," or "There is no information available." This is not true.

Although there are admittedly far fewer journal articles and research studies on the use of different medicines in camelids, there are many in the peer-reviewed literature. We know less about how doses should be adjusted for different age groups or disease states to account for variations in physiological status.

Safety of Medicines in Camelids

As mentioned above, no medicines are licensed for use in camelids. Licensing in a particular species entails the medicine undergoing a whole barrage of pharmacokinetics, safety and efficacy testing before going to market. Since medicines aren't licensed specifically for camelid species, these studies have not been done. They will have been completed for the species for which they are licensed and tested for the specific uses listed on the label.

So where does that leave us for using medicines in Camelid species? In general, drugs that are used safely in a wide range of different species and have a wide margin of safety in those species are also likely to be relatively safe in camelids. In addition, where doses used are similar across a range of species, those doses are *likely* to be similar (but not always) in camelids. An example of this would be penicillin.

Other drugs may have known toxicity issues and are more safely used based on pharmacologic study data. A drug that has known severe adverse consequences in some species would not be a drug to consider using off-label in camelids. One example is tilmicosin (e.g. "Micotil," Elanco Animal Health). This product bears a warning in the datasheet that it should not be administered to horses, goats or pigs and that "injection of the product in goats and pigs has been fatal." The label also says, "INJECTION OF THIS DRUG IN HUMANS HAS BEEN ASSOCIATED WITH FATALITIES." Despite this, due to its widespread and successful use in cattle for pneumonia, some clinicians have used tilmicosin in alpacas – and in some cases, it has been fatal. In one unpublished study, it killed 4 out of 8 alpacas treated with it. Therefore, it would clearly be best to avoid this drug in camelids!

Tilmicosin is a macrolide antibiotic. Two closely related drugs to tilmicosin, which are also macrolides, are gamithromycin, marketed as "Zactran" (Boehringer Ingelheim) and tulathromycin (Draxxin, Zoetis). I am aware of anecdotal reports of fatalities in alpacas administered tulathromycin but not specifically for gamithromycin. A recent study found that gamithromycin concentrates effectively in lung and white blood cells, making it potentially useful for treating pneumonia. Although camelids are less prone to pneumonia than cattle, one of the six treated alpacas in the study developed colic.[1] The study's authors recommended using it with caution until further investigations could be done about side effects. At this time, I am not comfortable recommending the use of any of these drugs in camelids without a pharmacokinetic and safety study. To date, this is not available.

Lutalyse (Zoetis) is a medicine with known toxicity in camelids.[2] Lutalyse contains dinoprost and is a natural prostaglandin used to treat retained corpora lutea or control reproduction. It has caused serious reactions in camelids, including respiratory distress and death, therefore is best avoided. Instead, we usually use cloprostenol, which is a synthetic form of prostaglandin.

Multimin (Virbac) has caused multiple deaths in alpacas due to selenium toxicity. This is thought to be a problem with products containing sodium selenate or selenite. Other brand-name products containing the same ingredients may also be toxic, so read the label on any selenium supplements you use. Long-acting products such as Selovin LA contain barium selenate and are safe; however, long-acting selenium products are banned in the EU for food-producing animals. If you are in the UK and wish to use these products, you can only do so legally by ensuring treated animals *never* potentially enter the food chain. This commitment must be passed on to any future owners. In any case, always check selenium concentrations before supplementation. Otherwise, I suggest using only oral products for supplementation in the UK.

Ionophore antibiotics are also known to be toxic to camelids. This was seen in a death outbreak that occurred in alpacas fed Land o' Lakes Camelid feed in 2003, in Ohio in the US.[3] In this case, the feed had been accidentally contaminated with salinomycin and other ionophores. The use of ionophores as growth promotion agents has been banned in the EU since 2006, but some are still used in poultry feed as coccidiostats. Therefore, it is recommended that camelid feed is not produced in mills that also produce poultry feed.

Efficacy of Medicines in Camelids

When deciding whether to use a particular drug, I will look for evidence of pharmacokinetics studies showing that a specific drug is absorbed effectively at the dosage and route listed and that it should reach therapeutic concentrations in camelids. Just because a drug is licensed via a particular route in a different species does not mean that it will be adequately absorbed to be effective in camelids – even drugs licensed for cattle and sheep. Most medicines, although not all, are ineffective via the oral route because dilution and inactivation occur in the first stomach fermentation chamber, resulting in poor bioavailability. A big exception is for anthelmintics (wormers), which are usually given orally and don't necessarily need to be absorbed to take effect.

Some groups of drugs, such as non-steroidal anti-inflammatory drugs (or NSAIDs), vary massively from species to species in terms of efficacy, including route of administration used, and also in terms of potential adverse side effects. For example, we know that flunixin (e.g. Finadyne, MSD Animal Health or Banamine, Merck Animal Health USA) should be dosed similarly to the dose for horses (1 mg/kg) or half the label dose for cattle. It should also be given as an injectable to be effective, as the oral formulation is not absorbed.[4]

Phenylbutazone ("Bute"), which is commonly used for horses with arthritis, is useless when given to camelids as it has a very short half-life and is not absorbed from the gut to be effective.[5] Note that it is also banned in food-producing animals because residues remain in the meat for a very long time. Meloxicam (e.g. "Metacam", Boehringer Ingelheim Ltd) is known to be safe and effective when given orally and can be useful in cases requiring a long-term anti-inflammatory or painkiller such as animals with arthritis.[6] It can also be used as an injectable.

Several antibiotics have been studied in camelids including ceftiofur, trimethoprim sulpha, ampicillin, amoxicillin, gentamicin, enrofloxacin and florphenicol. These studies give us useful information about therapeutic dosages, routes of administration and potential toxicities. Here are some key findings and conclusions from these studies:

- Multiple studies show the oral form of trimethoprim sulpha (TMP-S) is not absorbed in camelids.[7 8] With this drug given orally, all you will likely achieve is disruption of the normal gut flora. Injectable TMP-S can be used effectively as a broad-spectrum antibiotic, but it has been known to cause reactions if used in IV.
- Amoxicillin trihydrate (e.g. Synulox or Clamoxyl, Zoetis) needs to be used at 15 mg/kg, while the label dose for all species it is licensed for is 7 mg/kg.[9] It can be used once daily for highly susceptible organisms or twice daily for less susceptible organisms. This should be differentiated based on culture and sensitivity results.
- Ceftiofur should be used at 2.2 mg/kg twice daily (compared with 1 mg/kg for cattle and 2 mg/kg for horses).[10] Note that this is a critically important antimicrobial in human medicine, so it should not normally be used as a first-line antibiotic except in certain circumstances.
- Ceftiofur crystalline free acid ("long-acting ceftiofur") should be avoided except for highly susceptible microorganisms, based on culture and sensitivity results.[11] It is licensed for very specific uses in cattle (foot root and metritis) and is popular because it is long-acting. However, in camelids, this drug needs to be used more frequently than in cattle (every 2–3 days) and isn't the solution to treating an alpaca that can't be handled for more frequent administration of a more appropriate drug.
- Florfenicol can be used at a dose of 20 mg/kg IM. The higher label dose of 40 mg/kg used subcutaneously in this study should be avoided.[12] This study also demonstrated bone marrow suppression in alpacas treated with repeated dosing. Another study in llamas confirmed daily dosing at 20 mg/kg IM. It warned against the potential for adverse reactions associated with prolonged administration and the potential for accumulation in the tissues. A third study showed that IM dosing achieved higher and more reliable tissue concentrations of florfenicol than subcutaneous dosing and again confirmed a recommendation of daily IM dosing at 20mg/kg to provide sufficient concentrations.[13]
- Gentamicin should be used at 5 mg/kg IV once daily[14] (compared with 6.6 mg/kg for horses) – not to be used in animals intended for human consumption. Also, gentamicin can result in kidney problems in animals that aren't properly hydrated. Therefore, its use is likely minimal in the field unless monitoring can be done.
- Enrofloxacin. Based on pharmacokinetic studies, this is the only antibiotic known to be effective orally in camelids.[15] As a fluoroquinolone, it is also a critically important antimicrobial in human medicine, so its use should be avoided

where possible. Note that this drug has a fairly narrow therapeutic spectrum and should only be used in cases following results of culture and sensitivity.

Most of the literature talks about the correct therapeutic dose of penicillin being 22,000-44,000 IU/kg (equivalent to 13.2 mg/kg) intramuscularly once or twice daily, depending on the formulation. However, even higher doses and frequencies are recommended for clostridial diseases, and this would normally be done using a formulation that could be given IV.[16,17] Despite this, label dosing for large animals is often based on doses of 10 mg/kg (16670 IU/kg), which is approximately 75% of the doses typically recommended, or in the US, even at 6 mg/kg (equivalent to 10,000 IU/kg). Underdosing is a concern regarding reaching the minimum concentration needed to kill bacteria, as this would induce antimicrobial resistance. Therefore, re-assessment of label dosing recommendations is necessary in large animals. Two studies established the effectiveness of the 22,000 IU/kg dose rate in horses.[18,19] There are no efficacy studies in camelids to date. Increasing the dose is particularly concerning due to drug residues in animals entering the food chain, as approved limits are based on drugs used at label doses. Using a dose that is not licensed would violate the law. Where camelids are not treated as food-producing animals, however, and where they are not entering the food chain, doses higher than this are acceptable. It should preferentially be used to treat bacterial infections properly.

Penicillin-streptomycin combinations should be avoided entirely, but they are commonly used in some parts of the world because they are very cheap. Usually, the penicillin component is desired. To avoid the toxicity of streptomycin, penicillin has to be dosed at low concentrations, which is likely to result in ineffective treatment and the possibility of developing antibiotic resistance. In pen-strep combinations, the dose achieved is only 8 mg/kg at label dose, which is only 60% of the recommended dose.

Stewardship of Medicines

When using medicines, we must always consider that they are a privilege. If we misuse them by using the wrong dose, route of administration, or duration, we may inadvertently increase the likelihood of developing drug resistance. This is especially true for antibiotics and anthelmintics (wormers), which is why you should not use them without proper authorisation from your vet, based on clinical testing or evaluation, or as part of a properly thought-out parasite control programme.

Anthelmintic Use

In my opinion, the emergence of resistant parasites is the biggest threat to camelid farming. We already have extensive resistance to ivermectin and doramectin globally. Multi-drug resistant parasites have been reported in the southern US[20,21] and Australia.[22] In German alpaca herds, resistance to macrocyclic lactones (ivermectin and possibly moxidectin) was documented alongside a high level of resistance genes in *Haemonchus* larvae.[23] In the UK, I run a faecal testing service and have documented some resistance to fenbendazole and, more recently, to moxidectin. This developing resistance is in addition to longstanding resistance to ivermectin and doramectin, which is extremely worrying.

Camelid owners are particularly prone to reliance upon wormers, and this may be for several reasons. First, camelid owners may have come from a background of small animal ownership where routine wormer use is standard practice. Second, in the absence of other information, they may have felt this was the most appropriate method to control worms and were unaware of other options. Lastly, there is a tendency among new owners to adopt the "strategy" of other breeders, possibly without consideration of their own particular circumstances or consulting with their vet.

Awareness has improved considerably over the previous 10 years or so, with breeders adopting a far more holistic approach to parasite control strategies. However, some breeders still rely on old-fashioned techniques such as routine prophylaxis and wormer rotation. Thus, breed societies and breeders need to stress the importance of parasite control to new owners and encourage sustainable parasite control strategies that do not rely purely on drug use. Our advice constantly updates as new information about resistance and how to avoid it becomes available. Therefore, it is crucial to keep up to date to keep one step ahead of the parasites.

How Does Parasite Resistance Develop?

"Resistance" is when a susceptible population of worms responds less to treatment with a wormer than previously. Complete resistance occurs when there is zero response at all. It is heritable and, therefore, genetic within the worms. Resistant worms survive exposure to an anthelmintic and can then pass this resistance gene on to their offspring. Resistance can develop due to the following factors:

1. Anthelmintics are often used at doses lower than recommended, either because the correct dose for camelids is not known or because sufficient wormer is not given due to weight underestimations or poor technique. Underdosed worms have a greater chance of surviving.

2. Frequent use of the same group of anthelmintic or frequent and continuous use of a single drug. Each time a drug is used, we are selecting for resistance because susceptible worms are killed, and only resistant ones survive to breed and pass on their resistance genes.

3. Prophylactic mass treatment of animals. The only worms that survive on the pasture are the resistant ones!

The concept of refugia is relatively new in the world of veterinary parasitology, and failure to manage refugia is currently considered the most critical factor in the development of resistance.

The idea is that if you treat every animal with wormer, you kill all the susceptible worms and leave only those that are resistant. To decelerate the rate at which those resistance genes are passed on, you need to have some susceptible worms present on the pasture with which the resistant ones breed, such that future worming doses will kill a proportion of their offspring. Those susceptible worms are known as the "refugia population;" their presence slows down the development of resistance in parasites because they provide a pool of genes conferring susceptibility to anthelmintics and dilute the frequency of resistance genes.

To make use of refugia, you have to leave a proportion of the animals in any group or herd undrenched (or unwormed). Suggestions are to leave around 10–15% of the herd undrenched. An even better idea is to drench only when needed based on faecal egg counts (FECs). This strategy is known as "targeted selective worming." For larger herds where individual FECs of all animals are not feasible, perform faecal screening and drench only when a problem is detected, and then concentrate on dosing the worst performing animals, such as those who've lost weight or have poor BCS or pale mucous membranes. Leave those in the best condition untreated. With refugia management, it is also important that you don't always drench animals and then move them to clean ground, as you need the worms that survive dosing to come into contact with the susceptible worms still present on the "contaminated" pasture.

As detailed in Chapter 10, there are three main steps of parasite control strategies that help reduce our dependence on medicines.

These are:

1. Management of the Pasture
    - Removal of faecal material
    - Stocking density
    - Resting pastures
    - Quarantine
2. Monitoring
    - Body condition scoring and mucous membrane colour
    - Periodic faecal screening
3. Medications
    - Use of anthelmintics and anticoccidials as required
    - Targeted and based on faecal testing results

The use of anthelmintics and anticoccidials intentionally comes last on the list because the first two steps must be in place before using medications. It's also important to advise caution when newer drugs enter the market. They should be tested in camelids first, and dosing regimens should be confirmed. This is because using wormers at inappropriate doses is one of the quickest ways in which resistance is encouraged to develop. One example is the most recent wormer, Zolvix (containing monepantel). This drug is only effective at reducing egg counts by greater than 95% (the accepted standard in faecal egg count reduction tests) if used at *three times* the label dose! [24]

Some promising future directions in parasite control may complement our other tools in the parasite control toolbox. Genetic testing for parasite resistance in the livestock industry (sheep and cattle) has been possible for some years. It allows farmers to identify parasite-resistant stock that can be bred for that characteristic. This technology has potential in the camelid industry, but we need data, research funding and willingness to pursue the research. Plants high in condensed tannins have been shown to reduce worm egg counts in grazing livestock, but further work is required (e.g. Sainfoin, trefoil, chicory, sericea lespedeza). Finally, antiparasitic vaccines have had some encouraging results. A vaccine has been developed to help control *Haemonchus contortus* (Barber Pole Worm) in sheep. It is safe in alpacas and has shown promise under field conditions.[25 26]

Antibiotic Use

It has been impossible to avoid headlines over the last few years about the use of antibiotics in human and veterinary medicine, specifically on how to limit the emergence of antibiotic-resistant bacteria. This concern is a global one and of massive importance for both animal and public health. One cannot have failed to notice sensationalist headlines in recent years about multi-drug-resistant strains of bacteria such as MRSA (methicillin-resistant *Staph aureus*). On the 17th November 2011, the European Commission unveiled its "action plan against antimicrobial resistance: 12 concrete actions for the next five years" to limit the spread of resistance and develop new antimicrobials. November 2015 was the first World Antibiotic Awareness Week, while in March 2016, members of the European Parliament voted to back proposals that ban the collective and preventive use of antibiotics in animals, supporting restrictions on the use of existing antibiotics. The O'Neill Commission (UK) published a report in December 2015 recommending the reduction of antibiotic use in food production and restrictions on antibiotics considered important for human use. In September 2023, the World Organisation for Animal Health released a report showing a global decrease in antimicrobial use in animals – 13% in just 3 years.[27] In the UK alone, the reduction was 59% over the 8 years from 2014 to 2022.[28] Although the use of antibiotics in humans is thought to be responsible for most drug resistance, animal use is often blamed most loudly. Consequently, perhaps, more of the "actions" proposed govern control over the use of antibiotics in animals than in humans.

Politicians' decisions can drastically affect antibiotics vets and animal owners may use in the future. It is increasingly likely that antibiotics will *only* be available for use in animals when prescribed by a vet. In other European countries, certain antibiotics, including ceftiofur, are no longer available for use in animals. We have a vital role to play in ensuring that the antibiotics we have at our disposal remain useful, both to ourselves and to the animals that we treat. Our ability to prescribe antibiotics to camelids could be particularly at risk since all the drugs we use are used off-label since there are no licensed drugs for use in camelids. We could be in trouble if legislation is created that restricts antibiotics to licensed uses only. Licensing of medicines in camelids is unrealistic. At the end of the day, we have a responsibility to use drugs appropriately to safeguard their use in the future.

What Can You Do to Minimise Antibiotic Resistance?

- **Minimise infection risk.** Have good biosecurity and infection control.
- **Use antibiotics only under veterinary guidance.** Vets are trained to have an integrated understanding of medicine, surgery, microbiology, pharmacology and animal management, regardless of whether or not your vet is particularly knowledgeable about alpacas. They are the best people to decide whether the use of antibiotics is appropriate in any particular case. It may be very tempting to grab whatever antibiotic you have saved in your drug cupboard, but antibiotics are not always necessary, and the antibiotic you choose may be inappropriate for the problem. If an animal is sick enough for you to think about using antibiotics, it's sick enough to have a vet visit!
- **Base antibiotic choice on sensitivity testing.** Wherever possible, conduct testing to determine the most effective antibiotic.
- **Follow dosing instructions completely.** This includes the dose and frequency of administration as well as using the full duration of treatment prescribed. If you're having trouble administering the antibiotic, speak to your vet. They may be able to suggest a solution.
- **Weigh animals so that accurate doses can be used.** Doing so allows you to dose animals properly, based on weight, not guesstimates. Knowing the exact weight of an animal prevents their overdosing on a drug that may be toxic, or you underdosing a drug so that it is less effective or ineffective for them. Underdosing also increases the chances of causing antibiotic resistance.
- **Use antibiotics that are known to be effective in camelids.** Many antibiotics have been subjected to pharmacokinetic research in camelids so that we know they are safe in camelids and at what doses they should be used.
- **Follow directions for storage and use of antibiotics.** For example, they must be kept at the correct temperature, which might be in the fridge. Most medicines must be thrown away after 28 days once the bottle is opened. After that time, the effectiveness of the antibiotic cannot be guaranteed and may be harmful. Remember to write the date on the bottle when you open it so that you know when it should be thrown away. Some antibiotics have a shorter shelf-life than this, so always check the label. Always use a clean needle and syringe when drawing antibiotics from the bottle. Re-use is false economy and can introduce bacteria into the bottle. Return partially used bottles to your veterinarian for safe disposal.

MONITORING

This section of the pentagon covers regular observations to spot signs of illness, so you can step in early to help ensure their welfare. Monitoring includes body condition scoring, checking mucous membrane colour, checking toenails, faecal testing and

A few years ago, I visited a farm, and at one point, the owner had wandered off somewhere to do something. I had a peek inside a cupboard, and I was quite shocked to find seven different antibiotics on the medicine shelf (Figure 2). Some had been opened, but not all, suggesting they'd been acquired for "future" (not prescribed) use. One bottle had an open date from eight months earlier. While I acknowledge that this was some years ago, it's worth noting that there were two critically important antibiotics in there: ceftiofur and marbofloxacin. The ceftiofur should have been in the fridge. Also inside was oxytetracycline, two different types of amoxicillin and trimethoprim sulfa.

Recently, an owner with a previous liberal use of antimicrobials lost several crias to a highly drug-resistant strain of staphylococcus. While the loss of the crias is devastating, these owners also expose themselves to highly drug-resistant bacteria on the farm. If they personally get sick from those bacteria, it could potentially kill them. So do not underestimate the importance of this problem. Please do not self-prescribe, and don't hold onto bottles from previous cases to shove into something later. Also, do not demand bottles of antibiotics from your vets to have "just in case." If an animal is sick enough for antibiotics, it's sick enough for a vet visit.

Now, go clean out your cupboards and throw away any medicine bottles that have been opened for over 28 days!

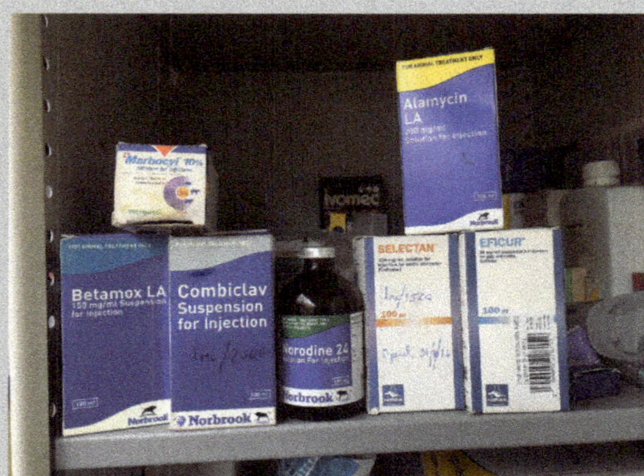

Figure 2. The inside of one owner's medicine cupboard. This is NOT a good look for antimicrobial stewardship!

observation of behaviour. These were all covered in detail in Chapter 3 on routine herd health activities.

MANAGEMENT

This aspect of responsible ownership is all about the day-to-day care you provide your animals. These were all covered in detail in Chapters 2 to 4. It includes ensuring that you provide your animals with a safe and appropriate environment, a balanced diet, access to fresh, clean water, vaccinations to prevent diseases prevalent in your part of the world, toenail trimming as needed, shearing and vitamin D supplementation.

MEAT

While this might not be a favoured topic for many in the camelid Industry, the fact is that some camelids will enter the food chain, whether you approve or not. The food-producing livestock industry is subject to additional controls where animals enter the food chain to protect the consumer from harmful drug residues. All medicines used in food-producing animals have a meat withdrawal period specified by the manufacturer, which is specific to the dose and route of administration of the medicine used. Some drugs, such as gentamicin, phenylbutazone and chloramphenicol, are banned from being used in food-producing animals because residues can be present for a long time or can cause specific reactions in humans exposed to them. For antibiotic use, failure to observe meat withdrawal periods can lead to antimicrobial resistance.

If you are a supplier of camelid meat into the food chain or think that you ever might, you must keep good records of all medicines used and observe meat withdrawal periods. These are not specified for camelids since all medicines are used outside of licensing. Therefore, default periods must be specified by your vet when supplying medicines, and the rules on this will vary depending on where you are in the world, so ask your vet for details. If you use any medicines by a different route, this may also affect the meat withdrawal period. For example, using antibiotics subcutaneously instead of intramuscularly can increase their persistence and withdrawal period.

Meat entering the food chain is subject to testing for drug residues. If residues are found, there will be an investigation, and ignorance will not be a valid excuse for putting people's lives at risk.

A Final Thought

In recent years, the internet has greatly facilitated global trade. It is quite easy to find what you want anywhere online, and you only have to pay for shipping to get it here! However, depending on what you buy, there are regulations on imports, and these include taxes and duties, of course. However, there are also specific restrictions on veterinary medicines.

A Veterinary Medicinal Product (VMP) is legally defined as any substance or combination of substances presented as having properties for treating or preventing disease in animals. So, this will include any medicine you would typically get from your veterinarian and things like wormers. Vets here in the UK can import products that are not available here, but to do so, we need to obtain authorisation from our regulatory body, the Veterinary Medicines Directorate. It is an offence to import a VMP without authorisation or to have an unauthorised VMP without a certificate granted under the Veterinary Medicine Regulations 2011. In other words, do not buy drugs yourself on the internet from a retailer outside of the UK because it could get you in trouble. There will almost certainly be similar or more restrictive regulations elsewhere. The regulations are there to protect the consumer as well as the animals who may be given these drugs. Depending on the source and manufacturer, quality control processes may not be as rigorous outside your country, and the drugs may be inferior. They may contain less active ingredients or harmful preservatives, for example. Remember that veterinarians have earned their license to prescribe medicines over many years spent at university learning how to do what they do in a load of different species. We have to pay for that privilege to prescribe. You will not do your animals any favours by trying to beat the system.

Key Takeaways

Having animals means having legal, ethical, and animal health-related responsibilities. My Pentagon for Responsible Camelid Ownership can help you remember your five areas of responsibility. The five points are mandate, medicines, monitoring, management and meat.

- Find out what your legal responsibilities are in your country, and consult with your veterinarian if you need help determining where to start.
- Before using medicines in camelids, we need to know if they are safe and effective and what dosing regimen should be used. Use medicines responsibly under the direction of your vet, particularly antibiotics, and do not self-prescribe. Make sure you have a parasite control strategy that minimises your use of anthelmintics and anticoccidials to ensure they are available when needed.
- Ensure you have an action plan for regularly monitoring your animals for illness and covering all their husbandry needs.
- Finally, if you think your animals might enter the food chain, be prepared by having adequate drug records that you can refer back to ensure consumer safety.

Conclusion

It's natural to feel a bit daunted after reading a book like this, where we cover the essentials of camelid care and the many potential issues that could arise. This can sometimes feel overwhelming for new or prospective owners and even raises doubts about whether owning alpacas or llamas is the right choice. However, most serious problems with these animals require professional veterinary care and are not something you'll need to manage alone. Your vet is an essential partner in keeping your animals healthy and will be equipped to diagnose and treat complex issues. That said, having a solid understanding of common conditions and health challenges can help you guide your vet's investigation, especially if working with a veterinarian with limited camelid experience.

Throughout this book, I've outlined what to expect as you begin and continue your journey with alpacas or llamas. I have provided insights into the daily management routines and health measures needed for a well-cared-for herd. You'll find practical guidance on feeding, disease prevention and establishing effective health routines. The latter half of this book focuses on common health issues, helping you recognise, address and prevent them.

This book is not a substitute for your veterinarian's expertise. Vets dedicate years to training and possess the skills and tools needed to address complex health issues that require professional intervention. Instead, the goal of this book is to empower you to identify potential health risks in your animals' environment, recognise early signs of illness, and know when to seek veterinary support. Acting promptly not only protects your animals' health but can also make treatment easier and potentially less costly.

My journey with alpacas began long before I became a veterinarian, giving me a unique understanding of the challenges owners face. Like you, I am captivated by these remarkable animals – caring for them is not only my profession but also my passion. I am deeply committed to improving the health and welfare of camelids everywhere, and sharing my knowledge with owners like you is a vital part of that mission. By expanding your understanding of camelid care, I hope to help you prevent health issues before they arise and feel confident when challenges do occur. With a strong foundation of knowledge, you'll feel more secure and capable as a camelid owner.

I encourage you now to assess any herd health plans you already have and identify areas that may need attention or improvement. Set up a schedule for your routine herd health activities and make a point of adding these dates to your calendar so they don't slip through the cracks. Life can get busy, and essential tasks can be easily overlooked without clear planning. For services that require extra preparation, like shearing, plan ahead—shearers may need to be booked up to six months in advance. Similarly, map out your yearly vaccination schedule, giving special consideration to groups with unique needs, such as pregnant animals and crias. Consider reviewing your plan with your veterinarian to ensure it best suits your herd. Finally, maintain detailed and organised records. Whether you use a notebook, spreadsheets or software, the key is having a reliable system so that vital information is easily accessible whenever you need it.

Remember, you don't have to navigate this path alone. There is a vast network of fellow owners and enthusiasts who are just as eager as I am to see your animals thrive. Local or regional camelid groups and online communities can be wonderful resources for camaraderie, advice and support. However, please make your veterinarian your first point of contact for any medical concerns with your animals. Professionals like myself are available to support you and your vet with challenging cases, and modern video conferencing makes it possible to consult with me from anywhere in the world.

To further support your journey, I offer a course for owners called Intensive Camelid Health Care, covering many topics from this book in a structured, online and on-demand format. You can take this course at your own pace and join live sessions where I'll answer your questions directly. Participants also gain access to my private online community on Facebook, where they can connect with like-minded individuals who share this foundational training. Additionally, I offer the Camelid Reproduction & Cria Care Intensive Course, a comprehensive course on breeding management, birthing, and newborn cria care.

For those interested in advanced nutritional management for camelids, my colleague Dr Robert Van Saun, teaches an Advanced Camelid Nutrition Masterclass. Dr Van Saun is an unparalleled expert in camelid nutrition, and his course provides invaluable insights for dedicated owners. You can find our resources and further information about these learning opportunities at www.ukalpacavet.com.

Finally, don't forget that you can get access to the free supplementary PDF resources that accompany this book at **camelidhandbook.** thealpacavet.com.

As you move forward with your herd of alpacas or llamas, remember that knowledge and preparation are your most valuable tools. By understanding the fundamentals of camelid care, recognising signs of illness and knowing when to seek help, you're already doing an incredible service to your animals. Each step you take to improve their health and well-being strengthens your bond with them and enhances the quality of life you can offer. With the guidance of this book, your expanding skills, and the support of a dedicated community, you are well-equipped to provide a fulfilling and healthy life for your herd. Embrace the journey! You're ready for it, and your animals will thrive because of your commitment.

"Forewarned, forearmed; to be prepared is half the victory."
– Miguel de Cervantes, 16th Century Spanish novelist

Glossary

Word	Definition
Acaricide	A substance that is poisonous to mites or ticks.
Acute / acutely	A word that describes medical issues that develop quickly and require immediate attention.
Anaemia	A condition where the body doesn't have enough healthy red blood cells or haemoglobin to carry oxygen to the cells and tissues.
Anamnestic response	A bodily defence reaction that occurs when the body encounters an antigen (foreign agent like a bacterium or virus) for the second time, resulting in a rapid production of antibodies. This is the basis for the 2nd dose of a vaccination primary course and results in the production of circulating antibodies ready to respond in case of an infection.
Anthelmintic	This is another word for a worming medication.
Anticoccidial	This is an umbrella term for medication used to deal with coccidia.
Biosecurity	Procedures or measures designed to protect the population against harmful biological agents.

Word	Definition
Body condition scoring	A non-negotiable husbandry skill. You must learn how to do this.
C1, C2, C3	First, second and third stomach compartments.
Camelidynamics	A particular approach to handling camelids that uses techniques developed by Marty McGee Bennett. This approach aims to minimise stress caused by handling.
Carpus / carpal joint	Often called the "front knees," as camelids will kneel on these.
Chronic	Indicates that something has been going on for some time.
Coccidia	A family of protozoal organisms that cause weight loss and diarrhoea in crias.
Deciduous teeth	Baby teeth.
Dry matter	The proportion of a feedstuff that is not water, expressed as a percentage.
Eimeria	The Latin group name for protozoan organisms called coccidia.
Eimeria macusaniensis; E mac	A particular type of coccidia affecting camelids only. This coccidia has a long life cycle and is associated with causing weight loss.
Enterotoxaemia	A condition caused by an overgrowth of toxin-producing bacteria in the intestines.

Word	Definition
Epg	Eggs per gram – used to quantify egg counts on a faecal test.
Faeces	Proper term for poop!
Fluke	A type of parasite (flatworm) that migrates to the liver and causes liver damage in the process.
Haemonchus	A type of strongyle worm that causes anaemia by sucking blood from the lining of C3. Also called the "Barber Pole Worm."
Husbandry	The practice of looking after animals.
Lesion	An area of tissue that has become damaged through injury or disease, such as an ulcer, bruise, cut, wound, tumour, abscess, etc.
Mineralysis	Analysis of mineral levels, usually done via a blood test.
Mucous membranes	The moist lining inside the mouth, nose, eyelids, vagina and intestinal tract. Mucous membranes produce mucus that keeps them moist.
Nematodirus	A roundworm that has a very large egg on faecals. Low egg producer so quite low levels can be significant.
NSAID	Non-steroidal anti-inflammatory medication such as flunixin or meloxicam.
Oocyst	Coccidia produce oocysts rather than "eggs."

Word	Definition
Pathogenic	Causing or capable of causing disease.
Packed Cell Volume (PCV)	The proportion of red cells in the blood as a whole. Serum and white cells make up the rest of the blood.
Photobiosynthesis	The act of making something that is induced by light.
Refugia	The susceptible worms in a population of worms.
Stifle	The knee joint on the hind leg.
Stocking Density	The number of animals in a specified area.
Strongyles	A large group of worms that includes *Haemonchus, Ostertagia, Teladorsagia, Cooperia, Bunostomum and Trichostrongylus.*
Trichuris	A whipworm. Also pathogenic at quite low egg counts. Can cause anaemia, weight loss and colic signs.
Volatile fatty acids	These are acids produced by the microbes in C1 and used as a source of energy.
Worming/deworming	Using an anthelmintic medication (wormer) to treat worm burdens. Worming and deworming are actually the same thing!
Zoonosis / zoonotic	A disease that is capable of transmission from animals to humans.

References

Chapter 2

1. Dulphy JP, Dardillat C, Jailler M, et al. Comparative study of forestomach digestion in llamas and sheep. Reprod Nutr Dev 1997;37:709-725.
2. Data from the World Bank, Climate Change Knowledge Portal (2024). URL: [https://climateknowledgeportal.worldbank.org/]. Date Accessed: 15/6/2024.
3. World Bank, Climate Change Knowledge Portal (2024). URL: [https://climateknowledgeportal.worldbank.org/] Date Accessed: 15/6/2024.

Chapter 3

1. Rosadio R, Maturrano L, Perez D, et al. Enterotoxemia: new evidence on pathogenesis and prevention of the number one cause of neonatal alpaca mortality in South America. In: World Alpaca Conference. Sydney, Australia: 2008:50-55.
2. Wallace RM, Niezgoda M, Waggoner EA, et al. Serologic response in eight alpacas vaccinated by extralabel use of a large animal rabies vaccine during a public health response to a rabid alpaca in South Carolina. J Am Vet Med Assoc 2016;249:678-681.
3. Kutzler MA, Baker RJ, Mattson DE. Humoral response to West Nile virus vaccination in alpacas and llamas. J Am Vet Med Assoc 2004;225:414-416.
4. Byers S. Vaccinations in Camelids, [https://www.midwestshearing.com/articles/vaccinations] (accessed 25th July 2024).

Chapter 4

1. Whitehead CE, Newman AJ. Investigating predisposing factors and heritability of hindlimb toenail deviation in a herd of alpacas. In: 2013.
2. Smith BB, Van Saun RJ. Seasonal changes in serum calcium, phosphorus, and vitamin

D concentrations in llamas and alpacas. Am J Vet Res 2001;62:1187-1193.
3. Smith BS, Wright H. Relative contributions of diet and sunshine to the overall vitamin D status of the grazing ewe. Vet Rec 1984;115:537-538.
4. Judson GJ, Feakes A. Vitamin D doses for alpacas (*Lama pacos*). Aust Vet J 1999;77:310-315.
5. Ross R, Care AD, Robinson JS, et al. Perinatal 1,25-dihydroxycholecalciferol in the sheep and its role in the maintenance of the transplacental calcium gradient. J Endocrinology 1980;87:17-18.
6. Wittek T, Salaberger T, Palme R, et al. Clinical parameters and adrenocortical activity to assess stress responses of alpacas using different methods of restraint either alone or with shearing. Vet Rec 2017;180:568.
7. Blache D, Maloney SK. Castration methods and welfare of alpacas: towards an appropriate solution. In: Industries AE, ed. Australia: 2017.
8. Wheeler JC. Aging llamas and alpacas by their teeth. In: Llama World 1982:12-17.

Chapter 5

1. Van Saun RJ. Feeding fundamentals for South American Camelids. In: International Camelid Health Conference, Columbus, OH 2006.
2. Ancco EG, Hinostroza MG, Quispe CE, et al. Niveles de nitrógeno ureico sanguíneo y su relación con la preñez en alpacas. Revista de Investigaciones Veterinarias del Peru 2018;29:1372-1376.
3. Nutrient requirements of small ruminants. Washington, D.C.: National Research Council, National Academies Press; 2007.
4. Van Saun RJ. Feeding and nutrition. In: Niehaus A, ed. Medicine and Surgery of Camelids, 4th ed. Hoboken NJ: Wiley-Blackwell; 2022:55-107.

Chapter 6

1. Van Saun RJ. Nutritional requirements and assessing nutritional status in camelids. Veterinary Clinics: Food Animal Practice 2009;25:265-279.
2. Zhang X, Dong X, Wanapat M, et al. Ruminal pH pattern, fermentation characteristics and related bacteria in response to dietary live yeast (*Saccharomyces cerevisiae*) supplementation in beef cattle. Anim Biosci 2022;35:184-195.
3. Ancco EG, Hinostroza MG, Quispe CE, et al. Niveles de nitrógeno ureico sanguíneo y su relación con la preñez en alpacas. Revista de Investigaciones Veterinarias del Peru 2018;29:1372-1376.

Chapter 7

1. Forestry Commission and Animal and Plant Health Agency, "How

Biosecurity Can Prevent the Introduction and Spread of Tree Pests and Diseases," Gov.uk, first published 26 September 2018, last updated 15 October 2024, [https://www.gov.uk/guidance/prevent-the-introduction-and-spread-of-tree-pests-and-diseases] (accessed 21 October 2024).

2. Cebra CK, Heidel JR, Cebra ML, et al. Pathogenesis of *Streptococcus zooepidemicus* infection after intratracheal inoculation in llamas. Am J Vet Res 2000;61:1525-1529.
3. Hewson J, Cebra CK. Peritonitis in a llama caused by *Streptococcus equi* subsp. *zooepidemicus*. Can Vet J 2001;42:465-467.
4. Jones M, Miesner M, Grondin T. Outbreak of *Streptococcus equi* ssp. *zooepidemicus* polyserositis in an alpaca herd. J Vet Intern Med 2009;23:220-223.
5. Corpa JM, Carvallo F, Anderson ML, et al. *Streptococcus equi* subspecies *zooepidemicus* septicemia in alpacas: three cases and review of the literature. J Vet Diagn Invest 2018;30:598-602.
6. Fondevila NA, Marcoveccio FJ, Blanco Viera JB, et al. Susceptibility of llamas (*Lama glama*) to infection with foot-and-mouth-disease virus. Zentralbl Veterinarmed B 1995;42:595-599.
7. Wernery U, Kinne J. Foot and mouth disease and similar virus infections in camelids: a review. Rev Sci Tech 2012;31:907-918.
8. Morris CA. A review of genetic resistance to disease in *Bos taurus* cattle. Vet J 2007;174:481-491.
9. Woolaston RR, Barger IA, Piper LR. Response to helminth infection of sheep selected for resistance to *Haemonchus contortus*. Int J Parasitol 1990;20:1015-1018.
10. Barrington GM, Allen AJ, Parish SM, et al. Biosecurity and biocontainment in alpaca operations. Small Rumin Res 2006;61:217-225.
11. Barrington GM. Biosecurity. In: Cebra C, Anderson DE, Tibary A, Van Saun RJ, Johnson LW, eds. Llama and Alpaca Care, Medicine, Surgery, Reproduction, Nutrition and Herd Health, 1st ed. St Louis, MO: Elsevier; 2014:1-5.
12. Jones M, Boileau M. Camelid herd health. Vet Clin North Am Food Anim Pract 2009;25:239-263.
13. Carr J. Biosecurity beyond the boot dip. In: London Vet Show, London 2014.

Chapter 8

1. Kapil S, Yeary T, Evermann JF. Viral diseases of new world camelids. Vet Clin North Am Food Anim Pract 2009;25:323-337.
2. Twomey DF, Collins R, Cranwell MP, et al. Controlling tuberculosis in a llama (*Lama glama*) herd using clinical signs, tuberculin

skin testing and serology. Vet J 2012;192:246-248.

3. Dean GS, Crawshaw TR, de la Rua-Domenech R, et al. Use of serological techniques for diagnosis of *Mycobacterium bovis* infection in a llama herd. Vet Rec 2009;165:323-324.
4. Rhodes S, Holder T, Clifford D, et al. Evaluation of gamma interferon and antibody tuberculosis tests in alpacas. Clin Vaccine Immunol 2012;19:1677-1683.
5. Bezos J, Casal C, Alvarez J, et al. Evaluation of the performance of cellular and serological diagnostic tests for the diagnosis of tuberculosis in an alpaca (*Vicugna pacos*) herd naturally infected with *Mycobacterium bovis*. Prev Vet Med 2013;111:304-313.
6. Foreyt WJ. Veterinary Parasitology Reference Manual, 5th edition, Iowa State University Press; 2001.

Chapter 9

1. Palmer DG, McCombe IL. Lectin staining of trichostrongylid nematode eggs of sheep: rapid identification of *Haemonchus contortus* eggs with peanut agglutinin. Int J Parasitol 1996;26:447-450.
2. Rashid MH, Beveridge I, Vaughan JL, et al. Worm burdens and associated histopathological changes caused by gastrointestinal nematodes in alpacas from Australia. Parasitol Res 2019;118:1031-1038.
3. Bauer C, Hirzmann J, Petzold J, et al. First detection of autochthonous *Lamanema chavezi* infections in llamas (*Lama glama*) in Europe. Vet Parasitol Reg Stud Reports 2024;47:100948.
4. Gliga DS, Kramer A, More G, et al. Early Detection and Management of *Lamanema chavezi* infection in a llama (*Lama glama*) in Switzerland. Vet Res Commun 2024.
5. Jarvinen JA, Whitley EM, Kreuder AJ, et al. Identification of *Lamanema chavezi* Becklund 1963 infection in a llama (*Lama glama*) in the United States. J Vet Diagn Invest 2014;26:178-183.
6. McKenna PB, Morley C, Koning M, et al. Confirmation of the occurrence of the nematode parasite *Lamanema chavezi* Becklund , 1963 in South American camelids in New Zealand. N Z Vet J 2009;57:395-396.
7. Cafrune MM, Aguirre DH, Rickard LG. First report of *Lamanema chavezi* (Nematoda: Trichostrongyloidea) in llamas (*Lama glama*) from Argentina. Vet Parasitol 2001;97:165-168.
8. Mitchell S, Hopkins B, Corfield C. *Nematodirus lamae* identified in an alpaca in the UK. Vet Rec 2016;178:271-272.

9. Hinkson J. Investigations into common farm management practices and diseases on alpaca farms in New Zealand. In: Massey University; 2015.
10. Welchman DdB, Parr JG, Wood R, et al. Alpaca and llama nematodes in Britain. Vet Rec 2008;162:832.
11. Rashid MH, Vaughan JL, Stevenson MA, et al. Epidemiology of gastrointestinal nematodes of alpacas in Australia: I. A cross-sectional study. Parasitol Res 2019;118:891-900.
12. Fowler ME. Medicine and Surgery of South American Camelids, 2nd ed. Ames: Blackwell Publishing; 1998;549.
13. Cheney JM, Allen GT. Parasitism in llamas. Vet Clin North Am Food Anim Pract 1989;5:217-225.
14. Guerrero CA. Coccidia (Protozoa: Eimeriidae) of the alpaca *Lama pacos*. J Protozool 1967;14:613-616.
15. Guerrero CA, Hernandez J, Bazalar H, et al. *Eimeria macusaniensis* n. sp. (Protozoa: Eimeriidae) of the alpaca *Lama pacos*. J Protozool 1971;18:162-163.
16. Schrey CF, Abbott TA, Stewart VA, et al. Coccidia of the llama, *Lama glama*, in Colorado and Wyoming. Vet Parasitol 1991;40:21-28.
17. Palacios CA, Perales RA, Chavera AE, et al. *Eimeria macusaniensis* and *Eimeria ivitaensis* co-infection in fatal cases of diarrhoea in young alpacas (*Lama pacos*) in Peru. Vet Rec 2006;158:344-345.
18. Foreyt WJ. Veterinary Parasitology Reference Manual, 5th ed Iowa State University Press; 2001.
19. Foreyt WJ, Lagerquist J. Experimental infections of *Eimeria alpacae* and *Eimeria punoensis* in llamas (*Lama glama*). J Parasitol 1992;78:906-909.
20. Jarvinen JA. Prevalence of *Eimeria macusaniensis* (Apicomplexa: Eimeriidae) in midwestern Lama spp. J Parasitol 1999;85:373-376.
21. Ballweber LR. Ecto- and endoparasites of new world camelids. Vet Clin North Am Food Anim Pract 2009;25:295-310.
22. Tzipori S, Ward H. Cryptosporidiosis: biology, pathogenesis and disease. Microbes Infect 2002;4:1047-1058.
23. Chen XM, Keithly JS, Paya CV, et al. Cryptosporidiosis. N Engl J Med 2002;346:1723-1731.
24. Duff JP, Maxwell AJ, Claxton JR. Chronic and fatal fascioliasis in llamas in the UK. Vet Rec 1999;145:315-316.
25. Hamir AN, Smith BB. Severe biliary hyperplasia associated with liver fluke infection in an adult alpaca. Vet Pathol 2002;39:592-594.
26. Harwood D, Nuttall J, Bidewell C. Fasciolosis in camelids. Vet Rec 2008;162:424.

27. Puente GL. Acute and subacute Fasciolosis of alpacas (*Lama pacos*) and treatment with triclabendazole. Trop Anim Health Prod 1997;29:31-32.
28. Klein D, Prosl H, Thaller D, et al. Diagnosis of a *Dicrocoelium dendriticum* infection in New World Camelids: a case report. Veterinarni Medicina 2012;57:154-162.
29. Dadak AM, Wieser C, Joachim A, et al. Efficacy and safety of oral praziquantel against *Dicrocoelium dendriticum* in llamas. Vet Parasitol 2013;197:122-125.

Chapter 10

1. Wikipedia. United Kingdom weather records, [https://en.wikipedia.org/wiki/United_Kingdom_weather_records] (accessed 14th October 2024).
2. Wormboss. How long do larvae take to die? 2022, [https://wormboss.com.au/tests-tools/grazing-management-sheep/how-long-do-larvae-take-to-die/] (accessed 14th October 2024).
3. Ehsan M, Hu RS, Liang QL, et al. Advances in the Development of Anti-*Haemonchus contortus* Vaccines: Challenges, Opportunities, and Perspectives. Vaccines (Basel) 2020;8.
4. Roeber F, Jex AR, Gasser RB. Advances in the diagnosis of key gastrointestinal nematode infections of livestock, with an emphasis on small ruminants. Biotechnol Adv 2013;31:1135-1152.
5. Maqbool I, Wani ZA, Shahardar RA, et al. Integrated parasite management with special reference to gastro-intestinal nematodes. J Parasit Dis 2017;41:1-8.
6. Agriculture & Horticulture Development Board. Grazing strategies for worm control, 2020, [https://ahdb.org.uk/news/grazing-strategies-for-worm-control] (accessed 15th October 2024).
7. Cebra CK, Stang BV. Comparison of methods to detect gastrointestinal parasites in llamas and alpacas. J Am Vet Med Assoc 2008;232:733-741.
8. Rashid MH, Stevenson MA, Waenga S, et al. Comparison of McMaster and FECPAK(G2) methods for counting nematode eggs in the faeces of alpacas. Parasit Vectors 2018;11:278.
9. Paras KL, George MM, Vidyashankar AN, et al. Comparison of fecal egg counting methods in four livestock species. Vet Parasitol 2018;257:21-27.
10. Gruntman A, Nolen-Walston R, Parry N, et al. Presumptive albendazole toxicosis in 12 alpacas. J Vet Intern Med 2009;23:945-949.
11. Dadak AM, Asanger H, Tichy A, et al. Establishing an efficacious dose rate of monepantel for treating gastrointestinal nematodes in

llamas under field conditions. Vet Rec 2013;172:155.

12. Thomas SM, Morgan ER. Effect on performance of weanling alpacas following treatments against gastro-intestinal parasites. Vet Parasitol 2013;198:244-249.
13. Smith WD. A commercial vaccine for Barber's pole worm - further development. In: Moredun Research Institute; 2014:209.
14. VanHoy G, Carman M, Habing G, et al. Safety and serologic response to a *Haemonchus contortus* vaccine in alpacas. Vet Parasitol 2018;252:180-186.
15. Carman MK, Lakritz J, Cheng TY, et al. Efficacy of a *Haemonchus contortus* vaccine under field conditions in young alpacas. Vet Parasitol 2024;331:110242.
16. Ballweber LR. Ecto- and endoparasites of new world camelids. Vet Clin North Am Food Anim Pract 2009;25:295-310.

Chapter 11

1. Ogawa Y, Kinoshita M, Shimada S, et al. Zinc and Skin Disorders. Nutrients 2018;10.
2. Cremers HJ. *Chorioptes bovis* (Acarina: Psoroptidae) in some camelids from Dutch zoos. Vet Q 1985;7:198-199.
3. D'Alterio GL, Jackson AP, Knowles TG, et al. Comparative study of the efficacy of eprinomectin versus ivermectin, and field efficacy of eprinomectin only, for the treatment of chorioptic mange in alpacas. Vet Parasitol 2005;130:267-275.
4. Plant JD, Kutzler MA, Cebra CK. Efficacy of topical eprinomectin in the treatment of *Chorioptes* sp. infestation in alpacas and llamas. Vet Dermatol 2007;18:59-62.
5. D'Alterio GL, Callaghan C, Just C, et al. Prevalence of *Chorioptes* sp. mite infestation in alpaca (*Lama pacos*) in the south-west of England: implications for skin health. Small Rumin Res 2005;57:221-228.
6. Hill FI, McKenna PB, Mirams CH. Demodex spp. infestation and suspected demodicosis of alpacas (*Vicugna pacos*) in New Zealand. N Z Vet J 2008;56:148-149.
7. Ferreyra HDV, Rudd J, Foley J, et al. Sarcoptic mange outbreak decimates South American wild camelid populations in San Guillermo National Park, Argentina. PLoS One 2022;17:e0256616.
8. Gomez-Puerta LA, Pacheco JI, Angulo-Tisoc JM, et al. Prevalence and molecular characterization of *Sarcoptes scabiei* from vicunas (*Vicugna vicugna*) from Southern Peruvian Andes. Parasitology 2021:1-6.
9. Escobar LE, Carver S, Cross PC, et al. Sarcoptic mange: An emerging panzootic in wildlife. Transbound Emerg Dis 2022;69:927-942.

10. Roberson JR, Baird AN, Pugh DG. Disease of the integumentary system. In: Pugh DG, Baird AN, eds. Sheep and Goat Medicine, 2nd edW. B. Saunders; 2012:256-290.
11. Rashmir-Raven AM. Disorders of the skin. In: Reed SM, Bayly WM, Sellon DC, eds. Equine Internal Medicine, 4th edW.B. Saunders; 2018:1159-1216.
12. Paterson S, Coumbe K. An open study to evaluate topical treatment of equine chorioptic mange with shampooing and lime sulphur solution. Vet Dermatol 2009;20:623-629.
13. Rosychuk RA. Llama dermatology. Vet Clin North Am Food Anim Pract 1994;10:228-239.
14. Scott DW, Vogel JW, Fleis RI, et al. Skin diseases in the alpaca (*Vicugna pacos*): a literature review and retrospective analysis of 68 cases (Cornell University 1997-2006). Vet Dermatol 2011;22:2-16.

Chapter 12

1. Vaughan JL, Lonsdale RA, Jackson G, et al. Congenital caudal vertebral malformations in the alpaca (*Lama pacos*). Aust Vet J 2000;78:412-415.
2. Alderson P, Roberts I. Corticosteroids for acute traumatic brain injury. Cochrane Database Syst Rev 2005;2005:CD000196.
3. Barker WH, Witte TH, Driver CJ, et al. Dorsal laminectomy for treatment of cervical vertebral stenotic myelopathy in an alpaca. J Am Vet Med Assoc 2015;246:1122-1128.
4. Talbot CE, Mueller K, Granger N, et al. Diagnosis and surgical removal of brain abscesses in a juvenile alpaca. J Am Vet Med Assoc 2007;231:1558-1561.
5. Chalkley MD, Kiupel M, Draper AC. Pituitary null cell adenoma in a domestic llama (*Lama glama*). J Comp Pathol 2014;151:51-56.
6. Gilsenan WF, Habecker PL, Coyne TM, et al. Neurologic disease attributed to a pituitary adenoma in an alpaca. J Vet Intern Med 2012;26:1073-1077.
7. Garlick DS, Doherty TJ, Paradis MR. Gemistocytic astrocytoma in a one-month-old llama. J Am Vet Med Assoc 1990;196:2009-2010.
8. Hill FI, Mirams CH. Intracranial teratoma in an alpaca (*Vicugna pacos*) in New Zealand. Vet Rec 2008;162:188-189.
9. Fielding A, Minuto J, Mazan M, et al. Intracranial embryonal neoplasm in an alpaca. J Vet Diagn Invest 2023;35:777-781.
10. Tsur I, Harmelin A, Dvir I, et al. Meningoencephalitis and brain abscessation due to *Escherichia coli* in a 2 week old alpaca cria. Aust Vet J 1996;74:437-438.
11. Franz S, Hogler S, Gumpenberger M, et al. Intracranial abscess

formation in an adult alpaca: a case report. BMC Vet Res 2019;15:183.

12. Soulsby E. Genus: *Parelaphostrongylus*. In: Soulsby E, ed. Helminths, arthropods and protozoa of domesticated animals, 7th ed. Philadelphia: Lea and Febiger; 1982:275-276.
13. Prestwood AK. Neurologic disease in a white-tailed deer massively infected with meningeal worm. J Wildl Dis 1970;6:84-86.
14. Presidente PJA. *Elaphostrongylus* in Deer. In. Australian Government Department of Agriculture, Fisheries and Forestry.
15. Rickard LG, Smith BB, Gentz EJ, et al. Experimentally induced meningeal worm (*Parelaphostrongylus tenuis*) infection in the llama (*Lama glama*): clinical evaluation and implications for parasite translocation. Journal of Zoo and Wildlife Medicine 1994;25:390-402.
16. Whitehead CE, Anderson DE, Saville WJA. Retrospective analysis of 185 occurrences of clinical neurological signs in 181 South American camelids. Journal of Veterinary Science and Animal Husbandry 2018;6.

Chapter 13

1. Drew ML, Ramsay E, Fowler ME, et al. Effect of flunixin meglumine and cimetidine hydrochloride on the pH in the third compartment of the stomach of llamas. J Am Vet Med Assoc 1992;201:1559-1563.
2. Christensen JM, Limsakun T, Smith BB, et al. Pharmacokinetics and pharmacodynamics of antiulcer agents in llama. J Vet Pharmacol Ther 2001;24:23-33.
3. McKenzie EC, Seguin B, Cebra CK, et al. Esophageal dysfunction in four alpaca crias and a llama cria with vascular ring anomalies. J Am Vet Med Assoc 2010;237:311-316.
4. Butt TD, MacDonald DG, Crawford WH. Persistent right aortic arch in a mature llama. Vet Rec 2001;148:118-119.
5. Watrous BJ, Pearson EG, Smith BB, et al. Megaesophagus in 15 llamas: a retrospective study (1985-1993). J Vet Intern Med 1995;9:92-99.
6. Thompson JM, Habrun CA, Scully CM, et al. Locally Transmitted *Trypanosoma cruzi* in a Domestic Llama (*Lama glama*) in a Rural Area of Greater New Orleans, Louisiana, USA. Vector Borne Zoonotic Dis 2021;21:762-768.
7. Cebra C. Disorders of the digestive system. In: Cebra C, Anderson DE, Tibary A, Van Saun RJ, Johnson LW, eds. Llama and alpaca care: medicine, surgery, reproduction, nutrition, and herd health, 1st ed. St Louis, Missouri: Elsevier Inc; 2014:477-536.

Chapter 14

1. Smith BB, Timm KI, Reed PJ, et al. Use of cloprostenol as an abortifacient in the llama (*Lama glama*). Theriogenology 2000;54:497-505.
2. Gordon E, Cebra CK, Stang BV, et al. Plasma pharmacokinetics, pulmonary disposition, and safety of subcutaneous gamithromycin in alpacas. J Vet Pharmacol Ther 2022;45:283-290.
3. Navarre CB, Ravis WR, Nagilla R, et al. Pharmacokinetics of phenylbutazone in llamas following single intravenous and oral doses. J Vet Pharmacol Ther 2001;24:227-231.
4. Edmondson M, D'uran SH, Passler WR, et al. Pharmacokinetics of intravenous and oral flunixin in alpacas. In. Alpaca Research Foundation.
5. Kreuder AJ, Coetzee JF, Wulf LW, et al. Bioavailability and pharmacokinetics of oral meloxicam in llamas. BMC Vet Res 2012;8:85.
6. Drew ML, Johnson L, Pugh D, et al. Pharmacokinetics of ceftiofur in llamas and alpacas. J Vet Pharmacol Ther 2004;27:13-20.
7. Kreil VE, Ambros L, Montoya L, et al. Pharmacokinetics of sodium and trihydrate amoxicillin after intravenous and intramuscular administration in llamas (*Lama glama*). Small Rumin Res 2011;102:208-212.

Chapter 15

1. Gordon E, Cebra CK, Stang BV, et al. Plasma pharmacokinetics, pulmonary disposition, and safety of subcutaneous gamithromycin in alpacas. J Vet Pharmacol Ther 2022;45:283-290.
2. Smith BB, Timm KI, Reed PJ, et al. Use of cloprostenol as an abortifacient in the llama (*Lama glama*). Theriogenology 2000;54:497-505.
3. Kosal ME, Anderson DE. An unaddressed issue of agricultural terrorism: a case study on feed security. J Anim Sci 2004;82:3394-3400.
4. Edmondson M, D'uran SH, Passler WR, et al. Pharmacokinetics of intravenous and oral flunixin in alpacas. In. Alpaca Research Foundation, [https://www.alpacaresearch.org/resources/dyn/files/317408z9554febd/_fn/flunixin-poster.pdf] (accessed 4th November 2024).
5. Navarre CB, Ravis WR, Nagilla R, et al. Pharmacokinetics of phenylbutazone in llamas following single intravenous and oral doses. J Vet Pharmacol Ther 2001;24:227-231.
6. Kreuder AJ, Coetzee JF, Wulf LW, et al. Bioavailability and pharmacokinetics of oral

meloxicam in llamas. BMC Vet Res 2012;8:85.
7. Chakwenya J, Lakritz J, Tyler J, et al. Pharmacokinetics and bioavailability of trimethoprim-sulfamethoxazole in alpacas. J Vet Pharmacol Ther 2002;25:321-327.
8. Snook CS, Poppenga RH, Rudik I, et al. Plasma concentrations of trimethoprim and sulfamethoxazole in llamas after orogastric administration. J Vet Pharmacol Ther 2002;25:383-386.
9. Kreil VE, Ambros L, Montoya L, et al. Pharmacokinetics of sodium and trihydrate amoxicillin after intravenous and intramuscular administration in llamas (*Lama glama*). Small Rumin Res 2011;102:208-212.
10. Drew ML, Johnson L, Pugh D, et al. Pharmacokinetics of ceftiofur in llamas and alpacas. J Vet Pharmacol Ther 2004;27:13-20.
11. Dechant JE, Rowe JD, Byrne BA, et al. Pharmacokinetics of ceftiofur crystalline free acid after single and multiple subcutaneous administrations in healthy alpacas (*Vicugna pacos*). J Vet Pharmacol Ther 2013;36:122-129.
12. Holmes K, Bedenice D, Papich MG. Florfenicol pharmacokinetics in healthy adult alpacas after subcutaneous and intramuscular injection. J Vet Pharmacol Ther 2012;35:382-388.
13. Pentecost RL, Niehaus AJ, Werle N, et al. Absorption and disposition of florfenicol after intravenous, intramuscular and subcutaneous dosing in alpacas. Res Vet Sci 2015;99:199-203.
14. Lackey MN, Belknap EB, Greco DS, et al. Single intravenous and multiple dose pharmacokinetics of gentamicin in healthy llamas. Am J Vet Res 1996;57:1193-1199.
15. Gandolf AR, Papich MG, Bringardner AB, et al. Pharmacokinetics after intravenous, subcutaneous, and oral administration of enrofloxacin to alpacas. Am J Vet Res 2005;66:767-771.
16. Davis JL. Pharmacologic Principles. In: Reed SM, Bayly WM, Sellon DC, eds. Equine Internal Medicine, 4th edW.B. Saunders; 2018:79-137.
17. Papich MG. Penicillin G. In: Papich MG, ed. Saunders Handbook of Veterinary Drugs 4th edW.B. Saunders; 2016:613-616.
18. Lallemand EA, Bousquet-Melou A, Chapuis L, et al. Pharmacokinetic-pharmacodynamic cutoff values for benzylpenicillin in horses to support the establishment of clinical breakpoints for benzylpenicillin antimicrobial susceptibility testing in horses. Front Microbiol 2023;14:1282949.
19. Ferran AA, Roques BB, Chapuis L, et al. Predicted efficacy and

tolerance of different dosage regimens of benzylpenicillin in horses based on a pharmacokinetic study with three IM formulations and one IV formulation. Front Vet Sci 2024;11:1409266.

20. Gillespie RA, Williamson LH, Terrill TH, et al. Efficacy of anthelmintics on South American camelid (llama and alpaca) farms in Georgia. Vet Parasitol 2010;172:168-171.
21. Dart A. Commentary: Pre weaning morbidity in llamas and alpacas. Aust Vet J 2009;87:4.
22. Rashid MH, Vaughan JL, Stevenson MA, et al. Anthelmintic resistance in gastrointestinal nematodes of alpacas (*Vicugna pacos*) in Australia. Parasit Vectors 2018;11:388.
23. Hinney B, Wiedermann S, Vaneev X, et al. High rates of benzimidazole-resistance-associated alleles in *Haemonchus contortus* and detection of resistance against macrocyclic lactones in strongylids from German alpaca herds. Parasit Vectors 2024;17:296.
24. Dadak AM, Asanger H, Tichy A, et al. Establishing an efficacious dose rate of monepantel for treating gastrointestinal nematodes in llamas under field conditions. Vet Rec 2013;172:155.
25. VanHoy G, Carman M, Habing G, et al. Safety and serologic response to a *Haemonchus contortus* vaccine in alpacas. Vet Parasitol 2018;252:180-186.
26. Carman S, Carr N, DeLay J, et al. Bovine viral diarrhea virus in alpaca: abortion and persistent infection. J Vet Diagn Invest 2005;17:589-593.
27. World Organisation for Animal Health. New Report reveals global decrease in antimicrobial use in animals, 2023, [https://www.woah.org/en/new-report-reveals-global-decrease-in-antimicrobial-use-in-animals/] (accessed 12/11/2024).
28. UK-VARSS. UK Veterinary Antibiotic Resistance and Sales Surveillance Report. In. New Haw, Addlestone: Veterinary Medicines Directorate; 2022.

www.ingramcontent.com/pod-product-compliance
Lightning Source LLC
LaVergne TN
LVHW070849210926
848482LV00016B/900
9781068357206